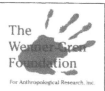

The
Wenner-Gren
Foundation
For Anthropological Research, Inc.

Plagues and Epidemics

WENNER-GREN INTERNATIONAL SYMPOSIUM SERIES

· ·

Series Editor: Leslie C. Aiello, President, Wenner-Gren Foundation for Anthropological Research, New York.

Since its inception in 1941, the Wenner-Gren Foundation has convened more than 125 international symposia on pressing issues in anthropology. These symposia affirm the worth of anthropology and its capacity to address the nature of humankind from a wide variety of perspectives. Each symposium brings together participants from around the world, representing different theoretical disciplines and traditions, for a week-long engagement on a specific issue. The Wenner-Gren International Symposium Series was initiated in 2000 to ensure the publication and distribution of the results of the foundation's International Symposium Program.

Prior to this series, some landmark Wenner-Gren volumes include: *Man's Role in Changing the Face of the Earth* (1956), ed. William L. Thomas; *Man the Hunter* (1968), eds Irv DeVore and Richard B. Lee; *Cloth and Human Experience* (1989), eds Jane Schneider and Annette Weiner; and *Tools, Language and Cognition in Human Evolution* (1993), eds Kathleen Gibson and Tim Ingold. Reports on recent symposia and further information can be found on the foundation's website at www.wennergren.org.

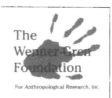

The
Wenner-Gren
Foundation
For Anthropological Research, Inc.

Plagues and Epidemics

Infected Spaces Past and Present

Edited by

D. ANN HERRING AND ALAN C. SWEDLUND

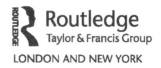

Routledge
Taylor & Francis Group

LONDON AND NEW YORK

First published 2010 by Berg Publishers

Published 2020 by Routledge
2 Park Square, Milton Park, Abingdon, Oxon OX14 4RN
605 Third Avenue, New York, NY 10017

Routledge is an imprint of the Taylor & Francis Group, an informa business

Library of Congress Cataloging-in-Publication Data

A catalogue record for this book is available from the Library of Congress.

British Library Cataloguing-in-Publication Data

A catalogue record for this book is available from the British Library.

ISBN 13: 978-1-8478-8548-7 (hbk)
ISBN 13: 978-1-8478-8547-0 (pbk)

Typeset by JS Typesetting Ltd, Porthcawl, Mid Glamorgan

Contents

Illustrations

Acknowledgments

Preparing this book has been a delightful experience for us because of the steadfast encouragement, support, and plain hard work of many people who sustained the project from start to finish. The book would not have been possible without the generous financial and intellectual support of the Wenner-Gren Foundation for Anthropological Research. Leslie Aiello, president of the Wenner-Gren Foundation, enthusiastically embraced the idea for our symposium on the subject of plagues and carefully shepherded it through the incomparable Wenner-Gren process. In the early stages of the symposium's formulation, Shirley Lindenbaum graciously gave her time and wisdom to help develop the framework for discussions. Laurie Obbink found an exquisite setting for our meeting in the Hacienda del Sol in Tucson, Arizona, and anticipated, with warmth, kindness, and great efficiency, our every need before, during, and after our week of meetings there.

The symposium participants, who authored the chapters in this book, displayed the best qualities of academic collegiality: respectful listening, vigorous debate, willingness to entertain and embrace new and opposing ideas, and generosity of spirit without sacrifice of intellectual rigor. We learned a lot from each other. Christianne Stephens, a doctoral candidate in the Department of Anthropology at McMaster University at the time of the symposium (now a Social Sciences and Humanities Postdoctoral Research Fellow at the University of Western Ontario), took on the grueling role of raporteur to the symposium participants. Her brilliant summary captured the essence of our daily discussions.

Victoria Malkin, Foundation Anthropologist at Wenner-Gren, kept us on track as we struggled to make manuscript deadlines. At Berg, Anna Wright and Emily Medcalf provided expertise and advice, always with good humor, and ensured that the volume reached bookstore shelves. Without Jane Kepp, our assiduous and meticulous copy editor; there would be far more errors in this book, because her scrupulous attention exceeded the usual bounds of grammar and language. Any errors that remain are ours and ours alone.

Our deepest thanks and gratitude to you all.

Ann Herring and Alan Swedlund

Contributors

Warwick Anderson, Department of History, University of Sydney, Australia

Ron Barrett, Department of Anthropology, Macalester College, USA

Charles L. Briggs, Department of Anthropology, University of California, Berkeley, USA

Linda Bryder, Department of History, University of Auckland, New Zealand

Arachu Castro, Department of Global Health and Social Medicine, Harvard University, USA

Marcos Cueto, Director, Instituto de Estudios Peruanos, Lima, Peru

Steven M. Goodreau, Department of Anthropology, University of Washington, USA

D. Ann Herring, Department of Anthropology, McMaster University, Canada

James Johnston, University of British Columbia, Canada

Mary-Ellen Kelm, Department of History, Simon Fraser University, Canada

Yasmin Khawja, Albert Einstein College of Medicine, Yeshiva University, USA

Katherine Lepani, College of Medicine, Biology and Environment, Australian National University, Australia

Shirley Lindenbaum, Department of Anthropology, City University of New York Graduate Center, USA

Judith Littleton, Department of Anthropology, University of Auckland, New Zealand

Stacy Lockerbie, Department of Anthropology, McMaster University, Canada

Ilana Löwy, CERMES, CNRS Paris, France

Andrew Noymer, Department of Sociology and Program in Public Health, University of California, Irvine, USA, and Health and

Global Change Project, International Institute for Applied Systems Analysis, Austria

Julie Park, Department of Anthropology, University of Auckland, New Zealand

Lawrence A. Sawchuk, Department of Anthropology, University of Toronto, Scarborough, Canada

Merrill Singer, Departments of Anthropology and Public Health, University of Connecticut, USA

Alan C. Swedlund, Department of Anthropology, University of Massachusetts (Emeritus), Amherst, and Santa Fe Institute, USA

James Trostle, Department of Anthropology, Trinity College, USA

Plagues and Epidemics in Anthropological Perspective

D. Ann Herring and *Alan C. Swedlund*

We live in a time obsessed with killer germs (Tomes 2000). People worldwide feel a growing sense of vulnerability and uncertainty with respect to infectious diseases as an expanding list of pathogens— referred to as "emerging infections"—becomes visible to investigators in conjunction with an increasingly lower technoscientific threshold for detection that reveals more diseases and their agents than ever imagined (Kilbourne 2006). As knowledge about pathogens is produced in laboratories and disseminated through various media to enter public consciousness (Briggs 2005), anxiety is rekindled about mortality on the scale of historic plagues such as the fourteenth-century Black Death in Europe. The anxiety spurs ever more research into conditions favoring the eruption of plagues today (Morse 1993).

In concert with a new language about emerging infections, an epidemiological story line has come to dominate discussions of the threat of infectious disease. Set against the certainty that "a tsunami is coming" (*Nature* 2009: 9), it describes scientists' discovery of a threatening infection, its travel through global networks, and medical projects that culminate in its control (Wald 2008). Whiffs of plague emanate from the story in the form of affliction, contagion, external threat, and dangerous relations; the crisis is resolved through appropriate moral behavior, expressed as medical intervention and effected through changes in cultural practices. In the wake of the story, the people among whom the disease has been made visible are often pathologized and tainted by that association through medical profiling (Briggs 2005; Briggs with Mantini-Briggs 2003). The emotive qualities of plague persist through memory, individual experience, and the social, economic, and political processes through which the story itself becomes a complex object that is mapped out, communicated, and perpetuated. The global reaction to the identification in 2009 of a new swine-flu-related H1N1 strain of influenza exemplifies the extent to which the story has become highly contagious and come to infect the world.

In September 2007 a group of anthropologists and scholars from allied fields met in Tucson, Arizona, to discuss the much publicized problem of infectious disease in the twenty-first century. Our symposium, generously funded by the Wenner-Gren Foundation for Anthropological Research, brought scholars engaged in the science of modeling and quantifying epidemics together with scholars engaged from historical, interpretive, critical, and metaphorical standpoints. Anthropologists are relative latecomers to the study of epidemics (Lindenbaum 2001: 378). Our aim was to encourage a conversation and exchange of ideas among researchers who, because of the Balkanization of academic thought and divisions in anthropology departments today, might not otherwise be aware of the richness of each other's work or of what each could contribute to and learn from the others. We wanted to breach the persistent gulf between the branches of anthropology to bring to bear the full power of our discipline's broad vision of humanity to address the issue of infected spaces, epidemics, and plagues.

We therefore chose not to organize the meeting around geographical regions or to ensure that particular infectious diseases were discussed. Rather, we were interested in convoking an unusual mix of scholars who brought qualitative and quantitative approaches in historical and contemporary settings to the same disease (such as HIV/AIDS) or issue (such as colonial medicine) and who represented a spectrum of research experience, from recently graduated PhDs to professors emeriti. Some readers of this collection may be disappointed by the omission of major historical plagues, such as the Black Death and syphilis, and of case studies from geographical areas such as the African continent. This is not because anthropologists are not offering new insights into these classic epidemics and infected spaces. The composition of scholars at our Wenner-Gren conference was determined not by their new findings about particular diseases but by the interesting and novel ways in which they were thinking about epidemics and plagues as *ideas* (see Ranger and Slack 1992) and about the political, cultural, and biological configurations they take.

Past and Present

Our project for the Tucson meeting and this volume was not only to explore anthropological thinking about epidemics but also to slice the discipline in order to lay bare the ways in which historical research speaks to contemporary ethnographic research, and vice versa. Current thinking about epidemics is rooted in past experience, and past experience, in turn, is reinterpreted through the imagination of the present.

Studies of the classic symbol of plague, bubonic plague (*Yersinia pestis*), illustrate the complex reticulations between past and present interpretations of disease. When bubonic plague erupted in India in the late nineteenth century, a concentrated international research effort was undertaken to determine its etiology. A group known as the Indian Plague Commission was formed because of mounting dread that the medieval levels of mortality associated with the Black Death would return (Cohn 2002: 13) and because of "anxiety that this was Armageddon" (Chandavarkar 1992: 239). The commission discovered much of what is known about the epidemiology of bubonic plague (Chandavarkar 1992: 204), and its findings in turn informed interpretations of the Black Death. The medieval historian Samuel Cohn Jr. contends, however, that this knowledge was misapplied to the Black Death, which he claims could not possibly have been caused by rat-based bubonic plague (Cohn 2002: 1). "Historians and scientists have taken the epidemiology of the modern plague and imposed it on the past, ignoring, denying and even changing contemporary testimony, both narrative and quantitative, when it conflicts with notions of how modern bubonic plague should behave" (Cohn 2002: 2). Whether or not Cohn is correct, the debate over which pathogens actually caused the Black Death underlines the involuted process by which interpretations of epidemics in the past and present become entangled and mutually sustaining.

A thorough understanding of contemporary epidemics, moreover, requires attention to the short- and long-term circumstances that have converged to provide the soil in which the seed of an epidemic can thrive. In the absence of a historical framework, it is impossible to grasp, for example, the processes through which HIV/AIDS spread to Haiti, HIV-related disorders came to dominate its disease profile, and the disease itself became integrated into ways of understanding illness (Farmer 1992). Even avian influenza, a relatively recent disease problem, can be viewed through epidemiological transition theory as part of ancient recursive processes that have shaped human disease patterns from the earliest origins of our species (Barrett, this volume; Barrett et al. 1998). Among the challenges of historical research are the difficulties of interpreting ever-changing "grammars of death" (Anderton and Hautaniemi Leonard 2004) and evaluating how certain explanations or frameworks come to dominate the theoretical positions of researchers themselves (Rosenberg 1989), sometimes waxing and waning in significance at different times of their lives (Anderson, this volume). Our discussions in Tucson and the chapters in this book reflect this historical and life-cycle sensibility.

Epidemics and Plagues

In pursuing ways of thinking about infection in the twenty-first century that reflect the broad concerns of anthropology, we also sought to stretch the constraints of conventional public health definitions and approaches to infectious disease. Although all the participants in our Tucson conference can be said to study epidemics, our research has taught us that the label *epidemic*—"the occurrence in a community or region of cases of an illness, specific health-related behavior, or other health-related events clearly in excess of normal expectancy" (Last 2001: 60)— has multiple meanings for individuals and communities experiencing the phenomenon, and these understandings change through time. The technical term *epidemic*, however, tends to homogenize, erase, and belie the diversity of experiences of people who are suffering or have suffered through what we call epidemics. The authoritative and seemingly neutral statistical language of *counting*, so fundamental to the definition of "epidemic," often overwhelms *accounts* of direct and indirect human encounters with epidemics, which are essential elements in much historical and contemporary anthropological research.

Many of the chapters in this volume present the perspectives of people who have been engulfed in experiences of infectious diseases labeled epidemics but having the hallmarks of plague: cycles of shame and blame, stigmatizing discourses, isolation of the sick, fear of contagion, and end-of-the-world scenarios. Plague, it would seem, is still among us, but its dimensions are frequently disguised by medical statistics that tailor not only the ways in which diseases are perceived but also the local and international policies designed to control them (see Briggs with Mantini-Briggs 2003: 256–268; Trostle, this volume). Epidemics can be made to disappear through the hiding or discounting of cases, because states have vested interests in their images, and epidemics call attention to government failures (Nichter 2008: 119–131; Trostle, this volume). Epidemics may be created where none exists (Herring and Lockerbie, this volume; Lepani, this volume). Diseases themselves may be made to disappear as a consequence of medical disputes (Löwy, this volume) and shifts in nosologic systems (Duffin 2005).

Complexity

Anthropologists are increasingly adding social and historical texture to research on epidemics by employing sophisticated models—advanced analytical tools grounded in mathematics, social theory, and fieldwork— that make it possible to explore how complex networks of human relationships influence the dynamics of epidemics such as that of HIV/ AIDS (Sattenspiel and Castillo-Chavez 1990; Sattenspiel et al. 1990). Here the mathematical language of counting and accounting refers generally to quantification and to statistical associations, respectively. Although the meanings attached to plague reside outside the purview of modelers, their methods imbue people in the models with qualities, refer to them as actors, allow them to make choices, and position them in intricate social networks shaped by the behavioral decisions of individuals and pairs and by the cultural, political, and economic contexts that constrain those decisions. When an epidemic is studied in this way, "everyone's risk is jointly affected by the behavior of everyone else in a complex feedback system" (Goodreau, this volume). The modeling of epidemics makes it possible to probe the "what ifs" of social life and behavior in the midst of a crisis and to uncover some of the complexity hidden by the term *epidemic*.

The hazard of delineating each epidemic as a distinct event that can be isolated in time and space recurs as a theme in these essays. When do epidemics begin and end? What are their borders? The concept of *syndemics* is particularly useful for drawing attention to the labyrinthine nature of epidemics. The syndemic approach requires that researchers look beyond individual infections to consider how they may be capacitated by the presence of other diseases and conditions and sustained by social inequity and the unjust exercise of power, which channels and sustains damaging disease clusters in disadvantaged populations (Singer 2009; Singer and Clair 2003). The key to syndemic thinking involves unraveling historical connections, both social and biological, that are woven into the fabric of ill health and give shape to infected spaces and epidemics. A direct link exists, for instance, between childhood Chagas' disease (American trypanosomiasis) and adult onset rheumatic heart disease (caused by *Streptococcus pyogenes* infection) among poor, rural children in Latin America (Löwy, this volume). Chagas' disease remains untreated because of lack of access to health care, and untreated Chagas' disease increases the probability that affected people will die from congestive heart failure in early adulthood (Singer et al. n.d.).

Similar co-occurrences characterized the once forgotten (Crosby 1989) but now highly publicized 1918 influenza pandemic. The very name of that pandemic cloaks the well-known observation that most of its excess mortality resulted from synergistic interactions between influenza and co-occurring bacterial infections such as those caused by *Streptococcus*, *Staphylococcus*, and *Mycobacterium tuberculosis* (Pearl 1919). Even the year 1918 in the pandemic's label needs to be reconsidered, in view of the fact that many people with tuberculosis who died from influenza in 1918 had acquired their tuberculosis infection decades before, making their demise that year a consequence of earlier life experience (Noymer, this volume). Although diseases may be tied biologically and socially to specific historical moments (Scheper-Hughes and Lock 1987), their spatial and temporal borders are fuzzy, and the edges of safety are unclear. A syndemics framework recognizes historical contingencies and interactions that are not readily apparent, allowing scholars to explore larger environments of risk and historically contingent social structures that converge to produce disproportionately infected spaces for some, but not all, members of society.

Anthropology, Epidemics, and Plagues

The essays in this volume reflect the broad expanse of anthropological inquiry and our stimulating, sometimes contentious, discussions in Tucson. Regardless of the perspective presented in each essay, the collection is strongly theorized, grounded in empirical research and specific case studies, and focused on probing into broad questions and themes in the subject of epidemics and plague. The authors have worked in many of the places in which emerging infections are said to be erupting. They take us into "the field," to places in which diseases have not yet arrived but are expected to take a heavy toll of human life and in which an epidemiological discourse has often arrived before the disease itself. They take us into the minds and memories of people who experienced plagues in their lifetimes. They transport us to places where plagues are waning and places where plagues are things of the past. They explore the ways in which researchers think about plagues and deploy their ideas in their work. They illuminate the way contemporary thinking about epidemics is anchored to images of plagues in the past and show how essentializing discourses, characteristic of the colonial period, continue to pathologize people who experience epidemics today. They study the way epidemic models are made and the ways in which they capture the complexity of human behavior, interactions, and cultural settings. They take us into public health bureaucracies and into the political arenas that control and disseminate information, where the power resides to make decisions about what is and is not an epidemic or a plague. They look back into deep history on a global scale to chart long historical disease trends, and they look ahead to the twenty-first century as a time of expanding and enhanced plagues in the context of climate change.

Frameworks

Merrill Singer, in chapter 2, invites us to think more deeply about circumstances in the twenty-first century that create new contexts in which infections can surge and interact in dynamic fashion. Building on the concept of syndemics described earlier, he argues that global processes that produce epidemics and plagues can be understood in terms of *ecosyndemics.* The emergence, spread, and interaction of diseases are being enhanced by climate change, human action, decision making, and the unequal and often oppressive structure of global social relations. It is important, therefore, to identify the strong, mutually reinforcing, and synergistic connections between large-scale environmental circumstances and the local health and social effects that are embedded in them. Major anthropogenic environmental changes, such as deforestation, agricultural intensification, dam construction, the industrialization of food production, increased population nucleation, and crowding in urban settings, are accelerating in tandem with the emergence and reemergence of pathogens, climate change, and persistent, large-scale, inegalitarian social structures. The environmental catastrophe of Hurricane Katrina in the US city of New Orleans exemplifies the action of ecosyndemic processes mediated by local microsocial processes. Over and above the physical destruction of the city's infrastructure and social damage to its residents, Katrina exacerbated already high rates of chronic and infectious disease, especially among historically disadvantaged groups living there. Singer calls for fresh studies of these problems and for a better understanding of how best to limit the health consequences of ecosyndemics and the social conditions that give rise to them.

In chapter 3, Charles Briggs draws attention to the ways in which health and technoscientific information is reshaping biomedical and scientific objects, institutions, and daily life. He analyses the structures through which story lines about emerging disease emanate, with fully formed packages of meanings, from the offices of public health officials and epidemiologists, are communicated through policy papers and news briefs, and are taken up by news media ("mediatization"). The public is expected to accept the nest of meanings and transform their intimate daily habits such as eating, drinking, and defecating. Briggs's concept of "communicability" describes the unidirectional process by which health professionals inform the public about new knowledge. Today, epidemics are "mediated objects from the get-go," Briggs writes, internalized through the media before they are experienced bodily by the public. Using two examples—cholera in Venezuela and West Nile virus in San Diego, California—he demonstrates how diseases that have not yet been reported take on particular biological, social, and political shapes in keeping with epidemiological projections, policy briefs, and news accounts communicated about them, and how public health officials and journalists collaborate in creating plagues. He challenges anthropologists to investigate sites of "epidemic struggle," the places where competing, complex understandings of diseases or epidemics are reduced to simple, reductionist narratives.

Jim Trostle, in chapter 4, considers how epidemics come to be defined in the first place, taking up the issue of who in fact has the power to observe and report on epidemics in the making. In "contested epidemics"—situations in which the existence of an epidemic is debated—particularly close attention is paid to enumeration and statistical estimation, central tools in epidemiological research. Trostle illustrates the concept by discussing the contested epidemic of civilian deaths during the current war in Iraq. He highlights the conflict that can arise between an epidemiologist's counts, which identify an epidemic of violence (or anything else deemed contrary to the interests of the state), and the state's view that it has the right to make its own claims about the legitimacy of that violence (or anything else involving public policy). Trostle calls for more research into the ways in which states remember and remain silent and in which epidemics can be made to appear or disappear.

Ron Barrett takes the long view of plague and in chapter 5 reviews the basic understanding of epidemiological transitions on a global scale, in deep history. Many scholars now argue that at least three major transitions have taken place in human health and disease profiles, in conjunction with significant shifts in subsistence, social organization, and demographic patterns (Barrett et al. 1998). The first, for example, occurred among people who participated in the shift from a nomadic foraging economy to a Neolithic pattern of sedentism, agriculture, and animal domestication. Barrett provides caveats about the generalizability of global epidemiological transition theory, especially because the experiences of impoverished versus affluent societies can vary widely with respect to the timing and process of the transitions themselves. It is against this deep historical background that emerging diseases such as avian influenza need to be understood, because their behavior as emerging diseases is modified and influenced by new global demographic and epidemiological conditions. Although socioeconomic inequalities have always played a major role in dictating who suffers most in an epidemic, Barrett proposes that globalization has changed the landscape of epidemics. Today, rich and poor are more closely connected, in terms of disease risk, than ever before.

Infection and Time

Defining the temporal and spatial limits of an epidemic and answering the question "When is an epidemic an epidemic?" are contingent not just on official, state recognition and publicity but also on the way in which a disease is interpreted, remembered, or understood, because epidemics are not solely about counts of deaths. In his essay (chapter 6), Larry Sawchuk points to the importance of perceptions and the temporal context in which an epidemic occurs by evaluating the effects of a series of cholera epidemics on the civilian population of nineteenth-century Gibraltar. Applying a sophisticated life table methodology that parallels Rosenberg's (1992a) narrative for epidemics, he considers mortality before and after each epidemic. Even though cholera is understood to be a "shock" disease, the cholera epidemics were not universally devastating. Some cholera epidemics, Sawchuk shows, produced a dramatic change in life expectancy (a drop of as much as twelve years), whereas others produced virtually none. After the severe epidemic of 1865, indeed, the life expectancy of survivors rose, whatever their age. In other words, the demise of the "frail" segment of the population left a residual population that was healthier and longer lived. Yet with good reason, the fear of cholera remained. Even minor visitations of cholera that had little effect on life expectancy had substantial effects on the lives of Gibraltarians, because the disease was infused with the meanings of plague, alive in memory and fed by prior experience.

The emotive qualities of plague are not confined to earlier times but continue to characterize reactions to epidemics today. In chapter 7, Judith Littleton and her colleagues unravel some of the ways in which the aura of plague can adhere to a disease even when it is no longer a major threat to health. They consider the case of tuberculosis (TB), a disease that has a low incidence and is on the wane in New Zealand but that has historical connections to ideas of affliction, moral taint, and external threat. TB retains its symbolic power and capacity to create stigma, isolation, and circles of blame and fear, especially because it has become associated with foreign-born residents. Attitudes that were prevalent when TB was at its peak reverberate through the convergence of individual experience, mediatization of the disease, and publicly expressed concerns of government institutions. In the midst of multiple understandings of TB, it has come to be construed both as a familiar and recurrent enemy and as a new and emerging threat requiring that borders be policed. Even though most migrants to New Zealand who develop active TB disease do so *after* screening and arrival, the policing of borders dominates public discourse, rather than concern about identifying the conditions that allow TB to blossom there in the first place. The assumption that TB is a disease of outsiders who bring it to New Zealand has other practical public health consequences. Some Pakeha (New Zealanders of European descent) delay diagnosis because they do not feel vulnerable to the disease.

If tuberculosis in New Zealand in the twenty-first century offers a glimpse of the end of a plague, then Andrew Noymer's study of the 1918 influenza epidemic (chapter 8) suggests that it is difficult to determine the boundaries of an epidemic and when, if ever, its influence ends. The true impact of a plague can be viewed only in the long term, Noymer argues, because many plagues play out over decades, interacting with a shifting matrix of diseases and within new demographic configurations, simply because the populations that survive a plague are not the same as those that existed before it. Noymer demonstrates that the effects of the 1918 pandemic were experienced more widely and deeply over time because influenza interacted with other diseases. People who were already suffering from other infections, particularly tuberculosis, were more likely to die during the 1918 pandemic. Although the idea that diseases are interrelated is not new (see Singer, this volume), Noymer shows compellingly how the death rate from tuberculosis in the United States changed during and following the 1918 flu. In effect, influenza exacerbated the already deteriorating lung function and hastened the deaths of some TB-infected persons who might otherwise have lived longer. For this reason, tuberculosis deaths actually declined in the aftermath of the 1918 flu epidemic, and the histories of the two diseases are inextricably entwined. Noymer's study also offers an important challenge to the presumption that major plagues such as the 1918 flu are indiscriminate with regard to socioeconomic status and ethnicity (see also Swedlund, this volume). Tuberculosis mortality demarks social boundaries and economic status; the predisposition of tubercular individuals to die during the 1918 flu tightens the connections between that pandemic and social inequalities (Mamelund 2006).

Alan Swedlund, in chapter 9, traces the progression of the 1918 influenza epidemic through a cluster of small towns in Massachusetts located several miles from the sites of the first appearance of the epidemic in the United States, in Charlestown and Camp Devens, Massachusetts, but sufficiently close to be overwhelmed by the flu's effects within a matter of days. Swedlund probes the everyday experiences of people exposed to the epidemic, with a view to gauging their reactions and anxieties and evaluating Crosby's (1986) conclusion that the pandemic has been forgotten. Using a highly localized context in which to study the effects of the 1918 flu, Swedlund consults newspapers, local narratives, and documents prepared by municipal and state authorities to assess perceptions of the threat and effects of the epidemic. He points out that other serious infectious diseases, including poliomyelitis, measles, and causes of infant mortality, competed for health professionals' attention in 1918. These competing concerns, coupled with the relatively short duration of the epidemic in any one place, served to dampen local panic except in the hardest-hit cities. A medical discourse founded on positivism and the optimistic claims of the Progressive Era prevailed at the time. Newspapers reported that the next week would be better than the last, and the public may have been inclined to believe them. In the months, years, and decades after the epidemic, perceived medical progress and advances in antibiotic therapies probably further dispelled fear for many citizens. Given these observations, Swedlund asks whether it is not the specter of a new, twenty-first-century influenza epidemic, and our contemporary angst, that makes it difficult for us to understand the partial loss of memory and coping mechanisms of the past.

Infected Spaces

In chapter 10, Ann Herring and Stacy Lockerbie look at the current experience of avian influenza in Vietnam from the perspective of the global discourse about "the coming pandemic." They chart the recent history of avian influenza and describe how few human cases have actually been identified, whereas several outbreaks have occurred among fowl, primarily in Asia. They use the fact of a relatively small number of confirmed human cases and deaths to illustrate how the current global fear of avian influenza is at odds with the actual experience of the disease. They propose that the fear of avian influenza far exceeds its actual threat and that anxiety about the coming plague is situated in a climate of viral panic ramped up by highly publicized links of avian influenza to Southeast Asian farms and markets, by worries about the nature of the pathogen itself—anchoring avian influenza to the destruction of the 1918 pandemic and to bioterrorism—and, ironically, by the very process of planning for the pandemic. The discourse of this plague-yet-to-be has serious repercussions for people living at the epicenters of the disease, such as Vietnam. Those most affected by international efforts to prevent "the coming plague" are impoverished rural farmers whose livelihoods and health are undermined by the protocols of international organizations such as the World Health Organization that order that their flocks be destroyed in the name of humanity. These farmers are in a real sense being plagued by the idea of plague and by the package of meanings that infiltrate the policies of international organizations and are put into practice by local governments.

Aboriginal people in Canada, too, have been saddled with stigmatizing images that impede public health programs. Mary-Ellen Kelm shows in chapter 11 how old notions of Aboriginal communities and people "as spaces of pathogenic behavior and Aboriginal bodies as highly mobile vectors of transmission, always on the verge of destruction," are imbedded in contemporary medical thought and writing about HIV/AIDS. HIV/AIDS was anticipated to appear in Aboriginal communities for two decades before it was actually identified, prompting increased public health surveillance. Health researchers raised the level of concern about HIV/AIDS by anchoring it to the history of devastating epidemics in the Americas, referring to AIDS as the "new smallpox." This sounded alarms about an epidemic of AIDS that had yet to arrive. HIV/AIDS incidence rates in Aboriginal and Native American populations in Canada and the United States, however, remain low in the context of the worldwide pandemic. Instead of asking what has constrained the spread of infection, researchers concluded that the disease was underreported and that the low numbers stemmed from poor surveillance or classification errors. Kelm counters that many Aboriginal communities, particularly those with a strong sense of culture, have been proactive in responding to the threat of HIV/AIDS. This contrasts with the historical stereotype of Aboriginal people as apathetic in the face of disease, a view that seems to be informing public health approaches. Kelm suggests that "reading against the grain" offers a methodology for avoiding the pitfalls and stereotypes of the past and for moving toward a postcolonial epidemiology. Researchers can read against the grain by using histories of medicine that situate Aboriginal interactions with Western medicine or by focusing on culturally protective factors and community strengths. By rejecting the stereotypes of the past and focusing on the successes of the present, "we begin to refuse the legacies of history." Essentializing discourses that focus on risk factors and link AIDS with Aboriginal bodies or culture discourage the very project in which public health is engaged: prevention.

Looking at infected spaces in a different way, Steven Goodreau invites us in chapter 12 to consider how anthropologists and other social scientists model epidemics in rigorous, quantitative ways without losing sight of the intimate details of diverse cultural contexts. Before the 1980s, epidemic modeling fell mostly within the purview of applied mathematicians and parasitologists. The explosion of sexually transmitted diseases (STDs) and large-scale computing in the 1980s stimulated the growth of epidemic modeling by social scientists, notably Lisa Sattenspiel's path-breaking research in anthropology. As more social scientists publish their work on epidemic modeling, the role of cultural practices is increasingly built into the models. Agent-based modeling, which represents each person in the population of interest and allows those persons to interact in dynamic social networks, makes it possible for modelers to explore complex social processes that underlie and sustain epidemics. Goodreau shows what can be learned from mathematical and statistical modeling when it is guided by ethnography, and he illustrates the way epidemiological approaches, specifically agent-based modeling, can reveal unexpected outcomes and test hypotheses about the transmissibility of HIV/AIDS.

Drawing on his research on HIV in Lima, Peru, among men who have sex with men (MSM), Goodreau addresses one of the most important tests to which modeling has been applied: the situation in which MSM have multiple sexual relationships simultaneously, rather than serially, and its effect on the spread of HIV. This practice can elevate the spread of infection significantly. Role preference in MSM relationships is important to the process and may act as a barrier to viral transmission. The selection of sexual role is deeply symbolic and enmeshed in personal webs of wealth, age, class, power, and desire. Against a backdrop of the globalization of gay identity, the selection of sexual role is changing in Peru, which may in turn influence the spread of HIV. Agent-based modeling makes it possible to build in and examine the effects of such changes in identity and role behavior on the spread of infection. As knowledge producers, Goodreau argues, modelers must take care to contextualize their results and not lose insights or readership by remaining at a level of abstraction that denies the costs of an epidemic in human suffering and lives.

In chapter 13, Arachu Castro and colleagues unravel the history of dengue fever—a disease with roots in the eighteenth-century South Asian slave trade—and the circumstances that have allowed it to become the most important mosquito-borne viral disease in the global environment of the twenty-first century. A legacy of failed projects to control mosquito-borne diseases, its contemporary distribution is linked to historical movements of people, goods, and *Aedes aegypti* mosquitoes and to ecosyndemic conditions (Singer, this volume) that encourage dengue to spiral and spread in Latin American cities today. Increasing diversity in the viral strains present in Latin America and growing concentrations of urban poor living under appallingly inadequate sanitary conditions have propelled the more severe forms of dengue to the forefront, especially among children. The collapse of public health infrastructure and inability to sustain dengue control programs, coupled with marked inequalities in access to health care, have allowed *Aedes aegypti* mosquitoes and dengue to thrive. The relationship between dengue and poverty is complicated, however; some people are exposed to dengue "because they have no running water and must collect it haphazardly, and ... others because they have plenty with which to water the plants in their balconies." But whereas the opportunity to be *exposed* to the virus may cross social divides in Latin America, social inequality channels its human toll disproportionately toward the poor through indirect mechanisms such as unequal access to health care and sanitary-social services.

Accounting and Recounting

In chapter 14, Warwick Anderson considers the processes through which we think about and account for epidemics and plagues. He provides a brief synopsis of the way environmentalist and contagionist theories, refined to concepts of "configuration" and "contamination," have been proffered as explanations for epidemics in the past. To illustrate the way these can play out in field epidemiology, Anderson takes us into the mind and fieldwork of the microbiologist Carleton Gajdusek as he and his collaborators study rare, lethal diseases in New Guinea, Guam, and Siberia. In each case Anderson illustrates how the training of investigators, methodologies deployed, and prior assumptions tended to favor one realm of explanation (configuration or contamination) over others. In doing so he draws out the crucial role of the anthropological insights of Robert Glasse and Shirley Glasse Lindenbaum (configuration) to the eventual explanation of kuru in Papua New Guinea (see also Lindenbaum, this volume). Yet Gajdusek was subsequently prone to focusing on the microbiology (contamination) and less on the cultural configurations that were the key to kuru's patterns of infection. Anderson provides a compelling account of the way one researcher's thinking about plague influenced the field of microbiology and the discovery of slow viruses, for which Gajdusek was awarded a Nobel Prize.

Ilana Löwy, in chapter 15, examines the way the presence of plagues shaped the representation of tropical regions of Latin America during the colonial period and how indigenous people came to be pathologized and essentialized through this process. Yellow fever, hookworm, and Chagas' disease each signaled that the tropics were dangerous places populated by dangerous inhabitants. Yellow fever took its toll of soldiers, colonial agents, and would-be entrepreneurs and therefore constituted a grave threat to the colonial project. Attempts to eliminate "tropical diseases" were tightly coupled with colonial ideologies and projects involving the social development and improved productivity of indigenous groups. Hookworm and Chagas' disease thus were interpreted as evidence for "backwardness" and were attributed to the "laziness" of the indigenous inhabitants. Löwy illustrates the ways in which medical investigators approached these diseases and attempted to follow infinitesimal traces of evidence to make their hidden reality "visible" and, in the case of Chagas' disease, to make it disappear entirely as a nosologic entity.

Marcos Cueto takes up several of these themes in his essay on malaria eradication efforts in Mexico (chapter 16). This far-reaching program, inaugurated in the 1950s, involved the US State Department and western European agencies working in coordination with the World Health Organization and the precursor to the Pan American Health Organization. Injected with a strong dose of American cold war foreign policy, the program aimed to foster economic development in Mexico by eliminating malaria and thereby both raising a "backward" country toward the path of a modern state and discouraging communistic tendencies feared to be festering among the rural poor. It was an opportunity to demonstrate the power of Western technology in the form of DDT, the "magic bullet" that would wipe out mosquitoes carrying the malarial parasite. Cueto illustrates how the program failed on many levels. Medical anthropologists who in the early years of the program argued for cultural sensitivity and recognition of diverse local practices were largely ignored. The propaganda campaign, heavily tinged with military metaphors and technical bravado, did not resonate with the largely rural population that was targeted. Language barriers and conceptualizations of malaria from traditional medicine were not addressed, and the agents who came into the communities and households to spray DDT and draw blood samples failed to grasp the diversity of the indigenous residents of the areas in which they worked. Despite the understanding of the effects of DDT that came years later, the project was a classic case of lost opportunities and failures.

Several contributors to this volume take issue with the practice of studying epidemics as single, bounded events. In chapter 17, Katherine Lepani's analysis of HIV/AIDS in the Trobriand Islands of Papua New Guinea (PNG) illustrates how epidemics are better understood as multiple, overlapping phenomena with many meanings. Much like Native Americans in North America, Trobriand islanders have been inundated with a discourse from the outside, well before much evidence for HIV/AIDS has appeared among them. The eroticized identity of the "Islands of Love," a legacy of anthropological investigation, inscribes the Trobriands and their inhabitants with the epidemiological label of "high risk" for HIV because of the standard, international checklist of sexual risk behaviors. HIV/AIDS is represented as a looming plague, brought on by alleged sexual excess and transgression. And although the images and explanations of global science have penetrated PNG, the resources and local capacity to test for and treat HIV/AIDS have not.

Lepani shows how epidemiological models of risk make little sense in the Trobriands. Sexuality is not a risk behavior but a life-affirming antidote to the destruction and death associated with supernatural beings. Sexual practice is influenced by place identity, relationality, and collectivity, not by numbers of partners. It is part of being "steady with custom," of behaving in ways that are in keeping with Trobriand identity. Epidemiological terminology that employs militaristic metaphors about impending doom and battles against disease—and that link the concept of risk to sexuality and cultural practice, making HIV "a plague of promiscuity"—will not work in the Trobriands. An approach that focuses on the way Trobriand culture can effectively be engaged is more likely to succeed as a public health campaign.

The final essay in this collection, written by Shirley Lindenbaum, weaves together many of the threads that connect the other chapters and in many ways captures the cosmopolitan essence of our discussions in Tucson. Lindenbaum considers how three sets of actors explained kuru, a plague of the past that once threatened the survival of the Fore people of the eastern highlands of Papua New Guinea. For the Fore, kuru was both an epidemic (involving the authority of numbers and counting) and a plague (laden with connotations of chaos, suffering, morality, and a "different kind of social work"). The actors in Lindenbaum's essay each presented ideas about the cause of the epidemic, explanatory frameworks that reflected the actors' cultural and historical assumptions about disease causation, their different relations to the object of study (kuru), and their relationships to each other. Lindenbaum cleverly works on two levels, in "double dialogical mode": One trio consists of medical people, anthropologists, and the Fore collectively; the other consists of three Fore men's views of the epidemic at its end.

Medical accounts in the 1950s established a framework for clinical and epidemiological research. Through the language of medicine and science, kuru was portrayed as an epidemic of Creutzfeldt-Jakob disease (CJD) caused by a slow virus of the central nervous system. Anthropologists working among the Fore in the 1960s (Robert Glasse and Shirley Glasse, now Shirley Lindenbaum) used the language of medicine but also portrayed Fore beliefs and experiences on the basis of long-term field research and a knowledge of Fore society and history. Understanding Fore rules for the consumption of human flesh allowed them to identify the key connection between kuru and cannibalism; later, experiments with laboratory-infected chimpanzees confirmed the presence of the transmissible agent associated with CJD. The Fore, too, sought knowledge about the cause of kuru and wanted to arrest its toll of sickness and death. They used the methods of epidemiology (identifying and counting cases) as well as the language of plague to express their worries about unseen, secret actions used to afflict others with kuru. For the Fore, there was no monolithic explanation for kuru: it was simultaneously an epidemic and a plague, which they sought to understand in terms of sorcery and sickness. Lindenbaum's three "men in the middle" had different accounts of kuru, reflecting their personal histories since the 1960s, the social relations within which their knowledge of it developed, and their particular roles in helping bring an end to kuru. The fullest historical understanding of kuru—more widely generalizable to the understanding of any epidemic—is achieved when *all* styles of explanation are combined.

Epidemics and Plagues in Anthropological Perspective

Public health policy makers in the late twentieth century successfully moved infectious disease forward on the health agenda after several decades during which interest in the subject languished because of the belief that epidemics were controllable, at least in a Western bio-medical context, and less important than chronic, degenerative diseases (Berkelman and Freeman 2004; Omran 1971). Despite a long history of collaboration and theoretical affinities with epidemiologists (Janes, Stall, and Gifford 1986) and the emergence of the anthropology of infectious disease as an area of inquiry (Inhorn and Brown 1990), anthropologists have been relatively slow to respond to the new agenda surrounding emerging infectious disease research galvanized by the HIV/AIDS pandemic (Lindenbaum 2001: 378). The essays in this volume offer a small sample of the kinds of questions anthropologists are probing to enrich the current debate.

Certainly there is more thinking to be done about how epidemics come to be defined in the first place (counting) and about the biopolitical processes through which they, and even whole disease categories (see Löwy, this volume), can be made to appear or disappear (accounting and recounting), depending on the interests of the state or investigators. If anthropologists are to have a place in the discussion of contested epidemics, they must pay attention to and be conversant in the statistical processes normally used to define and evaluate epidemics as events worthy of attention (or not), and they must inform through ethnographic detail the models being generated to explore the shapes epidemics may take. Renewed theorizing of the epidemic concept in anthropology calls for studies of syndemic and ecosyndemic problems in historical perspective, with a view to developing recommendations on how best to limit their health consequences.

It is evident from several contributions to this volume (Löwy, Cueto; see also Farmer 1992; Nichter 2008) that many of the failures that characterized the history of colonial medicine and the study of "tropical disease" are being perpetuated and reproduced in the representation of epidemics and the people vulnerable to them today. Because of their long-term fieldwork programs, anthropologists are well placed to write accounts of epidemics and to offer counternarratives ("writing against the grain") to the contagious stories that circulate through the power of the media and through the aegis of international bodies. How do other explanations become forgotten and pushed aside, such as occurred for West Nile virus in San Diego? What are the pathways through which agreed-upon explanations come to be put in place? How do the explanations, loaded with meaning, then work their way through chains of institutions and governing bodies, both global and local, into the everyday practices of ordinary people? Historians have explored the making of germ panic in America (e.g., Humphreys 2002; Tomes 2002), but as several contributors to this volume show (e.g., Lepani), less is known about how Western and indigenous explanatory frameworks interact in the face of epidemics, real or imagined, and with the discourse that often precedes them.

Anthropologists can play an important role in this regard by scrutinizing the communicability of health and technoscientific information and subjecting to analysis places where competing, complex understandings of epidemics are rendered into simple reductionist narratives. Because of the view afforded by long-term fieldwork, anthropologists are also in a position to explore epidemics from the vantage point of community strengths and successful community mobilization. By focusing on community successes instead of inappropriate lists of behavioral risks, it may be possible to engage local communities in meaningful public health campaigns instead of alienating them.

Finally, as demonstrated by our discussions in Tucson and by Lindenbaum's account (this volume) of the various ways in which kuru can be understood, it is important to marshal the full range of anthropological inquiry, theoretical frameworks, and methods to reveal the complexities of infected spaces in the past and in the present.

Ecosyndemics
Global Warming and the Coming Plagues of the Twenty-first Century

Merrill Singer

As is characteristic in big city hospitals, the emergency room at Toronto's Scarborough Grace Hospital on the night of 7 March 2003 was "overwhelmed and understaffed" (Frank 2003). Yet when a Chinese-Canadian patient showed up with a fever and a cough, he caught the immediate attention of the harried ER personnel. Having a hard time catching his breath and clearly frightened, the patient was admitted and placed in a corner bed of the ER's observation ward, separated from other patients only by sliding cloth curtains.

The patient, forty-three-year-old Tse Chi Kwan, reported to nurses that his seventy-eight-year-old mother, Sui-Chu Kwan, a diabetic, had died at home two days earlier after suffering from a chest infection. The doctors' initial suspicion was that Tse had tuberculosis, a common disease in the ethnically diverse Toronto neighborhood where he lived. This diagnosis was soon in doubt because of the rapid decline in Tse's condition. Six days after entering the hospital, he, too, was dead. His wife died as well. Two of his siblings got sick but recovered. Lying next to Tse in the observation ward was Joseph Pollack, seventy-six, who suffered from a heart arrhythmia condition. After exposure to Tse, Pollack began coughing and registering a fever. He, too, died. So did James Dougherty, a patient who was in the ER being treated for congestive heart problems. Within a few days, a number of Scarborough Grace Hospital staff began showing up at the ER as patients exhibiting fever and respiratory symptoms.

Amid growing panic and uncertainty, Severe Acute Respiratory Syndrome (SARS) had arrived in Toronto. Eventually, at least 129 probable and suspected cases of Toronto's short-lived but painful SARS epidemic were traced directly back to exposure to Tse and his mother. The patients ranged in age from twenty-one months to eighty-six years; 60 percent were female. Seventeen of these people died, producing a case-fatality rate of 13.3 percent (Varia et al. 2003). Overall, between February and September 2003, Health Canada reported 438 probable and suspected cases of SARS, primarily in the greater Toronto area, resulting in forty-three deaths (Borgundvaag et al. 2004). Notably, unlike during the flu pandemic of 1918, which tended to take the lives of younger, healthier individuals, co-morbidity with diabetes (relative risk 3.1) was found to be associated with SARS deaths and poorer outcomes, including intensive care unit (ICU) admission and need for mechanical ventilation, an association also found at other sites around the world that were hard hit by SARS. Persons with cardiopulmonary disease were also at heightened risk if they were infected with the coronavirus that causes SARS (Chan et al. 2003). SARS, in other words, did not exact its toll alone; its worst effects were the result of interactions with other diseases. Suffering from diabetes or cardiopulmonary disease has been established as an independent predictor of mortality and level of morbidity in SARS patients (Yang et al. 2006).

As we now know, SARS first appeared in Guangdong, in the south of China, although the outbreak was concealed by the Chinese government. A Chinese physician, Liu Jianlun, from Zhongshan University, was among those who began treating the first cases, which were thought to be a form of atypical pneumonia. In late February 2003, Dr. Liu made a short trip to Hong Kong, where he stayed in room 911 of the Metropole Hotel (now renamed the Metropark Kowloon) in the Kowloon district, a popular shopping area and one of the most densely populated places on the planet. Also in the hotel and also staying on the ninth floor were Kwan Sui-chu Kwan and her husband, visiting as tourists from Toronto. It is believed that through some chance encounter with Liu in the hotel, Sui-chu Kwan was infected with SARS, for Liu died of the disease on 4 March.

Analyzing the Third Epidemiological Transition

With the emergence and rapid spread of SARS from Asia to North America and the infection within eight months of more than eight thousand people, the feared new era of disease that had been signaled by the appearance and worldwide spread of AIDS in the early 1980s had clearly arrived. This new stage in the human encounter with disease, sometimes called the "third epidemiological transition" (Armelagos, Barnes, and Lin 1996; Barrett, this volume), has been described as a return to a time of infectious disease or, as Crosby (2003: 131) vividly characterized the change, "the nineteenth century was followed by the twentieth century, which was followed by the ... nineteenth century."

The defining feature of this period from a public health perspective is the appearance in rapid succession of a series of emerging and reemerging infectious diseases. Since about 1975, previously unknown infectious diseases have surfaced at the astonishing pace of one per year, mostly caused by newly discovered viruses (Cohen 1998; Epstein, Chivian, and Frith 2003). The concept of "emerging infectious diseases" has itself emerged as a new medical and research specialty. A Medline keyword search for "communicable diseases, emerging," for example, found that five times more medical journal articles were written on emerging infectious diseases during the preceding four years than during the previous one hundred years (Geger 2006). In recognition of the significant biosocial shift that was occurring—a shift away from the pre-HIV era, when infectious disease was believed to be declining as a health factor on the world stage, especially in its more developed sectors—the US Centers for Disease Control and Prevention (CDC) launched a new monthly journal, *Emerging Infectious Diseases*, in 1994. The introduction of this vehicle for accelerated scientific communication was propelled by recognition that public health was increasingly at risk because of the rapid appearance of "elusive, continuous, evolving, and global" new and renewed infections (CDC 2002).

In a sense, the history of the notion of "emergent infectious diseases" as a social conception (as well as that of global warming as a significant biosocial process with imperative health implications) parallels Rosenberg's (1992a) dramaturgic model of plague epidemics, characterized, like any stage drama, by a discernable social chronology. In such social events, the first act involves a slow, often painful, yet progressive recognition that the world has changed and there is no way to go back to the old days.

Although it is difficult, except in retrospect, to know where one is in an unfolding social process, because events are, so to speak, in the making, it appears that with reference to both emergent diseases and global warming, the first act has ended (or at least is approaching that point, if more so with health and climate-focused scientists than with politicians). The second act, Rosenberg argues, ushered in by acceptance of the striking change that has occurred, involves the emergence of a social framework for managing uncertainty. An important part of the story of this process with reference to emergent diseases has been the slow collapse of hope for the rapid arrival of the medical silver bullets that were to save us from further threat from the diseases of the past. As Armelagos and co-workers (1996: 1) observed, "today, with the increasing use of antibiotics, we are facing a third epidemiological transition, a reemergence of infectious disease, with pathogens that are antibiotic-resistant and have the potential to be transmitted on a global scale." A further component of the new global public health paradigm is recognition of the degree to which the factors underlying the third epidemiological transition reflect socioeconomic inequalities.

Rapid, almost instant, global transmission of new infectious diseases has been linked to the so-called second wave of globalism.[1] According to Waters (2001: 8), globalism involves the "creation of new economic, financial, political, cultural, and personal relationships through which societies and nations come into closer and novel types of contact with one another." Driving this worldwide change is a set of transnational capitalist economic processes. As Greaves (2005: 154) observed, "at its heart, globalization involves corporations, technology, and capital. More precisely, it is a process of rapid internationalization and integration of commercial enterprises, supported by global communication technologies and global deployment of financial capital." In a globalized world, things—including capital, technology, commodities, people, and infectious diseases—move quickly and widely. All these flows, and their entwinement, have significant consequences for human health and well-being.

My purpose in this chapter, in light of the earlier discussion of SARS, is to push for a recharacterization of key features of the third epidemiological transition. Although it is evident that new infectious diseases are appearing in quick order and that globalism is an important part of the social context for this change, a critical feature of the contemporary epidemiological era is not just new infections but the *interaction* of diseases both old and new, acute and chronic, with significant effects on human morbidity and mortality—an epidemiological dynamic known as a *syndemic*. More exactly, I am concerned with the ever-growing impact of climate change on the spread of disease and on the syndemic process, a development that I call here an *ecosyndemic*. The notion of ecosyndemic fits within the broader perspective of "ecohealth" (Forget and Lebel 2001), an approach that "recognizes that there are inextricable links between humans and their biophysical, social, and economic environments that are reflected in individual/communities' health" (Bonet, quoted in Lebel 2003: 2). In short, I argue that the plagues of the twenty-first century are not an isolated set of individual diseases appearing in the world but an ever more complex array of interacting diseases, the spread of which is being driven by the dual (and themselves interacting) forces of globalism and global warming, both of which are shaped by human action, decision making, and the unequal and often oppressive structure of social relations.

The third and fourth acts in Rosenberg's model of plague epidemics (1992a: 285)—the social negotiation of "decisive and visible community response" (Act 3) and the assessment of lessons learned (Act 4)—are issues addressed in the conclusion of the chapter with specific reference to the synergistic diseases of global warming.

Introducing the Syndemic Perspective

Influenced by a political ecological understanding of the interface between social structure and the environment, the syndemic perspective developed initially in medical anthropology (Singer 2009) and diffused to epidemiology and public health. The perspective emerged in specific response to the dominant biomedical conceptualization of diseases as distinct entities in nature, separate from other diseases and independent of the social and cultural contexts in which they are found. The multi-disciplinary political ecology approach incorporates political economy but, going beyond assessing the relationship of social inequality to health, takes into consideration the effects of social inequality on the environment and in turn, through human interactions, the effects of the environment on human health (Foster 2000). In its recognition and structural analysis of the fundamental role of social inequality as a critical factor in health, political ecology extends the concerns of medical ecology to the effects of human activity on the environment and the role of the environment on human health.

Within this expanded biosocial framework, the syndemic perspective is characterized by three features. First, it draws attention to the multiple and often complex interconnections that develop between co-morbid diseases and other health-related problems in a population, as well as in the bodies of individual sufferers at both the biological and social levels. Demarcating individual diseases, giving them unique labels such as "tuberculosis," and focusing intensely on understanding their specific nature, array of signs and symptoms, and immediate causes have allowed the development of modern pharmaceutical, surgical, and other biomedical treatments of disease. Nevertheless, it has become increasingly evident that diseases and other health conditions such as violence victimization do not exist in nature in isolation. Nor do they merely coexist with other diseases. Instead, diseases *interact synergistically* in substantial ways that affect individuals and populations.

A syndemic perspective is intended to allow a new way of thinking about disease in relational rather than categorical terms. In other words, instead of focusing an ever more powerful lens on the "part," as has been the case historically in biomedicine and public health, syndemics theory draws attention to the whole and to the connections among the parts, including the ways in which they promote and reinforce each other and thereby create complex health conditions. As Chadwick (2003: 119) explains about new ways of looking at the notion of species, if you look at them one way, "you see individual things; look the other way, you see processes, relationships—things together. This is the new level in understanding biology."

Second, syndemics theory points to the fundamental importance of the interacting social and environmental conditions that promote the spread of disease, as well as their health effects at the individual and group levels. In this regard, syndemics theory focuses attention on disease concentrations or clusters, the specific pathways and processes through which diseases interrelate biologically in individual bodies and in populations, and the ways in which these interactions increase disease burden. Significantly, in syndemics, the health effects of co-morbid conditions are not additive but multiplicative.

Finally, in keeping with its focus on connections and crossing points, syndemics theory conceptualizes disease in terms of the encompassing biosocial environment. Unlike in traditional environmental models, however, nature is not conceived of as natural, in the sense of being separate from and independent of human action, a reserve of nonhuman things. Rather, there is a strong concern in the syndemic perspective about the historical ways in which the "natural" environment, no less than the built environment, has been shaped and influenced by human action, intentional and otherwise. Of special concern are the ways in which affected environments reflect social inequalities within and across societies. The latter is important because (1) syndemics are found disproportionately among subordinated groups, precisely because of their social status; (2) the exercise of power in society shapes the human imprint on the physical environment; and (3) effective public health responses to syndemics (including ecosyndemics) require a focus on underlying causal factors. In this, the syndemic perspective transcends mere awareness or even investigation of disease co-morbidity as a health condition. As Krieger (2001: 674) commented, it is important to think "critically and systematically about intimate and integral connections between our social and biological existence—and ... to name explicitly who benefits from and is accountable for social inequalities in health."

Varieties of Disease Interactions

Interest in the syndemic perspective has been driven by growing evidence of the regularity of interactions among diseases and the recognition that these contacts influence disease course, expression, severity, transmission, diffusion, and response to treatment. Several kinds of interactions among diseases have been described, including both indirect interface (i.e., changes caused by one disease that facilitate another disease) and direct interface (i.e., several diseases acting together in causing ill health). In some syndemic interactions—such as the one between diabetes and SARS—changes in biochemistry or damage to organ systems caused by one disease, such as weakening of the immune system, promotes the progression of another (Rickerts et al. 2006). Similarly, evidence exists that periodontitis, the progressive loss of the soft tissues that surround and support the teeth, may be the consequence of a syndemic involving the promotion of one type of infection by another (Slots 2007).

A different type of syndemic relationship involves one disease enhancing the virulence of another (McKenny, Brown, and Allison 1995; Scheiblauer et al. 1992). There is evidence, for example, that herpesvirus has this effect on HIV infection, with progression to full-blown AIDS being significantly accelerated by co-infection with herpesvirus (Lusso et al. 2007). Alternatively, one disease can assist the physical transmission of another, as seen in syphilis and HIV co-infection (McClelland et al. 2005).

Direct interaction of diseases is seen in the case of gene mixing among different types of pathogenic agents, as has been described in various species, or even among different strains or clades of the same pathogen (Steain et al. 2004).

In some cases, co-infection may open up multiple syndemic pathways. A lethal synergism has been identified, for example, between influenza virus and pneumococcus, a likely cause of excess mortality from secondary bacterial pneumonia during influenza epidemics (McCullers and Rehg 2002). In other cases, syndemic interaction among diseases is apparent but the linkages have not yet been made clear (Decock, Verslype, and Fevery 2007).

Social Origins of Syndemics

The term *syndemic* points beyond interactive biology to the roles of social conditions and the structure of social relations in the development of disease concentrations, the frequency of disease interactions, and the health outcomes of synergistic disease interactions. In syndemics, the interface among diseases or other health-related problems commonly reflects a configuration of adverse social factors (e.g., poverty, stigmatization, health care disparities) that put subjugated individuals and groups at heightened risk for disease exposure while limiting their access to prevention and treatment. Additionally, as a result of various physical effects of being subject to discrimination, suffering social rejection, enduring stigmatization, and internalizing oppression (Baer, Singer, and Susser 2003; Dressler and Bindon 2000), as well as exposure to noxious living and working conditions, subordinated populations commonly encounter disease threats in less than optimal health and with potentially compromised immune and other body systems.

This pattern can be seen, for example, in the mortality and morbidity statistics for African Americans. Whereas average life expectancy at birth for white males in the United States is 76.7 years, for African American males it is only 67.8 years, a deficit of about eight years. Among white females, the average life expectancy is 79.9 years, compared with 74.7 years for African American females, a deficit of about five years. African Americans have been found to be at significantly greater risk of death, including premature death, than whites, among all people still alive at any given age. Most existing studies show a 30 percent higher age-adjusted risk of mortality among African Americans. Much of the difference, which reflects a greater disease burden, is explained by differences in the socioeconomic status (SES) of African Americans relative to whites. Analysis of several national studies by Franks and colleagues (2006) found that an additional mortality burden among African Americans after statistical adjustment for SES was a consequence of the health damage caused by being subjected to racism and related forms of discriminatory treatment, which resulted in adverse chemical changes in the bodies of stressed populations and caused health damage (Krieger and Sidney 1996).

Lower SES and being subject to racism have been found to interact, increasing the damaging health effects of each condition. Further, poor people in cities with smaller impoverished populations have been found to be at lower risk of dying than those in cities with large impoverished populations. In other words, the density of poverty in an area appears to be a crucial determinant of the health status of the poor (Budrys 2003). Studies of differences by location among the poor show that the "sociophysical" environment in which people live— that is, their conscious experience of their surrounding community, including issues of danger, stress, comfort, and appeal—is also an important determinant of their health. Feelings of hopelessness and powerlessness in a community have been found to be good predictors of health risk and health status. There is, in short, a biology of poverty and social injustice that puts subjugated populations at heightened risk (Leatherman and Goodman 1998).

A recent example of this pattern is seen in the case of antimicrobial drug–resistant *Staphylococcus aureus*. This staph strain, which can cause skin infections, usually mild but capable of developing into pneumonia, was first described in hospitals and nursing homes (Maree et al. 2007). It was, in fact, the first bacterium in which resistance to penicillin was discovered, just four years after the drug entered into mass production. A new study by Hota and co-workers (2007) found that the greatest risk factors of infection included prior experience with incarceration, being African American, and residence in public housing. Being poor and a member of a marginalized ethnic minority, in conjunction with the living conditions and experiences this entails—from overcrowding to a lack of sanitary conditions—has become a risk factor for what began as a disease of clinical settings.

In the same way, HIV, which was first observed among gay men, became a disease of the poor and of ethnic minorities in the United States. Freudenberg and colleagues (2006), for example, described a syndemic composed of HIV, tuberculosis (TB), and street violence among the inner-city poor in New York that began in the mid-1970s. This syndemic was produced by oppressive social conditions exacerbated by budget and policy decisions involving cuts to health and social programs intended, ostensibly, to save money for the city. Instead, they contributed to deteriorating living conditions, a 20 percent rise in the number of poor people in the city despite an overall population decrease of 10 percent, and a rise in the health burden of the poor. As a result, TB rates in New York began going up after a century of decline, producing an excess of more than fifty thousand TB cases beyond what was expected. AIDS cases, too, shot up, especially among drug users. By 1985 there were estimated to be 250,000 drug addicts in New York City, only 30,000 (12 percent) of whom were in drug treatment (CDC 2005). Rates of homicide in the city also began rising in the late 1970s and continued to climb through 1990, resulting in the deaths of more than twenty thousand people (Freudenberg et al. 2006). Research by my colleagues and I in Hartford, Connecticut (Singer 2009), identified the existence of what we called the SAVA syndemic, involving intertwined substance abuse, street and domestic violence, and AIDS and a second syndemic involving HIV, chlamydia, and gonorrhea among the inner-city poor. Similarly, Stall and co-workers (2007) described a syndemic involving HIV, drug use, and partner violence among men who have sex with men. As these examples suggest, an emergent disease such as HIV can come to be intertwined with several different diseases and other threats to health, forming various distributional clusters. In time, these independent syndemics may merge into what might be called a "supersyndemic," a dynamic that syndemic theory predicts is most likely in populations that suffer multiple structural disadvantages.

In addition to the examples already cited, a growing number of other syndemics have been described in the literature (Singer 2009). Indeed, syndemics are being identified around the world as researchers begin to focus on the nature of connections among diseases and the social context factors that foster disease interactions (e.g., Herring and Sattenspiel 2007; Marshall 2005). Moreover, and of primary concern for this chapter, the rate at which new syndemics develop and are identified is likely to be significantly increased by global warming.

Dynamics of Global Warming

Although there has been debate among scientists about global warming, a clear consensus has emerged in recent years, if not one pleasing to many who wield power (Montet 2007). Climate scientists generally agree that a significant global warming trend is occurring, and it is primarily a consequence of human activities. What has particularly startled researchers in the last several years is the unexpected pace and magnitude of global warming. Just as the twentieth century was the warmest century in the past millennium, so the last ten years of the twentieth century constituted the warmest decade of the millennium. The initial years of the twenty-first century have continued to set records as well.

Underlying this climate change is the buildup of so-called greenhouse gases, most notably carbon dioxide, which trap a blanket of warm air around the planet and produce a rapid heating up of the oceans, initially, and the land as well. Over the last half century the oceans have absorbed about 85 percent of this increased heat. Warmer seawater speeds the rate of evaporation, fueling heavier rains and more damaging storms. In recent years, heavy rains (more than two inches per day) have increased by 14 percent, and very heavy rains (more than four inches per day) have gone up by 20 percent (Groisman et al. 2004). Moreover, tropical cyclones are growing in their destructive power as a result of longer storm duration and higher winds, and the frequency of major storms parallels increases in ocean temperature.

Additionally, over the last fifty years, weather patterns generally have become increasingly variable, with growth in the frequency of occurrence of extreme events such as prolonged and more intensive heat waves and enduring droughts (Houghton, Ding, and Griggs 2001). Many climatologists expect that the earth's climate will continue to warm by as much as 2.5–10°F over the next century.

Correspondingly, there has been a rise in sea level. According to estimates by the US Environmental Protection Agency (2007), global sea level rose six to twelve inches over the last one hundred years, some of it because of melting glaciers and the remainder because as seawater grows warmer, it expands. Importantly, various feedback systems appear to be accelerating climate change.

In sum, "global climate change is beginning [to affect] every aspect of life" on earth (Epstein and Mills 2005: 5), including, of special concern here, human health and well-being. Further, it is now recognized that the effects of global warming can develop suddenly, producing "climate shocks" that likely will have grave consequences for human societies.

Anthropogenesis and Sociogenesis: Human Diseases and Human Behavior

A growing number of climate scientists, including climate anthropologists, have reached the conclusion that global warming is largely anthropogenic—that is, the result of human activities—particularly since the Industrial Revolution. As Fagan (2004: 250) observed, "with the Industrial Revolution, we took a giant stride into an era in which we are frighteningly exposed to potential cataclysm, enhanced by our own seeming ability to warm the earth and increase the probability of extreme climate events." The United States, home to only 4 percent of the world's population, produces 25 percent of the planet's greenhouse gases, more than most of the developing nations of Asia, Latin America, and Africa combined (although Canada actually has a somewhat higher per capita level of energy consumption than the United States) (Lindsay 2001).

Global warming is not only anthropogenic but also sociogenic. It is largely a by-product of social structures and patterns, namely, the self-serving belief held by global elites and powerful corporations that the world has unlimited resources and the wedding of that belief to a neoliberal governmental policy commitment to the unrestrained flow of capital, ever-increasing commodity production, and the promotion of consumption-based lifestyles. Ideologically, global capitalism "promotes ... a 'productivist ethic,' a belief that continual economic expansion is necessary, socially beneficial, and natural" (Baer 2007: 13). "Ultimately," notes Baer (2007: 6), "global warming ... is primarily a problem that is part and parcel of global capitalism with its drive for profits that results in a tread-mill of ever increasing production and consumption." Notably, as Patz observed, "those most vulnerable to climate change are not the ones responsible for causing it ... Our energy-consumptive lifestyles are having lethal impacts on other people around the globe, especially the poor" (quoted in Elperin 2005: 2).

As the poor migrate to megalopolises in search of a livelihood (as they will at even faster rates as global warming undercuts subsistence in various locales), vast, ever-growing, concentrated populations are created and placed at risk of swift-moving infections and other diseases. Some of the developing world's megalopolises are now Mumbai, India, with more than 13 million people; Karachi, Pakistan, which is approaching 12 million; and Sao Paulo, Brazil, which has 11 million. The sheer size of these urban population islands is staggering, as is the potential for syndemic disasters resulting from the interactions of poverty, global warming, and globalism. In this light, Moran (2006: 21) asks: "Do we recognize that business-as-usual threatens the end of life as we know it? Or are we so self-satisfied in our own material success that we cannot recognize overwhelming evidence when we see it?" Global warming and the movement of diseases are components of the evidence to which Moran refers.

Global Warming and the Movement of Diseases

That diseases move is not new; people have always carried their disease with them, and diseases have found ways to diffuse by air, water, and other means, including on and in the bodies of pets and livestock. But global warming has disrupted natural ecosystems and thereby contributed to the rapid movement of a growing number of disease-causing pathogens. This pathogenic migration is occurring at a time when the planetary population growth recently concentrated in megalopolises places an unprecedented number people at risk for new diseases. In particular, pathogenic species that previously were restricted in their distribution by seasonal temperatures have begun invading new areas as the climate changes. As Ostfeld observed, "we're alarmed because in reviewing the research on a variety of different organisms we are seeing strikingly similar patterns of increases in disease spread or incidence with climate warming" (quoted in CBS News 2002). Diseases that may be spread because of global warming include mosquito-borne maladies such as malaria, dengue, Rift Valley fever, West Nile disease, Chikungunya fever, and yellow fever (Epstein 2007).

Until recently, for example, dengue was not found above 3,300 feet above sea level, because climates above that elevation were inhospitable to the Asian tiger mosquito. Today, it is found at 7,200 feet in the Andes in Colombia and is beginning to show up at similarly high elevations in Indonesia (Martens et al. 1995). In the United States, the mosquito that carries the dengue virus has moved as far north as Chicago. McAllen, Texas, suffered a harsh outbreak of dengue fever in 1995 (Patz et al. 1998). Malaria, which in Kenya was previously limited to three districts, has now been identified in thirteen of the country's districts. In 2005, South Africa's environment minister warned that the country could face a quadrupling of malaria cases by 2020 (Struck 2006). As many as 100 million extra cases of malaria have been predicted to occur worldwide by the end of the century than would have occurred without global warming (Pennington 1995). Houston, Texas, experienced a malaria outbreak in recent years, and cases have been diagnosed as far north as Michigan. Similarly, West Nile virus, which was not found in North America until the end of the twentieth century, has infected more than twenty thousand people in the United States and Canada and killed more than eight hundred people in recent years. The cause is the spread of the *Cluex pipiens* mosquito. Also of concern is the climate-based spread of disease-bearing rodents such as those responsible for the outbreak of hantavirus in the US Southwest in 1993 and pneumatic plague in India the following year; the spread of disease-causing ticks that carry encephalitis and Lyme disease and of sandflies that transmit visceral leishmaniasis (Cross and Hyams 1996); and an increase in water-borne diseases such as cholera in ever warmer seas. Warmer climates have led to notable jumps in encephalitis rates in Sweden and to cases of dengue in the Netherlands. Since 1987, major outbreaks of encephalitis have been recorded in the United States in Florida, Mississippi, Louisiana, Texas, Arizona, California, and Colorado.

These disease movements are occurring at an alarming pace. As Epstein reported, "things we projected to occur in 2080 are happening in 2006.... Our mistake was underestimation" (quoted in Struck 2006). Beyond rapid migration, global warming has a direct effect on the metabolism of pathogenic organisms, resulting in increased rates of growth and cell division (Platt 1995). Epstein (2005) calculated that an increase in temperature of only four degrees Fahrenheit would more than double the metabolism of mosquitoes, leading to more frequent feedings and resulting opportunities for the transmission of infections.

Increased heat and ozone depletion resulting from global warming increase ultraviolet-B radiation exposure. Because microorganisms reproduce rapidly, they are capable of swift genetic change, allowing for ever more rapid development of pathogen resistance to the chemical arsenal of biomedicine. Additionally, the same factors that cause global warming—environmental pollution and the buildup of chlorinated hydrocarbons—suppress the effectiveness of the immune system. This is true as well of malnutrition, which warmer climates will promote in many parts of the world. It has been established that the absolute virulence of many pathogens is kept in check by the body's natural defense systems. If these are compromised by a deteriorating environment and diet, previously harmless pathogenic strains can become lethal.

Heat exhaustion brought on by global warming is also increasing as a stressor on human populations, further reducing their capacity to respond to a disease challenge. In 1995, for example, Chicago experienced a summer heat wave that killed at least seven hundred people (Whitman et al. 1997). It has been estimated that by the year 2020, global warming could cause up to a 145 percent rise in mortality in megalopolises such as New York City. The problem is not only an urban issue. Research on the health effects of global-warming-related drought on the Canadian prairie, for example, found that it is associated with a range of health problems, "from respiratory illnesses from inhaling dust or smoke to mental health concerns arising from economic stress," as well as with nutritional problems related to crop failure and lack of access to clean water (Smoyer-Tomic et al. 2004: 144). Conversely, in mountain regions, the health consequences of global warming, such as the spread of infectious diseases to new elevations, will be enhanced by the social stress of flooding. An assessment of the health consequences of global warming in the Hindu Kush–Himalayas by Ebi and colleagues (2007: 269) concluded that "climate change ... will, mostly negatively, influence mountains and the people who depend on the ecosystem services they provide. The impacts of climate change on human health will be direct, indirect, multiple, interacting, and significant."

One effect of a warming climate is that pollen production has gone up, triggered by higher levels of carbon dioxide in the air. Tests on ragweed (*Ambrosia artemisiifolia*), a potent producer of pollen allergens, indicate that heightened carbon dioxide produces taller plants, greater biomass, and more pollen. Warmer weather also results in greater pollen production (Epstein and Rogers 2004) and longer growing periods. As a result, another health consequence of global warming is an escalation in rates of allergies and asthma associated with plant pollens and increases in carbon dioxide in the atmosphere. Currently, allergic diseases constitute the sixth leading cause of chronic illness in the United States, affecting the lives of 17 percent of the population. Asthma affects about 8 percent of the US population, with notable increases in rates in recent years, especially in low-income, ethnic minority populations. Both conditions are adversely affected by global warming. Compounding the problem, airborne pollens have been found to attach themselves to diesel particles from truck and other vehicular exhaust floating in the air, resulting in heightened rates of asthma in places where busy roads bisect densely populated areas, most notably in poorer inner-city areas. Additionally, increased moisture produced by global warming facilitates the growth of mold and of respiratory and other health complaints associated with mold inhalation.

As Epstein and Rogers emphasized (2004: 11), these patterns repeat themselves at the international level: "For developing nations and poor communities, the health impacts may be significant. As developing countries incorporate modern technologies to cope with climate change (e.g., air conditioning, indoor plumbing) on a wider scale, the resulting problems associated with poor building construction and maintenance also increase."

A study by the World Health Organization (2002) concluded that more than 150,000 people a year were already dying from the effects of global warming, and this number was expected to go up, doubling by 2020. Given the accelerated rate at which the effects of global warming are appearing, this, too, may be a case of underestimation.

Toward a Model of Ecosyndemics

From a syndemic perspective, an issue of great concern is what happens to diseases as they spread to new environments. To what degree, for example, do they encounter and cluster with other diseases in new host populations? Precisely which other diseases do they come into contact with there? In what ways, if any, do they interact with these coterminous diseases? And with what consequences for human health? The term *ecosyndemic* is used specifically to label the dual and interconnected effects of economic (and resulting social) changes introduced and advanced by processes of globalism and the spread of infectious diseases and other health problems produced by global warming. In light of these influences on the present and future health of the world's population, there is a critical need to rethink the nature of the third epidemiological transition. This transition is marked not only by emergent diseases in a globalized, high-tech world of growing class and ethnic health disparities but also by a sociogenically transformed physical environment characterized by diverse syndemics, ecosyndemics, and supersyndemics—the coming plagues of the twenty-first century—with untold consequences for human health and well-being.

Conclusion

The third act in Rosenberg's dramaturgic model concerns social response; he notes that "recognition implies collective action" (Rosenberg 1992a: 285). From a research perspective, further advances in understanding the nature of syndemic processes under conditions of globalism and global warming require pursuit of several lines of inquiry. First, there is a need for studies of the precise physical and social processes by which syndemics emerge, including the sets of health and social conditions that foster the occurrence of multiple epidemics in populations and the way syndemics function to produce specific kinds of health outcomes. Increasingly, the forces and processes of globalism are a fundamental element in this regard. Second, there is a need to better understand pathways of interaction between various kinds of diseases as well as between diseases and other adverse health-related factors, such as malnutrition and toxic environmental exposure, that reflect oppressive social relationships. Third, there is a need for closer examination of the ways in which global warming enables the spread of diseases and otherwise affects human health and its consequences, particularly for subordinate populations. Finally, there is a need for a better understanding of how the public health and medical systems as well as communities and nations can respond to limit the health consequences of syndemics and the social conditions that cause them.

Beyond research, there is an ever pressing need for significant social action, including structural change toward a "global system [that is] ... committed to meeting people's basic needs, [and achieving] social equity and justice, democracy, and environmental sustainability" (Baer 2007:

21). Failure to act in this way portends, in Epstein's apt phrase (quoted in Reinberg 2007: 1), a "sick future." Our contemporary dilemma is rooted in our capacity to learn this lesson in advance in order to be able to look back (in what in Rosenberg's framework is the final, culminating act) on a global disaster that was averted, if not (very likely) without significant social cost. Alternatively, if the worst nightmarish fears of some climate and health scientists are realized, there will be no looking back or lessons learned.

Notes

An earlier version of this chapter benefited significantly from insightful comments from Pamela Erickson and Hans Baer, as well as from all the participants in the Wenner-Gren Foundation conference "Plagues: Models and Metaphors in the Human Struggle with Disease."

1. A number of potentially confusing chronological schemes are in play here, which, like a Chinese puzzle, fit historically (more or less) within each other. At the broadest level, there are the first and second waves of globalism, which helped create the contemporary world as we know it. Within this framework, the first epidemiological transition—the consequential movement from small-scale, mobile, dispersed human societies to larger, settled populations that controlled domesticated animals and as a result were subject to infectious diseases of animal origin—occurred prior to the first wave of globalism, that is, the era of European global expansion and colonialism. The second epidemiological transition—involving the shift from a period characterized by the dominance of acute infectious diseases to one characterized, at least in the developed world, by chronic conditions associated with a longer-living population less subject to early death from infection—was very much a product of social developments ushered in by the first wave of globalism. Similarly, the second wave of globalism (the contemporary development of a global market system and rapid as well as boundless transportation and electronic communication systems) has played an important role in ushering in the third epidemiological transition, involving the rapid appearance and spread of emergent and reemergent infectious diseases (and, as argued here, of the interacting diseases of global warming). Rosenberg's dramaturgic model of plague epidemics (1992a) is invoked with specific reference to social processes associated with the third epidemiological transition.

three

Pressing Plagues
On the Mediated Communicability of Virtual Epidemics

Charles L. Briggs

Charles Rosenberg (1992b) urged us to think of epidemics drama-turgically—that is, as structured by common sorts of narrative sequences that move from increasing revelatory tension to crisis and on to closure. Their "public character and dramatic intensity," he argued, enable them to expose and illuminate epistemologies, cultural assumptions, moral values, social relations, and institutional practices. I am with him so far, but he comes to a point at which I feel the need to push farther. He continues: "Just as a playwright chooses a theme and manages plot development, so a particular society constructs its characteristic response to an epidemic" (1992: 279). What happens when the response comes before the epidemic? I would like to reverse the directionality here: How might we see epidemics as responses to processes of representation? I am concerned in this chapter with the development of narratives of epidemics of West Nile virus in San Diego, California, and cholera in Venezuela—before any humans became infected. These virtual epidemics (surely the best kind) enable me to ask how a plague comes to have a "public character and dramatic intensity" in the first place. I believe that taking up these questions, even in a preliminary way, can help us think more broadly about what sorts of medical objects are emerging and what kinds of medical subjects we are becoming in the twenty-first century.

Science studies scholars have sparked growing interest in ethnographic studies of science, the effects of new scientific objects on contemporary life, and the ways in which they are imbued with value. As Kaushik Sunder

Rajan (2006) suggested, however, the cachet seems to lie in studying scientific concepts "upstream," following them to the laboratories and other sites in which they are made, named, disputed, normalized, and black-boxed. Interested in issues of scale (Latour 1988; Tsing 2005), here I look "downstream" at the way science and medicine seem to move from laboratories or the offices of epidemiologists to become spectacles. The news media play crucial roles in deciding when research findings will be transformed into widespread changes in biopolitical perspectives or when reports on pens of infected chickens, handfuls of patients in rural hospitals, and accounts of new influenzas, most recently H1N1, will set off global alarms. As the Latin American media theorist Jesús Martín Barbero (1987) poignantly argued, the media are not simply *in* society but shape concepts of self, social life, and our understandings of "society" itself, at the same time that the meaning and impact of media texts are shaped by active processes of reception.

Note the dual implications here. First, news coverage of epidemics and health in general has been marginalized in the anthropology of medicine and science, leaving us with little understanding of a key dimension of public discourse in these areas—let alone of the way health and science become news. Second, and perhaps most important, we have missed the "mediatization" of health and science, that is, the way these processes of representation are reshaping biomedical and scientific institutions.

One reason news coverage of biomedicine is generally sidelined is the reductionist way in which it is viewed by scholars and laypersons alike. Ideologies of communication that characterize it as the transfer of information generally lead to a focus on *content*. As Rosenberg suggested for epidemics, however, "framing and blaming are inextricably mingled" (1992b: 287). The role of the narrative content of news coverage of plagues in scapegoating stigmatized populations—and thus shaping the actions of public health authorities and clinicians—is crucial; I have worked on these issues myself (Briggs with Mantini-Briggs 2003). Nevertheless, we know much less about practices, about how biomedical objects—microbes, medications, devices, and diseases—are produced as communicative-biomedical hybrids, fusing our understanding of these objects with genealogies of the representations through which we learn about them.

My claim is that news coverage plays a crucial part not just in the way plagues get "covered" but in the way they come to be social and scientific phenomena in the first place. Mediatization does not begin simply when reporters enter the scene but in laboratories, clinics, and epidemiologists' offices as well. In order to grasp how epidemics emerge in news coverage, we need to pay close attention to issues of content, practices, and the ideological construction of the process, which I examine here by scrutinizing the virtual phases of epidemics of West Nile virus and cholera. To return to Rosenberg, I hope to show that epidemics are not simply metaphorically constructed as narratives, but their social lives are produced in part by a range of practices that we reductionistically envision as "news stories." Nevertheless, mediatized plagues spring not only from journalistic practices but also from the way biomedical institutions create images that are designed to be detached by journalists and reinserted in particular ways. I do not wish to make some sort of claim for an autonomous realm of representation or discourse—the power, I suggest, lies in the way microbes, mosquitoes, public health offices, antibiotics, and news reports intersect in consequential ways. Audiences, of course, have their own detachment practices that can reconfigure these images and structure their social and political effects. I propose that we need to study the way epidemics become mediatized, examining both ideologies and practices.

Covering Cholera in Venezuela, February–November 1991

My first example comes from news coverage of cholera in Venezuela between late January 1991, when the first cases were reported in Peru, and 4 December 1991, when the first case emerged in Venezuela. This was an ideal scenario from a health education and promotion point of view. The Venezuelan Ministry of Health and Social Assistance (MSAS) focused substantial energy and resources on "informing the public" about the disease and preventive measures. Founded in 1943, *El Nacional* had enjoyed decades as Venezuela's national reference newspaper (Bisbal 1994: 111; Giménez and Hernández 1988: 83). *El Nacional* published several articles a day on cholera, and its reporters considered themselves to be collaborators in this pedagogical project (Briggs 2003). Public awareness was high, and many Venezuelans were concerned about a possible epidemic. Co-researcher Clara Mantini-Briggs (a Venezuelan public health physician) and I collected nearly all the articles that appeared in *El Nacional* and several other national and regional newspapers between February 1991 and December 1992. We also interviewed public health officials, health education and promotion specialists, journalists, politicians, and laypersons.

With respect to content, we have detailed elsewhere (Briggs 2003; Briggs with Mantini-Briggs 2003) how press reporting merged images of a frightening, highly infectious disease with images of three populations "at high risk" for being infected with cholera and for infecting others: the poor; street vendors of food and drink; and indigenous people. Reporters and public health officials claimed to have empirical evidence of these groups' susceptibility, seemingly acquired by visiting poor homes and sidewalk stalls and pushcarts and discovering unhygienic conditions and biomedical ignorance. Since 59 percent, 40 percent, and 2 percent of the population, respectively, were classified as poor, as workers in the "informal" economy, and as members of indigenous groups, we could surmise that it was quite a feat of epidemiological detective work to have determined where cholera would be concentrated and how it would spread, even before any cases were reported in Venezuela. A more likely explanation seems to emerge from Stuart Hall's (1985) notion of "articulation," the way in which old categories are reinscribed in new crises and moral panics. Photographs, many of them archival shots, were placed alongside the newspaper articles, imbuing stereotypes with visual form and thus an air of authenticity and credibility. By the time *Vibrio cholerae* made its entrance in Venezuela, cholera had become a hybrid object—a fusion of biomedical pathogens and human "vectors."

Health reporters accommodated their everyday practices not to *Vibrio cholerae* (there wasn't any in the country for nearly a year) but to the dissemination of information about it. Health reporters attended press conferences held by the minister of health and the national epidemiologist. Isabel Machado, a reporter at *El Nacional* for more than twenty years, noted that "they really helped us out a lot, they gave us the bulletins, we called them every day. I had the cell phone number of the minister of health, I'd call, 'Look, what's new, has anything happened?' We had access to everybody . . . We had the advantage that they knew us already, we weren't just somebody who was calling them."

The ministry itself systematically reorganized its practices to meet the challenges offered by an impending cholera epidemic—the communicative challenges, that is. Relationships between ministry offices were defined, in the *Weekly Epidemiological Record*, in terms of the way cholera statistics were to be produced and circulated and who had the right to relay them beyond the walls of the institution (MSAS 1991). This communicative restructuring was designed to regulate which discourse about cholera would be produced, how it would move within the institution, and what would be publicly released; only a few persons could speak for the ministry.

This mediatization of institutional practices—their reorganization in order to control media representations of cholera—continued once the first cases were reported. In a letter dated 8 January 1992 (a month into the Venezuelan epidemic), Minister Páez Camargo decreed that "from this date on, information regarding 'Suspected Cholera Cases' will remain outside of the vocabulary of declarations to the media, treating doubtful cases as diarrhea until the 'positive' feces culture is in hand." Practices in the ministry concerned not only the production of mediatized information but also its reception. A minister of health who served during the cholera epidemic told me that his daily routine began at five in the morning; when his driver picked him up, he had all the major newspapers stacked on the seat beside him. In other words, the minister was one of the most avid consumers of health news coverage.

Public health officials and medical reporters whom we interviewed largely shared an ideological construction of how public discourse about cholera should be produced and circulated. Authoritative information about the disease emanated from the National Office of Epidemiology and the national reference laboratory, along with a number of international institutions that shape health policies and practices, particularly the Pan American Health Organization (PAHO) and the World Health Organization (WHO). This information was then projected as moving through three circuits. First, health professionals, particularly those employed by MSAS, received technical information from manuals, the *Boletín Epidemiológico Semanal* (Weekly Epidemiological Record), circulars, and the like. Second, the Division of Social Health Promotion circulated nontechnical information in forms such as posters and brochures to employees in other institutions, community leaders, and other laypersons. Some of this information also found its way to "the public" via the media. Finally, statements by the minister of health and the national epidemiologist, as articulated in press conferences and telephone calls, were relayed as news by reporters to their audiences. Journalists and public health officials characterized the way this information should be received—it should be comprehended, assimilated into ways of thinking about hygiene, disease, food procurement and preparation, and so forth, embodied in action, and then relayed to family members, co-workers, and neighbors.

This projection of the production, circulation, and reception of knowledge about health imagines a number of subject positions arranged hierarchically on the basis of their proximity to the "source" of the information. It constitutes a chronotope, imagining information as flowing outward in time and space from an institutional center. Each party has specific and limited communicative obligations. It is the professional obligation of institutional officials and reporters and the moral duty of members of "the public" to pass on the information in a way that retains its referential stability—that is, without "distorting" or "misunderstanding" it.

The process was, however, precarious. Reporters often criticized the minister and other officials for perceived failures to immediately transmit full, accurate information. Although reporters imagined themselves as partners in health education, public health officials complained bitterly that reporters "distorted" their words through ignorance of the biomedical facts, interest in selling newspapers or television advertising, and antagonism toward the state. Both saw "the public" as the weakest link, uninterested, ignorant, or resistant. Members of the three "high risk" categories were deemed to be virtually incapable of playing their proper role. Speaking of the immediate visibility of the hygienic shortcomings of the poor and workers in the informal sector, veteran *El Nacional* health reporter Marlene Rizk (1991) stated: "None of these measures is being complied with, and [to observe this] it takes only a trip through the center of the city [Caracas], where every day the number of street vendors increases, or a visit to any barrio, where the minimum hygienic conditions are missing." To be judged as failing to grasp "the message" properly was tantamount to being characterized as unsanitary subjects, people who did not relate to their bodies through biomedical epistemologies, adopt hygienic practices, or respect the monopoly of medical professionals over issues of disease. The implications for broader political and social rights were profound (Briggs with Mantini-Briggs 2003).

West Nile Virus in San Diego County

To further investigate the mediatization of health, media scholar Daniel Hallin and I conducted a study of news coverage of health in the United States, initially concentrating on the San Diego, California, area. Our original focus was the *San Diego Union-Tribune* (SDU-T), which has a paper circulation of 242,705 on weekdays and 309,571 on Sundays and 1.3 million electronic users, making it twenty-fourth largest in the United States.[1] Our initial corpus included all the health coverage from 2002 and the first half of 2003. We did a quantitative content analysis of the 1,205 stories that appeared in the first six months of 2002. We then interviewed individuals and organizations listed as sources, including hospital and health maintenance organizations, clinicians, medical researchers, public health officials, representatives of biotechnology and pharmaceutical corporations, trade groups, and media consultants. We also interviewed health reporters and their editors or producers and conducted interviews and focus groups with readers and viewers. We later compiled corpora from English- and Spanish-language television news and other print media. Our present work includes other media with larger circulations, such as the *New York Times* and CNN.

Within the San Diego County government, the Department of Environmental Health (DEH) and the Health and Human Services Agency (HHSA) split the state-mandated obligation to disseminate public health information, the former largely taking up clinical issues, and the latter, vector control, food safety, and other environmentally related health issues. Dr. Susan Norris is the public health officer for San Diego County, directing HHSA's Public Health Program.[2] Confident and poised, she had gained substantial experience with the press in the two and a half years she had served in this capacity by the time of the interview. DEH director Dr. George Murdoch, knowledgeable and self-assured, included two of his colleagues, Judy Evans and Art Smith, the directors of DEH's food safety and vector-borne disease programs, respectively. As we looked out at a beautiful view of the San Diego harbor, the three responded in a remarkably coordinated fashion, constructing cogent responses that, in the case of Evans and Smith, reflected their particular institutional foci. Following up on Norris's suggestion, I interviewed Traci McCollum, a media specialist in the Office of Media and Public Affairs (OMPA) who coordinates press relations for HHSA. McCollum had previously worked for fourteen years as a reporter in San Diego County, followed by three years in a for-profit health maintenance organization (HMO).

Ideologies of Mediatization

I begin by examining the way these officials constructed news reporting of health issues. Efforts to obtain and shape press coverage were a major way in which officials constructed the county government. As Murdoch put it, "I think we're fortunate in this county that this county's culture is: we need to work with the media to the maximum extent possible to get our message out, no matter what program it is." Note the invocation here of the classic sender-receiver mode of communication, involving a unilinear "transmission" of "a message," a bounded packet of information that is defined in terms of its referential content, from one party to another, both of whom are defined by their contrastive roles in the communicative "event." Murdoch ideologically constructed this media-centered institutional "culture" through the use of the sender-receiver model: "You know, we really rely on the media to help us get our message out, because we can only reach a limited segment of the population [with] anything organized that we may do. And the media is much more effective than we are in getting that out." Who, then, is the receiver? In reference to news coverage of "a large food-borne outbreak," Evans noted that DEH and HHSA joined forces to "provide the message to the public and to keep them informed about the progress of the investigation."

These officials constructed the desired process of public reception in both cognitive and behavioral terms. Cognitively, just as the county had a duty to "inform the public," so members of the public were expected to be informed by county-initiated press coverage and to change their cognitive maps of health issues to reflect the scientific evidence that, according to Norris, shaped what was placed in public circulation. Press coverage was needed to overcome a "lack of knowledge" on the part of the public. When asked what type of response should result from the reception of health news, Murdoch stated clearly and succinctly: "They should change their behavior." Evans added that "we may want them to take action." The concepts of knowledge and behavior are co-constitutive in this communicable lexicon—ignorance is defined in terms of behavior as the failure of "the public" to act in ways that county health officials deem necessary. In short, just as news coverage plays a key role in the way these officials construct county government, so it provides a key dimension in the way they imagine "the public" and the state.

Reporters, on the other hand, are neither "senders" nor "receivers" but parties whom health officials can "utilize ... to get [the] message out," as Murdoch put it. Many health reporters describe themselves similarly to public health professionals, as constituted through their efforts to "inform the public." Nevertheless, public health officials—even when they recognize that reporters embrace this ideological construction— contrast their own orientation toward "the public's" health with the "mission" of journalists: "to get customers," Norris said, that is, to sell newspapers or television advertising. Lacking knowledge of health issues and the proper orientation, reporters could adequately fulfill their function of providing a useful vehicle through which health officials could reach "the public" only once they became objects of a pedagogical process. Murdoch defined his agency's task as that of "trying to educate the uninformed reporter. So I'm going to go a little bit further to educate them, to get my message across."

County officials constructed their relationship with reporters as involving two distinct processes, which Smith referred to as "push" and "pull":

> There's two parts to that—some of it is we decide what we want to get out, and the other is someone else's pushing us to get something else out. Like the press is calling us, saying, "We just heard about" or "There's a story breaking in northern California or someplace else and is that happening here?" or "What's going on?" And vice [versa]—you know, West Nile virus or food safety stuff. We push it out. So there's a little push, a little pull.

The "pull" involves responding to reporters' requests for information, including those relating to health crises and accusations leveled against these agencies.

Ideologies of Mediatization and Biocommunicability

The manner in which these officials construct their interactions with the press and the process of "informing the public" in general illustrate what I refer to as *communicability* (Briggs 2007), meaning the sorts of everyday constructions of the way knowledge is purportedly produced, circulated, and received and the way individuals and institutions participate in this process. I term discursive acts and practices that focus on health and medical issues *biocommunicability* (Briggs 2005; Briggs and Hallin 2007). A perspective that relies on the concepts of communicability and biocommunicability stands in contrast to the functionalist approach, based in information theory and concerned with the effectiveness of the transmission of messages to individual patients or the mass public, which dominates most research in health communication and practices of health education and health promotion.

The concept I call biocommunicability draws on several theoretical perspectives. European critical discourse analysis envisions discourse both in Foucauldian perspective, as practices that produce the objects to which they purport to refer, and through Bourdieu's (1991) practice theory, as infusing symbolic forms with value, siting their acquisition within particular institutions, controlling access to them, and naturalizing their categories and inequalities ("misrecognition"). Linguistic anthropologists have stressed that language and communication are ideologically constructed; language ideologies are both shaped by and shape social relations, history, and political economy (Schieffelin, Woolard, and

Kroskrity 1998). Michael Silverstein (2004) suggested that discursive practices produce subjectivities and inequalities through the ongoing ideological construction of discursive events as they are unfolding.

I also draw on the post-Habermasian literature, specifically Michael Warner's attention to the way discourses create publics that are nevertheless characterized as preexisting. Warner (2002: 116) suggested that "the pragmatics of public discourse must be systematically blocked from view." This public (re)production, rather, seems to involve the cultural construction of ongoing discursive practices, rendering some dimensions visible and construing them in particular ways, erasing others, and imagining subjectivities, social relations, and forms of agency. My work with Hallin on mediatized health also has affinities with the work of Roddy Reid (2005), who explored the creation of neoliberal subjects in anti-smoking campaigns, and Eric Klinenberg (2002), who examined the ideological construction of the public health catastrophe that resulted from the 1995 Chicago heat wave.

Communicability is a central dimension of self-regulation—individuals structure schemes of self-surveillance and self-control, in part, as they are interpellated vis-à-vis categories, subjectivities, and discursive relations seemingly presupposed by communicative processes (I use *interpellation* to refer to the act of assuming the social position in which one is located by virtue of being designated as the "receiver" of a particular discursive act). Biocommunicability draws attention to the ways in which the constitution of social subjects is embedded in ideologies about the "flow" of health information, who generates biomedical knowledge, who is authorized to evaluate it and to speak about it, and through what channels it is assumed to "flow." Communicable cartographies do not automatically produce social subjects, nor do they necessarily reproduce or naturalize hierarchies of power neatly and without contradiction; they are produced in multiple ways by biomedical researchers, public health officials, journalists, and audiences.

The county health officials I interviewed provided similar cartographies of biocommunicability. Norris suggested that the "information" officials used in "informing the public" was evidence based—by analogy, it would seem, with current constructions of clinical and public health practice. Murdoch, Norris, and their colleagues then envisioned themselves as transforming specialized scientific and medical knowledge into messages comprehensible to reporters and in line with their notions of newsworthiness. The media made this "information" available to "the public," which became "informed," made needed "behavioral changes," and took the specified "actions." The informational process was thus unidirectional, constituting a flow from specialized, knowledge-rich sectors to sectors lacking this information or possessing erroneous beliefs and undertaking inappropriate behaviors and misguided actions. This is a classic example of what Hallin and I characterize as the biomedical, or "doctor's orders"/passive patient, cartography of biocommunicability, which contrasts with two other varieties that center on neoliberal constructions of active patient-consumers and public-sphere debates between citizens (Briggs and Hallin n.d.).

The Communicability of West Nile Virus

San Diego County's West Nile virus (WNV) "campaign" beautifully illustrates these social constructs in action, for a number of reasons. One is that the county's attempt to get press coverage of WNV is a locus classicus of "push" efforts, and it constitutes a key site for attempting to sustain biomedical-authority cartographies of communicability. Second, WNV emerged fairly recently as a health focus in California, in July 2003, enabling us to track its emergence. Third, both DEH and HHSA have made WNV a major focus of their media efforts.[3] Fourth, West Nile virus, unlike cholera, is imagined as a disease that affects broad populations rather than "targeting" particular demographic sectors; in other words, it "threatens" middle-class white residents as well as others. Finally, WNV is a hard sell: with relatively few human cases and no deaths in the county, it has been difficult to generate much interest in it on the part of reporters or audiences. WNV thus reveals the mediatization process by putting it to the test.

West Nile virus is a member of the Japanese encephalitis antigenic complex of viruses, generally transmitted by *Culex* mosquitoes, which infect humans, birds, horses, and other animals. In humans, the vast number of people infected are asymptomatic, 20 percent develop the flu-like symptoms of West Nile fever (fever, headache, body aches, nausea, and vomiting, as well as swollen lymph glands and skin rashes in some patients), and fewer than 1 percent develop severe symptoms that can lead to coma, convulsions, numbness, paralysis, and occasionally death. The disease was first reported in the United States in New York in 1999. Spread by migratory birds, it is now found in nearly every US state, Canada, Mexico, and other parts of the Americas. WNV was first documented in California in July 2003 (Reisen et al. 2004). By the end of 2004, the virus was reported in all California counties (at least in mosquitoes or animals), 830 people had been infected, and 28 people had died (County of San Diego 2004b).

The California Department of Health Services (CDHS) WNV program tests mosquitoes and compiles statistics by county on the number of birds, squirrels, horses, sentinel chickens, and humans infected and killed by West Nile virus. It also tracks the western equine encephalomyelitis (WEE) and St. Louis encephalitis (SLE) viruses. A "Be a West Nile Watcher" program invites members of the public to become amateur disease detectives by reporting dead birds and squirrels to toll-free telephone numbers or the Web site www.westnile.ca.gov. In keeping with the dominant biocommunicable model, nearly all WNV press releases specify the behaviors and actions that San Diego residents should take: "The public can protect against WNV by limiting outdoor activity at dawn and dusk, wearing long sleeves and pants, using insect repellant with DEET, removing standing water from the perimeter of your house, and ensuring that windows and doors have tight fitting screens, and holes in screens are repaired" (County of San Diego 2004a). Carrying out these "behavioral changes" and "actions" involves curbing some of the most popular activities in San Diego, such as gathering along the beach at sunset, wearing shorts and short-sleeved shirts, and leaving doors and windows open. It seeks to discipline bodies in an area that prides itself on freedom from climatic and social constraints on attire.

One of the duties of county public health departments in California is to disseminate WNV information, which is prominently displayed on their Web sites. WNV media efforts vary widely between counties, reflecting substantial differences in scale and resources. Smaller offices essentially repeat CDHS press releases, whereas those boasting metropolitan centers generate much more WNV press activity. These differences are not simply epidemiologically driven. As of May 2009, San Diego County had reported fifty-six human WNV cases and no deaths.[4] Nevertheless, the county public health office had generated substantial press coverage regarding WNV, revealing how attempts to regulate public discourse about health intersect with journalistic practices and how this process shapes both what can be said and what cannot be said in public discourse.

Months of planning prepared DEH, HHSA, OMPA, and their respective staffs for the periodic release of WNV "campaign" materials and for the first animal or bird case in the state or, especially, the county, for a sudden rise in animal or bird cases or deaths, for the first human infection, and for the possibility of a human death. Norris commented that "months before even the season was going to start, you know, we got the logo, the character, we had a lot of contingency stuff ready to go when the ... first isolate in California happened. Then we would go with all of this out to the media." Nevertheless, as Smith put it, getting the media to cover WNV was a hard sell: "Frankly, we can't get into the media right now, because it's not interesting enough... We've put out press releases, but you wouldn't know it because the media isn't really picking up on it."

Accordingly, the announcement of a possible human infection in San Diego County on 5 July 2004 caused quite a stir. Media specialist McCollum recounted how the event—the communicable event, that is—was sparked:

> A woman called the media and said, "I have the West Nile virus, I'm the first test case." ... If the person goes out in front of you and says, "I'm it!" to get the media's attention, that's not something that you're totally prepared for, and then as an agency you have to respond to that.... So that would be one where we would probably look at, we did everything we possibly could, but I wouldn't think that it would have portrayed us in the right light.

McCollum characterizes the situation as an embarrassing abnormality—from the perspective of the dominant biocommunicable cartography. Only particular public health officials, it seems, have the right to initiate press coverage, and the only appropriate source of information is a definitive test from a state laboratory, reported directly to Norris. McCollum surmises that lay challenges to this communicable monopoly could be motivated only by the desire "to get the media's attention," not by a shared concern with public health.

Murdoch and Norris successfully turned a potentially embarrassing "pull" into possibly the most effective "push" of 2004. Drawing on resources that had been created for just this sort of occasion, HHSA sent out a press release titled "First Possible Human Case of West Nile Virus Reported" shortly after the press covered the woman's auto-proclamation. As Geert Jacobs (1999) has argued, press releases are constructed in a complexly interdiscursive fashion in order to "preformulate the news," using features of style and content to distance the document from the person(s) and institution(s) responsible for writing it and to bring it nearer to the voice of the reporter, who will, it is hoped, reproduce it (with some modification) in his or her own voice. The press release from the San Diego County HHSA was a twofold pedagogical project, both providing specific WNV information and reinscribing the official biocommunicable cartography of epidemic information, laying out how and where authoritative information is produced, how it circulates, who has the right to convey it to the press, and how both reporters and "the public" should be interpellated and respond.

In this example, the opening sentence erases the woman's previous communicable position and recasts her anonymously as "a 45-year-old Escondido-area woman." The press release lodges the authority to assume the roles of speaker, author, and originator of the discourse in the institution, thereby monopolizing communicable agency:[5] "The San Diego County Health and Human Services Agency (HHSA) reports the first possible human case of locally acquired West Nile Virus (WNV) in San Diego County." The next sentence specifies the source of the information ("preliminary testing") and places communicable power specifically in Norris, who is referred to by both degree and institutional position. By quoting her directly in the third paragraph, the press release establishes its credibility by projecting itself as an iconic, direct extension of a performative utterance delivered by the county's highest public health authority. Even as she positions herself at the center of the communicable cartography, Norris distances herself, her agency, and the press release from the process by noting the preliminary nature of the results—the event might only seem to be of epidemiological significance.

This press release attempts to supplant the problematic communicable cartography, one that involves a test performed by a local hospital as announced to the press by the patient herself, with one that places sole authority to make public statements regarding epidemic diseases in the voice of the state. The map that is projected by the press release and attributed to Norris is located in a communicable chronotope (Bakhtin 1981) that extends from the Escondido area, in the northern part of the county, to Norris's downtown office to the CDHS in Sacramento. Norris projects the cartography upstream in time and space by declaring that the ground zero for the production of authoritative knowledge about WNV lies in "tests being done at the state level." In doing so, the press release not only specifies how reporters are to be interpellated but projects how and when the next communicable event can be initiated: "We have been told the results will be given to us after 4 p.m. today (July 6)." Thus, future press coverage must flow not from another statement by the possible WNV patient but from definitive knowledge provided by the state lab. Only an official report of the results of a viral test will resolve the dramatic tension—is this or it is not the long-awaited human index case in San Diego County? Norris constructs herself as the obligatory passage point (Latour 1988), the only legitimate conduit by which this information can reach San Diego reporters and audiences.

The press release then "pushes" this communicable cartography, suggesting that either positive *or* negative results will extend the standing communicable trajectory: "People in San Diego County need to be aware of the disease and ways to protect themselves against it." The next two paragraphs provide boilerplate statements regarding WNV transmission and the actions required on the part of "the public." The cartography is then projected into the future in terms of HHSA's and DEH's continuing communicable roles of WNV surveillance and research. Readers are invited to insert themselves into county communicability more directly by visiting its Web site—thereby avoiding the mediating role of reporters.

Just who, we might ask, are these readers? As Jacobs (1999) argued, press releases often use third-person self-reference (HHSA "reports"), direct quotations, and expert knowledge to replace a tone of possible bias or self-promotion with an objective, neutral, disinterested voice. Style and content project a journalistic voice that reproduces information provided by the state (which seems to stand outside the body of the press release) as information that is already in public circulation—not as provided by an institutional official to a reporter. This style not only makes it easy for reporters to incorporate material from releases directly into their stories but also casts the discourse as "information" that "the public" has a right and a need to know.

Biocommunicable Contradictions

It might seem as if Murdoch, Norris, and their colleagues project a seamless communicable model. I suggest, rather, that county officials structurally undermine their cartography through the generally negative way in which they construct reporters and "the public." Rather than ratifying the authority of health officials as public-minded embodiments of scientific knowledge, reporters, in the eyes of county officials, look for bad news that will cast health professionals as biocommunicable failures. "We're keenly aware that they would really like to catch us fumbling, stumbling, mumbling, making a mistake, because that's much more entertaining than doing the right thing at the right time," said Murdoch. The public seems to present even more frequent and problematic threats to official biocommunicability. Rather than being passive receivers of whatever information county officials deem to be medically important, they "tune in" only to particular channels of communication "that people find most credible"—meaning that they have their own canons of evidence for deciding what is authoritative and relevant. Even when the "information" is successfully conveyed and learned, people forget and must be periodically reminded. Moreover, what should be an automatic transfer from cognition to behavior and action is often fractured: "What people know and what people do are two separate things," commented Evans.

Indeed, we found no focus group participants who worried about West Nile virus. Rather, they seemed to take precisely an "evidence-based" approach, drawing on their failure to witness WNV cases and deaths in their own environments and on their interpretations of official statistics as evidence. They read the county health authorities' biocommunicable construction—that knowledge of health threats should lead automatically to behavioral changes and actions—in reverse, suggesting that it would be inappropriate to become worried about and defend themselves against a disease that had infected only a small number of San Diego residents and killed no one, when their lives were significantly affected by other, quite real health issues. This skepticism seemed to be strongest among working-class Latinos and Latinas, who, according to county, state, and federal statistics, bear much greater health burdens than other segments of the population and have the least access to health care. Among middle-class participants, criticism of WNV discourse seemed to be more closely associated with distancing from the biomedical authority/passive patient cartography of communicability that organized the county's WNV press practices; they identified more with the neoliberal type of cartography (see Briggs and Hallin 2007). They saw themselves as active consumers who were governmentally required to seek out and evaluate health information and choose between treatment options. Even the sudden onset of a life-threatening illness seemed to require an active consumerist orientation toward tapping multiple sources of information and making choices, rather than simply accepting biomedical authority.

By asserting the right to derive evidence from their own experience and their reading of news coverage, and by placing WNV discourse in relationship to other health issues, laypersons constructed different communicable cartographies and positioned themselves within them. Insofar as members of the public seemed to accept the dominant cartography, they turned it around, viewing county officials as failing to act in keeping with the scientific evidence that would render their discourse authoritative. In other words, some audience members could accept official cartographies but reject the way they were interpellated within them, repositioning health officials, reporters, and themselves in the proffered subject positions. Others exploited the fissures and changing relations between biomedical authority, patient-consumer, and public sphere types of cartographies in constructing their own maps.

Official constructions of "the public" point to the gap between official practices and communicable cartographies. If efforts to inform the public were guided primarily by scientific evidence, health officials might have focused less on a disease that at the time had infected fewer than sixty people in San Diego County and killed none, and more on the ten leading causes of death in the county that year (coronary diseases, cancer, cerebrovascular diseases, chronic lower respiratory diseases, unintentional injuries, diabetes mellitus, influenza, pneumonia, suicide, and renal disease; see County of San Diego Board of Supervisors 2004). The seemingly unidirectional flow of discourse from scientific research to health authorities and from the media to the public, constructed in press releases and conferences, broke down as officials commented on specific examples of press coverage. Their candor suggests that what gets "pushed" depends a great deal on institutional criteria, including the availability of funding and the agendas of county and state politicians. Political pressure can even lead to scientifically questionable public statements, thereby contradicting the closely held professional commitments and ideologies of these dedicated public officials. The communicable role occupied by public health officials can be just as precarious as that of "the public." After detailing the extent of his and his staff's efforts to educate reporters and the public, Murdoch noted bluntly: "I don't really have any way to evaluate whether it makes a difference or not. I mean I have—I just know that we're there and we try, as [Evans] said, to develop out message points so they're succinct and concise ... but I really have no way of knowing if it matters at all that we did that or not."

Conclusion

My point in this chapter is not that communicable cartographies are simply a ruse to mask efforts to impose state agendas on "the public"; indeed, this formulation would reify the very communicable constructions that I am tracing and erase their multiplicity, contradictions, and uncertainties. It would also reproduce an elitist view of public health officials, suggesting that they (and they alone) see through the ideologies to grasp the way the process "really" works and are able to transform their designs into communicable reality. In spite of their many insights, this is just what Edward Herman and Noam Chomsky did in their *Manufacturing Consent* (1988). It would also construct San

Diego County public health officials in ways that contradict their daily struggle to resolve contradictions between their commitment to public health premises and practices and the ideologies of race, immigration, class, gender, sexuality, and the state that have great force in a politically conservative border area with a strong military presence. Given my own theoretical orientation, I would hardly want to argue that the political economies of health and the media and the ways in which they come together are irrelevant. The problem, rather, is that both popular and academic critics of state and journalistic representations of plagues tend to share the same depoliticized ideologies of communication that imbue media accounts of plagues with power.

I think we might start, instead, with the premise that creating a plague involves creating communicable cartographies, drawing on ideologies of communication and media, science and medicine, class, race, sexuality, gender, and place, and inflecting them in terms of the way the disease and its epidemiological profile are constructed and according to institutional contingencies. Just as Venezuelan national health authorities in the 1990s and San Diego County officials in 2003 shared remarkably similar constructions of the way health gets mediatized, so their cartographies were shaped by particular social inequalities, institutional structures and threats, historical circumstances, and clinical and epidemiological constructions of cholera and West Nile virus.

Both the cholera and WNV examples suggest that communicable cartographies and epidemic diseases are parts of the same semiotic packages. Focusing on the way meanings get attached to the experience of plagues and the way plagues are rendered understandable would seem to put the cart before the proverbial horse. With few exceptions, plagues are mediatized objects from the get-go these days, and even people who experience them bodily have generally come to know them previously through the media. An interesting discussion between medical anthropologists and colleagues in the history of medicine and public health might emerge if we compared differences and similarities between, on the one hand, the role of newspapers, television, radio, the Internet, cell phones, and other technologies in constructing contemporary plagues and, on the other, the rise of newspapers, novels, the telegraph, and other media in the case of nineteenth-century epidemics. At the same time that we seek to better capture the complexities of plague (see Herring and Swedlund, this volume), we need to account for seeming simplicities, to examine how heterogeneous, competing ideologies and practices are transformed into amazingly reductive narratives: Cholera is coming to Venezuela, and the poor, the street vendors, and the indigenous people will be to blame.

I have tried to show that it is not just diseases and epidemics that become mediatized objects; public health institutions themselves become profoundly mediatized. Procedures for attempting to control the creation, circulation, and reception of public discourse structure the way knowledge is produced in public health institutions; they are structured in part around questions of who can legitimately say what to whom. The example of the Venezuelan Ministry of Health and Social Assistance suggests how state agencies reorganize themselves and their knowledge practices in anticipation of a plague. The production of biomedical knowledge about cholera in Venezuela—how cases were officially diagnosed, how statistics were compiled and analyzed—was organized around the moments in which the minister or the national epidemiologist reported statistics and other information to the press, as well as to the World Health Organization. Communicable imaginaries deeply shaped what sorts of subjects and objects could become part of biomedical discourse and clinical practices, as well as what could be said about the disease. After the health minister officially declared the 1991–1992 epidemic to have ended, pity the poor clinician who identified a case of acute diarrhea as cholera.

The communicable cartographies associated with cases I have discussed are different because of clinical and epidemiological differences, historical circumstances, political economies, economies of social difference, and the contours of states and their "publics." It would thus be unsafe to infectiously generalize from these two cases to plagues in general. I do think, however, that these examples can suggest some propositions that need to be scrutinized in a broad range of cases, contemporary and historical. For one thing, plagues tend to be constructed as mediatized objects in terms of the communicable cartographies associated with them. This process not only generally begins long before clinical or epidemiological data are locally available but also shapes what sorts of clinical and epidemiological imaginaries can emerge. The intense global media coverage of Ebola, swine flu, SARS, avian flu, and—even as I write these lines—the outbreak of A(H1N1) influenza in the spring of 2009 suggests how deeply distant or possible epidemics can create local and national economies of fear and structure the way public health dollars are distributed.

Plagues provide high-stakes scenarios for efforts to control these ideological constructs and the practices with which they are related in complicated ways. In most countries, epidemics bring into effect special laws and regulations that provide public health officials with unusual powers to control the production and circulation of discourse.

Epidemics of cholera, plague, and smallpox prompted a series of international sanitary conferences in the nineteenth century, for example, that generated global communicable cartographies associated with the dissemination of information about these diseases; many countries incorporated them into national public health legislation. Plagues—including virtual ones—continue to be key sites in which states construct themselves as holding special rights over the production, circulation, and reception of health discourse. They similarly help infuse biomedical-authority varieties of communicability with power, even as patient-consumer and public-sphere varieties become increasingly central in many countries. Indeed, constructing themselves as informing publics about epidemic diseases is a key means by which states continue to project themselves as remaining faithful to one of their constitutive tasks—defending the health of citizens—even as many of them withdraw from active participation in and regulation of health services.

Nevertheless, the literature on plagues is notoriously full of examples of resistance, of occasions on which people talk back to "the state" even as the latter claims that individual and collective survival depends on passive reproduction of dominant "messages." People can challenge dominant communicable models by refusing to be interpellated in subject positions projected by official cartographies, revising these ideological maps, and sometimes proposing alternatives. This is no simple act of "just saying no," as Nancy Reagan would have had it. For one thing, official cartographies are shot through with contradictions, declaring themselves to be the only route to health and well-being at the same time they project their own failure. For cholera in Venezuela, it was the communicable failure of the poor, of indigenous people, and of street vendors that would bring on the epidemic; nevertheless, state cholera messages were addressed not to them but to the good sanitary citizens who were not "at risk" for the disease. In the case of WNV, county officials projected themselves as providing evidence-based knowledge to an ignorant public, which in turn laughed at the state for disregarding epidemiological evidence regarding morbidity and mortality in San Diego County. Even as they fulfilled their institutional obligations to claim control over the production and circulation of public discourses of health, MSAS, DEH, and HHSA lost a great deal of public credibility. Meanwhile, however, public criticism often reproduced the communicable understanding that the state *should* produce authoritative knowledge about health and give it to "the public" and that scientifically based information *should* translate into particular types of behaviors and actions.

In the end, biocommunicability is not just about health or com-munication but about understandings of states, citizens, noncitizens, political agency, and knowledge. If plagues x-ray social relations, epist-emologies, and power, then communicable cartographies crucially structure these representational processes and affect biomedical, social, and political-economic practices. Because these cartographies form such important sites of epidemic struggle, it might behoove scholars to turn them into loci of research on plagues.

Notes

1. Circulation statistics for April–September 2009 are taken from www. signonsandiego.com/stories/2009/oct/26/us-newspaper-circulation-list-102609/ (print) and www.signonsandiego.com/news/2009/nov/01/signon-san-diego-gets-new-look-more-changes-ahead/ (electronic), both accessed 6 November 2009. The broader research project is also being carried out in Argentina, Brazil, Cuba, Ecuador, Mexico, and Venezuela.

2. The names of all interviewees are pseudonyms.

3. Having posed the question "What are the roles and responsibilities of local agencies with regards to WNV surveillance and case prevention?" the California Department of Health Services WNV Web site suggests that "your local mosquito and vector control agency" has the responsibility for produc-ing "targeted public education." Electronic document, www.westnile.ca.gov/wnv_faqs_basics.php#564, accessed 4 July 2007.

4. Figures are based on annual reports available at www.sdcounty.ca.gov/deh/pests/chd_wnv_casesbyzip.html, accessed 5 May 2009.

5. See Goffman 1981 for a discussion of these roles.

On Creating Epidemics, Plagues, and Other Wartime Alarums and Excursions

Enumerating versus Estimating Civilian Mortality in Iraq

James Trostle

In this chapter I examine whether social violence in wartime, resulting in civilian mortality, can be said to reach "epidemic" proportions. According to *A Dictionary of Epidemiology*, an epidemic can be defined as "the occurrence in a community or region of cases of an illness, specific health-related behavior, or other health-related events clearly in excess of normal expectancy" (Last 2001: 60). Although civilian mortality during war is not usually associated with the word *epidemic*, it is a "health-related event" that can be included according to this definition. The definition assumes and requires that both case occurrence and normal expectation of disease or death be measured, and it allows variability by community or region. Fifty cases of cholera in a week in Dhaka, Bangladesh, is not an epidemic, because it is within what is normally expected. Even five cases of cholera in Los Angeles, California, however, would certainly be labeled an epidemic. But how can one determine whether levels of violence or death exceed what might be normally expected during wartime?

Whether the word *epidemic* can be applied to social phenomena such as mortality from extreme violence is contested because it necessarily involves critics and defenders of certain political positions as well as interpretations of scientific data. By a "contested epidemic" I mean an

61

instance in which a definitional dispute exists concerning the measured occurrence of cases, what constitutes "normal expectancy," or both. Contested epidemics reveal important but often tacit understandings about evidence, proof, conventional wisdom, and the exercise of power. Like other anthropological projects that interrogate boundaries (of identity or "the state," for example), contested epidemics are therefore ripe for anthropological inquiry. Epidemics are individual diagnoses writ large; that is, they are outcomes of the bureaucratic process through which states acknowledge the existence of more cases of disease or death than one would expect to see in a population. (For ethnographic examples, see Briggs with Mantini-Briggs 2003; Farmer 1992; Lindenbaum 1979; Scheper-Hughes 1992. For historical examples, see Sawchuk, this volume; Swedlund, this volume.)

In this chapter I attend to the threshold at which the number of deaths exceeds expectation with respect to wartime civilian mortality in Iraq from 2003 through 2007.[1] Arguments about whether and for what purposes this mortality might constitute a plague—which we might define as a real or metaphorical excess that carries particular horror—are still being made and remade, so I am particularly interested in examining the ongoing struggles over which data will be admitted into evidence. What, indeed, constitutes "evidence"? This leads me to examine which data are allowed to enter the fray and how those data reverberate in society (see examples in this volume by Briggs and by Löwy).

I am more interested here in describing and explaining the conflicts over the magnitude of civilian mortality in wartime than I am in whether that mortality should specifically be labeled a plague. For most of us, the horror is clear. The Geneva Convention (Protocol I, Article 51, Section 1) states: "The civilian population and individual civilians shall enjoy general protection against dangers arising from military operations" (Trombly 2003). Civilian wartime mortality is *always* horrible because civilians are not lawful instruments of warfare. Military labeling of wartime civilian mortality as "collateral damage" dehumanizes that mortality and makes it appear to be a necessary or inevitable by-product of violence. Thus my title for this chapter emphasizes the drama and manipulation inherent in warfare. "Alarums and excursions" was the Elizabethan stage direction indicating warlike sounds or activity.

Contested epidemics are a bit like curious incidents involving Sherlock Holmes and dogs that "did nothing in the night-time" (Conan Doyle 1894). ("Gregory: "The dog did nothing in the night-time." Holmes: "That was the curious incident.") Their status as "might-have-beens" or "almosts" or "never-weres" allows one to attend especially to that which prevented them from appearing. Processes of evidence collection, interpretation, and refutation are particularly important to examine here, not to mention the subsequent repercussions for advocates of unpopular positions. Some contested epidemics include predicted epidemics that never came to be, such as the 1976 swine flu scare. That year, more than 40 million Americans were vaccinated, the epidemic never began, and the director of the US Centers for Disease Control lost his job (Krause 2006; Neustadt and Fineberg 1983). Contested epidemics also include accounts of "disallowed" or "postponed" plagues (HIV and smoking-related lung cancer in their early years; iatrogenic hospital mortality), which offer their own gripping dramas and revelations (see, e.g., Glantz et al. 1998; Institute of Medicine 2000; Shilts 1987; for analyses of this type of narrative form, see Lindenbaum 2001; Rosenberg 1992a).

In this chapter I concentrate on a particular contested epidemic of high mortality, namely, the number of civilian deaths in Iraq from the US invasion in 2003 until January 2008. Because this case is fraught with contemporary political significance, it helps highlight the roles that politicians, news media, and scientists play in measuring cases, deciding what is normal and expected, declaring epidemics, and deciding whether armed conflict can or should be framed in public health terms. All these groups could agree that some level of civilian mortality accompanied the US invasion of, and war in, Iraq. But how high was this mortality? Was it higher than that which might normally be expected in a time of war? Should it therefore have been labeled an epidemic and responded to with special attention, including that of voters or courts of international law? These questions arise within what has been called the "epidemiology of violence" or "epidemiology of conflict."

The sociocultural history of disease or mortality in populations can be thought of as marked by stages of exposure, epidemic onset, crisis recognition, intervention, and recovery or recrimination (Trostle 2005). Here I emphasize the stages of epidemic onset and crisis recognition. During these stages decisions are made about what constitutes an excessive number of cases, such that an epidemic can be declared, and whether said epidemic can be considered a crisis, so that resources can be invested above and beyond what might usually be marshaled. I examine the way a contested epidemic is represented in the news media, paying special attention to processes of enumeration and statistical estimation.

The Status of Violence as a Public Health Problem

Public health has only recently taken up the measurement of inter-personal violence and war as a legitimate subject for epidemiological analysis (Garfield and Neugut 1991). The word *violence* has been included as a search term for journal articles in the National Library of Medicine only since 1970. An important edited text titled *War and Public Health* was published by the American Public Health Association in the late 1990s (Levy and Sidel 1997). A public health review article in 2003 stated that "through efforts of the public health community since the early 1980s, violence is now widely accepted as a public health issue" (Mair and Mair 2003: 209). Most schools of public health offer courses on violence, hence acknowledging that it is an appropriate subject of study in the discipline. But the specific study of violence resulting from war and social conflict is less widely accepted. A news article in *Nature* described "the growing field of conflict epidemiology" (Giles 2006: 728), and an article in the *Bulletin of the World Health Organization* described it as an "emerging practice" (Thieren 2007). A Google search for the term *conflict epidemiology* provided only 119 Web sites, and a Google Scholar search returned 6, as of 1 August 2007. Six months later these numbers were 604 and 15, respectively. Thus it appears that the idea of an "epidemiology of violence" is relatively well accepted, whereas the field called "conflict epidemiology" is advancing but not yet common.

Those who argue that mortality from violence is an appropriate topic for epidemiological study argue in part that epidemiological techniques can be usefully and appropriately applied to the causes of any type of mortality. From this perspective, one can search for the distribution and determinants of mortality from violence just as readily as mortality from cancer or malaria. Durkheim's *Suicide*, now celebrated as a classic in social epidemiology, dates back more than a century. But because violence is a purely "social" phenomenon, some within and outside the discipline resist considering violence with tools that are more usually applied to "natural" (nonhuman) pathogens or modes of transmission.

Some politicians and state-level bureaucrats also resist the claim that epidemiologists can quantify state-sponsored conflict or violence. After all, the emergence of such a subfield could be viewed, at the least, as inconvenient to state policies, and possibly as detrimental or even antithetical. This is an area in which the "counting" of the epidemiologist can lead to an "accounting" by civil society. If epidemiologists label the violent or mortal outcomes of state policies as epidemics, does that not intrude upon a state's practice, if not right, to make its own claims about the legitimacy or illegitimacy of such violence or mortality? If state policies cause workplace mortality or infant mortality to increase, or if they increase mortality from environmental contamination, then epidemiologists contravene the state by labeling these events epidemics. So if state-sponsored civilian mortality during wartime is part of "normal expectancy," then epidemiologists' claims that the mortality is reaching "epidemic" proportions should be contested by the state.

To foreshadow just a bit, this is what I believe took place—and continues to take place—in the handling of data about civilian mortality during the Iraq war. The conflict is about the absolute numbers of dead but also about what number or proportion is expected, thus constituting a "normal" level during times of war. Some epidemiologists and anthropologists argue that most suffering, disease, and death is socially produced and differentially distributed across the population according to one's place in the social hierarchy (see, e.g., Baer, Singer, and Sussman 2003; Farmer 1992; Krieger 2007). Behind the conflict over the numbers lies the question of who has the power to articulate what level of disease or mortality is expected, thus defining what others should take to be normal.

Measuring Civilian Mortality

Measuring mortality among soldiers and civilians is a common way to assess the dubious progress of war. US citizens in the 1960s and 1970s were accustomed to hearing daily "body counts" of dead soldiers during the Vietnam war. Measuring civilian deaths is useful for other purposes, both to determine the possible misconduct of warring factions and to assess the impact of war on civil society. But measuring civilian mortality is especially problematic when it can interfere with the promulgated image of a "just war." When civilian casualties mount to the level of an epidemic ("more civilian deaths than would be expected in wartime"), questions can arise about the course, ethics, and even legality of the war, quite apart from any political costs to its sponsors.

The struggle for an accurate accounting of deaths in the Iraq war has been well documented. The US and Iraqi positions were described in an Associated Press report published on 7 September 2006:

> In December 2003, the [Iraq] Health Ministry stopped releasing civilian casualty figures for several months. Dr. Nagham Mohsen, the head of the ministry's statistics department, said at the time that the order ultimately came from the US-led occupation authority, which didn't want to draw attention to civilian suffering.

[Human Rights Watch researcher] Abrahams said there is no concrete
evidence that Iraqi officials are cooking the numbers. "But obviously,
the environment is very politicized and obviously the civilian casualties
figure is an important game and several groups will play that," he said.

Some officials believe that releasing death figures plays into insurgent hands, by undermining confidence in the government. "Do you
want me to give you numbers that would paint a smile on the face
of those terrorist dogs?" snapped Interior Ministry spokesman Brig.
Abdul Kareem Khalaf when asked for August death tolls. "Not going to
happen." (Associated Press 2006)

The absence of civilian casualty figures in the news is particularly
notable when contrasted with the care taken to count US military
casualties.[2] The news media pay particular attention to the casualty
count at moments when it acquires a new set of zeros, such as the 4,000
level reached in March 2008 (*New York Times*, 25 March 2008, A1).
Photographs of the faces of the most recent 1,000 military casualties
filled four pages of that newspaper in March 2008, and its Web site
contains a searchable database of photos of all soldiers killed in Iraq,
along with name, age, hometown, military branch, and date of death.[3]

But what about civilian casualties? Three methods are commonly
used to estimate the extent of civilian casualties during a war. Two
are based on counts of existing records and are therefore known as
"surveillance" estimates. The third is based on a sample survey and
is therefore known as a "population" estimate. Surveillance estimates
can be summed from government records of mortality, usually in
the form of death certificates or morgue body counts, or they can be
drawn from news reports of civilian casualties. Each of these sources
is predictably subject to miscounting: governments face incentives to
over- and understate their official tallies; citizens face incentives (and
disincentives) to register the loss of their loved ones through official
channels; media are unable to capture all incidents of mortality and
are likely to capture a greater proportion of mortality in some places,
among some people, and at certain times than others. Population
estimates are also subject to miscounting, but their miscounts are, at
least in theory, easier to trace and estimate: the steps of data collection and interpretation in a sample survey are open to critique and
analysis.[4]

Advocates of surveillance methods assert that their methods are as
accurate as possible: they are summing and constructing the burden
of "real" deaths in a census by counting all cases rather than creating

statistical portraits of "projected" deaths. So, for example, one of the directors of the surveillance Web site "Iraq Body Count" has posted this statement on the site: "In some—but still far too few—cases we know the name, ages, occupation, and exact circumstances of death. Information presented at this level of detail is the only way to arrive at once-for-all certainty, in a way that does justice to the victims, honours their memory, and provides the closure that only a full list, or census, can do satisfactorily" (Dardagan, Sloboda, and Dougherty 2006).

Census strategies applied to large populations invariably miss opportunities to count all cases of interest. But even though surveillance methods are likely to undercount, their consistent application can nevertheless show changes over time. In contrast, advocates of population methods assert that sample-based inferences are the only effective method for assessing general mortality at a time of conflict (Garfield 2005). Even if population methods involve statistical inference and projection, these techniques, it is held, are the only ones useful to estimate "real" magnitudes of disease or mortality at the scale of an entire nation. In a sense, then, the surveillance approach constructs its reality out of actual and officially reported deaths, even if it represents an incomplete count, whereas the population approach constructs its reality out of a limited number of official and unofficial deaths reported to interviewers and infers what is happening in the population on the basis of what has been reported in that sample of interviews.

It is obviously difficult to study wartime deaths, and especially difficult to do so among noncombatant civilians or among combatants not in uniform. Policy makers, government officials, and the public health community have usually chosen the population-based approach to estimating disease and mortality in times of conflict, despite its significant problems (Thieren 2005). Sample surveys have been used in more than twenty countries, from Darfur to Bosnia and East Timor, to estimate civilian mortality and disease burden during wartime. Surveillance approaches have rarely been validated with population surveys but are generally thought to include only a minority (anywhere from 5 to 50 percent) of actual wartime deaths.

In the rest of this chapter I examine a recent example of a contested epidemic in which researchers produced estimates of civilian mortality in Iraq. Those researchers were portrayed as either well intentioned or nefarious, and their estimates as either accurate or biased. I pay particular attention to where and how researchers and media examined the evidence and to the ways in which political and media interests interpreted the data. This type of analysis allows us to see not only how science is judged and disseminated but also which kinds of scientific explanations meet which kinds of receptions from different audiences.

A Contested Measurement: The Framework

In 2004 and 2006, Les Roberts, a medical doctor, and colleagues in the United States and Iraq published provocative articles on levels of civilian mortality in Iraq. Each of two studies, based on random cluster surveys, was peer reviewed and appeared in the prestigious British journal *Lancet* shortly before US federal elections. The first study (Roberts et al. 2004) estimated that 98,000 more deaths than expected had occurred among civilians in Iraq in the eighteen months following the US-sponsored war in March 2003, compared with fifteen months before the invasion. The 95 percent confidence interval around this estimate ranged from 8,000 to 194,000 deaths. The estimate was startling in part because it was so much higher than those from other sources. An antiwar group called Iraq Body Count had counted between 14,000 and 16,000 deaths mentioned in news articles during this period, and the Brookings Institute had estimated 10,000 to 27,000 (BBC News 2004). Even a political group in Iraq called the People's Kifah, or Struggle Against Hegemony movement, which might have been predicted to produce a high estimate, had counted "only" 37,000 deaths in the first nine months of the war (Janabi 2004).

The second study (Burnham et al. 2006) used much the same methods as the first. The authors stated that they wanted to address some of the critiques about sample size and precision that had been raised about their first study. Given the absence of other population-based studies, they also sought to update their estimates. They concluded that as of July 2006, there had been 654,965 civilian deaths in Iraq as a result of the US war, with more than 601,000 deaths attributable to violence, most often gunfire. The 95 percent confidence interval around their estimate of deaths was 426,369 to 793,663.

The methods used in each of these studies were those of multistage cluster surveys. In a truly randomized sample, every individual in a population has an equal chance of being included. Since assembling and managing national lists of inhabitants is obviously impossible during wartime, cluster surveys approach the ideal of true random selection through a staged series of steps. In the Iraq studies, the first step was to assign a number of clusters to each Iraqi province, proportional to its total population. Then each province's administrative units were listed by population and again chosen randomly, in proportion to size. Within each administrative unit, clusters of households were chosen randomly. In the first study this was done by using a global positioning unit; in the second it was done with random numbers assigned to streets or blocks. Once a street or block had been selected, a house was randomly chosen as a starting point, and the interviewers proceeded to interview in adjacent occupied dwellings until their household quota was reached. In the 2004 study, 33 clusters of 30 households each were chosen, and in the 2006 study, 47 clusters of 40 households each.

A Contested Measurement: The Stories

Both studies were met with extreme and contradictory reactions. Editorials appeared in journals such as *Nature* and *Science*, in newspapers such as the *New York Times* and the *Wall Street Journal*, and in a variety of Web sites and blogs. Commentators argued over whether the story was receiving too much attention or not enough. An editorial in the conservative *Wall Street Journal* on 19 October 2006, headlined "The 655,000 Fraud," said the article was everywhere: "Reporting on the Lancet study … has also been all over television and radio, as well as Internet sites such as Google and Yahoo news. All of which leaves us wondering if reporters and editors have enough sense anymore to ask basic questions about such enormous numbers, or whether they are simply too biased against the Bush Administration and its Iraq policy to do so."

On the other side, MediaLens, a liberal media blog, said the story had been buried: "The media coverage has been appalling—the words 'Lancet' and 'Iraq' have appeared in national UK newspaper articles some 30 times, with many of these mentions in passing. There has been no serious attempt to examine the Lancet's figures, to explain how they compare to earlier findings from different studies. Anyone aspiring to understand the issue could do so only by visiting the small, alternative Web sites" (MediaLens 2006).

Silencing

Whether overplayed or ignored by the media, the study's political reception was extreme. Asked about the Burnham et al. 2006 article at a news conference in October 2006, President George W. Bush dismissed both this study and the prior one as using "discredited" methods that "guessed" at the mortality. At the same time, he cited a mortality figure lower than most other prevailing estimates:

Q: A group of American and Iraqi health officials today released a report saying that 655,000 Iraqis have died since the Iraq war. That figure is 20 times the figure that you cited in December, at 30,000. Do you care to amend or update your figure, and do you consider this a credible report?

THE PRESIDENT: No, I don't consider it a credible report. Neither does General Casey and neither do Iraqi officials. I do know that a lot of innocent people have died, and that troubles me and it grieves me... No question, it's violent, but this report is one—they put it out before, it was pretty well—the methodology was pretty well discredited. But I talk to people like General Casey and, of course, the Iraqi government put out a statement talking about the report.

Q: The 30,000, Mr. President? Do you stand by your figure, 30,000?

THE PRESIDENT: You know, I stand by the figure. A lot of innocent people have lost their life—600,000, or whatever they guessed at, is just—it's not credible. Thank you. (White House 2006)

This statement by the president represents an official repudiation of both the number 655,000 and the methods used to reach it. It is an official attempt to claim instead that 30,000 is a reasonable, though lamentable, count of civilian casualties. But it also represents a claim ("No question, it's violent") that casualties of this magnitude are what we should accept as "normal" in wartime.

The British government had forcefully criticized Roberts and his colleagues two years earlier, in October 2004. The foreign secretary, Jack Straw, took the unusual step of releasing a ministerial statement responding to the study, although, unlike Bush, he did not dismiss it. Straw acknowledged that the cluster sample approach was a legitimate method, even as he criticized the result: "The design of the *Lancet* study and its statistical methodology passed the process of peer review before publication and is similar to that followed in cases where the data are difficult to obtain. But that should not mask the fact that any methodology critically depends on the accuracy of the data subject to its analysis" (Straw 2004). It is noteworthy that the British government commented that the cluster method was legitimate two years before the US president said it was "pretty well discredited" and before General Casey said that the total "seems way, way beyond any number that I have seen. I've not seen a number higher than 50,000. And so I don't give that much credibility at all" (*Boston Globe*, 12 October 2006, A16). The British newspaper the *Independent* reported in March 2007 that a BBC freedom-of-information request yielded documents about the second Iraq study showing that "the chief scientific advisor to the

Ministry of Defence, Roy Anderson, described the methods used in the study as 'robust' and 'close to best practice'" (Lawless 2007).

Straw's statement went farther than simply commenting on the accuracy of the data, by arguing that the government had no obligation to collect such data. It specifically disputed a claim from Roberts and co-workers that the Geneva Convention obligated the military to keep a count of civilian mortality. The Bush administration similarly claimed that it kept no data on civilian mortality, leaving this to the Iraqi government. A US Defense Department spokesman, quoted in the *Washington Post*, said that "it would be difficult for the US to precisely determine the number of civilian deaths in Iraq as a result of insurgent activity. The Iraqi Ministry of Health would be in a better position, with all of its records, to provide more accurate information on deaths in Iraq" (Brown 2006). Yet the Iraqi government claimed to be unable to provide accurate figures, either. The *New York Times*, citing an Iraqi government spokesman, said, "Though the government closely tracks deaths through the Interior and Health Ministries, he said it did not have a system in place for compiling a comprehensive figure" (17 January 2007). This, I think, is another manifestation of the attempt by the state to assert its right to determine what constitutes excess mortality and what constitutes normal mortality. The state claims the right to respond to criticism by impugning the methods of its critics, but it also claims the right not to maintain records that might validate—or invalidate—their criticisms.

Media Interpretations of Statistics and Confidence

Both the media and government accounts exacerbated the controversy over methods by focusing on a statistical tool known as the "confidence interval." While the confidence interval is a very informative tool in the hands of a statistician, it can be less so in the hands of a journalist or politician. Indeed, almost all media sources commenting on the *Lancet* Iraq mortality studies seemed to interpret the confidence interval itself as a piece of suspect data. A confidence interval is a statistical calculation used to compute the probability, usually set at 90 or 95 percent, "that the true value of a variable such as a mean, proportion, or rate is contained within the interval" (Last 2001). Health researchers rarely have the chance to study all the people (the population) who suffer from some particular malady. Instead, they measure a smaller sample from that population and then make inferences about the population based on the characteristics of their sample. When a researcher draws a sample from a population and calculates the sample's mean, proportion, or rate, the confidence interval around any of those statistical estimates shows, at a given calculated probability, the range of values that the population is likely to have.

Although the "true" (population) value can lie anywhere within a confidence interval, the fact that the values in that interval have their own probability distribution means that values closer to the point estimate are likelier to be the population value than those farther from that point estimate. Cluster sample procedures increase the width of a confidence interval (and thus reduce its statistical precision) in comparison with what the width would be with a simple random sample. In general, smaller sample sizes also increase the width of a confidence interval, because the smaller the sample, the larger the range of population values possibly represented by a sample estimate.

Foreign Minister Straw's statement about the 2004 Roberts article acknowledged this statistical convention but distorted its interpretation, making it sound as if the breadth of the interval itself lessened the importance of the estimate. As the statement put it: "In general they have noted that the data on which they based their projections was of '*limited precision*.' This limited precision is reflected in the very large range which they use for their estimate of excess mortality (8,000–194,000). Although the levels of probability vary across its range, any figure within this range is consistent with the data" (Straw 2004). "Limited precision" is a statistical term that does not mean "inaccurate" but rather "of less detail than the true value." By italicizing and quoting the words "limited precision," Straw's account gives a precise statistical term overtones of methodological sloppiness. In addition, the use of the word *consistent* is misleading, because it suggests that every value in the interval is as likely to occur as every other, and this thereby dilutes the power and importance of the point estimate. Straw's political statement seems to be suggesting that these scientists really know nothing at all if their estimate ranges from a number lower than that given by body counts to a number five times higher than the next highest estimate.

The *New York Times*'s interpretation of the confidence interval turned it from a statistical tool into an admission of error:

> Last year, a team of American and Iraqi public health researchers for the Johns Hopkins Bloomberg School of Public Health estimated that 600,000 civilians had died in violence from the 2003 American invasion until last summer, the highest estimate at the time for the toll of the war.

But it was *an estimate and not a precise count*, and researchers *acknowledged a margin of error* that ranged from 426,369 to 793,663 deaths. The study used samples of casualties from Iraqi households to extrapolate an overall figure of 601,017 Iraqis dead from violence between March 2003 and July 2006. (*New York Times*, 3 January 2007; my emphasis).

Emphasizing that the survey was "not a precise count" and calling the confidence interval "a margin of error" both served to label the study suspect. Other newspapers used words that made the confidence interval seem more like a wide array of guesses than a calculation of probability. The British paper the *Independent* said, "The researchers, reflecting the inherent uncertainties in such extrapolations, said they were 95 per cent certain that the real number of deaths lay somewhere between 392,979 and 942,636" (Lawless 2007). The *Los Angeles Times* said, "The study found that, with 95 percent certainty, 426,369 to 793,663 Iraqis had died violently since the US-led invasion in March 2003, with 601,027 statistically the most probable death toll" (Daragahi 2006). The *Boston Globe* called it a "confidence index," and the *Wall Street Journal* published the following as a correction on 12 October: "A Johns Hopkins survey of civilian casualties in Iraq, 'The Human Cost of the War in Iraq,' gave a 95 percent certainty to the number of fatalities being between 426,369 and 793,663 with the highest probability given to the figure of 601,027. A Politics & Economics article yesterday incorrectly said the study gave a 95 percent certainty to the 601,027 figure." These five newspapers quoted, then, described a 95 percent confidence interval as, respectively, a "margin of error," "95 percent certain," a "95 percent certainty," a "confidence index," and a corrected "95 percent certainty." Although the researchers had included the confidence interval to better inform their readers, the newspapers turned it into a weapon that seemed to generate more suspicion and criticism than understanding.

At the least, these terms represent very different types of discourse strategies from those used in science (see Briggs, this volume). But do they represent rhetorics designed to help readers better understand, and thereby interpret, scientific data, or do they represent skeptical rhetorics that persuade readers to reject scientific data?

Only one report paid specific attention to the media analysis of the confidence intervals used in the studies—this from the *Columbia Journalism Review* by way of a reporter for the *Chronicle of Higher Education*:

What's a reporter to make of such a broad range? The lower end of that range overlaps well with previous, nonscientific estimates, but the middle and upper range seem outrageous. True, had the researchers surveyed more houses in more neighborhoods, the interval would have been narrower. But each day spent traveling within Iraq for the study presented grave dangers to the American and Iraqi researchers.

Reporters' unease about the wide range may have been a primary reason many didn't cover the study. One columnist, Fred Kaplan of Slate, called the estimate "meaningless" and labeled the range "a dart board."

But he was wrong. I called about ten biostatisticians and mortality experts. Not one of them took issue with the study's methods or its conclusions. If anything, the scientists told me, the authors had been cautious in their estimates. With a quick call to a statistician, reporters would have found that the probability forms a bell curve—the likelihood is very small that the number of deaths fell at either extreme of the range. It was very likely to fall near the middle. (Guterman 2005)

This kind of news analysis is rare, both for its serious attempt to understand the meaning of a statistical term and for its critique of other media stories. Many of the other news reports recycled critiques from one another. One of the more egregious examples occurred when the writer of an op-ed in the *Wall Street Journal* claimed that the surveillance studies had included no demographic questions or analyses and were therefore unverifiable. This claim was patently false to anyone who had read the articles and seen their demographic analyses, but that did not stop the criticism from being repeated by the *Wall Street Journal* and other papers. Although the media had trouble correctly interpreting and conveying the statistical nuances of the study, they were not reluctant to assign suspect motives to the authors. This was visible in the way media analysts interpreted the timing of publication of the study and the way they described the political leanings of the study's authors. Reporting on Roberts et al. 2004, the *New York Times* was suspicious of the study's release date: "Editors of the Lancet, the London-based medical publication, where an article describing the study is scheduled to appear, decided not to wait for the normal publication date next week, but to place the research online Friday, apparently so it could circulate before the [Iraqi] election" (*New York Times*, 29 October 2004). The editors of *Lancet* retorted that they had not released the study early but rather had given it the same "fast track" processing they had given to other important research papers. Roberts said that having finished the study in mid-September, he was reluctant to wait until after the elections to publish: "I think in Iraq, a post-election publication in

2004 would have been seen as my colleagues knowing something but keeping it hidden" (MediaLens 2006).

The relationship between politics and science played an overt role in discussions about the validity of the Iraq mortality studies. Roberts told a reporter, "I was opposed to the war and I still think that the war was a bad idea, but I think that our science has transcended our perspectives" (CNN, 29 October 2004). The *New York Times* mentioned Roberts's political critique at the same time it described his study as objective: "The study is scientific, reserving judgment on the politics of the Iraqi conflict. But Dr. Roberts and his colleagues are critical of the Bush administration and the Army for not releasing estimates of civilian deaths" (*New York Times*, 29 October 2004). The reader is left to wonder whether "reservation of judgment" is an inherent attribute of science and under what circumstances a scientific study might legitimately and appropriately be critical of a presidential administration or an army. Because these numbers describe dead civilians, they carry heavy symbolic significance. Scientists who report such numbers cannot expect to remain immune from politics.

A New Population Survey

The *New York Times* of 10 January 2008 described a recently published Iraq civilian mortality study under the headline "W.H.O. Says Iraq Civilian Death Toll Higher than Cited." The article, on page A12, made clear in its first paragraph that this study by the World Health Organization was being compared with data from the "oft-cited Iraq Body Count." The Johns Hopkins survey was not mentioned until paragraph three, and in this fashion: "But another study by Johns Hopkins, which has come under criticism for its methodology, cited an estimate of about 600,000 dead." The article went on to quote the WHO study's point estimate of 151,000 civilian dead, with a "95 percent degree of certainty" that the number was between 104,000 and 223,000. It reviewed in some detail the strengths and limitations of the WHO study's methods and quoted conflicting opinions about the study's validity from two Iraqi senior officials.

The new study (Iraq Family Health Survey Study Group 2008) was published in the *New England Journal of Medicine* and used cluster survey methods similar to those employed in the Johns Hopkins study. The difference between the two lay not so much in method as in scale—that is, in number of clusters (1,086 as compared with 47 in Burnham et al. 2006) and number of households (9,345 as compared with 1,849 in

Burnham et al. 2006). Les Roberts, one of the coauthors of the Johns Hopkins study, described in an Internet blog the many similarities between his group's findings and those in the Iraq Family Health Survey (IFHS) and suggested that at least some of the differences between the two mortality estimates could have been caused by the underreporting of violent deaths in the IFHS. This he attributed to the IFHS's failure to confirm deaths with death certificates and to possible respondent fears of reporting violent deaths to Ministry of Health officials. He commented that "both studies suggest things are far worse than our leaders have reported."

Given the preceding discussion, two points are worth making about this newer study and its coverage. First, the article in the *New York Times* suggests that the baseline for comparison is "the oft-cited Iraq Body Count." This wording suggests that the familiarity of a source through frequency of citation is valued more than comprehensiveness, since the incomplete coverage of the Body Count is not mentioned. Second, the media continued to focus on the methods more than the significance of the estimates. Roberts's reference to leadership was an attempt to contrast the high estimates of mortality in the population studies with the low estimates of mortality in the surveillance data preferred by politicians who supported the war.

Conclusion

The controversy over civilian mortality in Iraq is not, for most scientists, about whether the American invasion caused excess civilian mortality but rather about whether the large mortality estimates provided in the Burnham et al. study are reasonable and defensible. Few epidemiologists would argue that record-based surveillance estimates of mortality in developing countries are better than sample-based inferences about a population. And fewer still would claim this about attempts to estimate wartime civilian mortality. So the debate is not really about *whether* an epidemic of mortality is taking place in Iraq but about *how large* that epidemic is.

Antiwar activists who are deeply suspicious of sample-based inferences acknowledge the rationale for these studies and even in their critiques never express doubt that the civilian mortality is excessive or that it should be called an epidemic. But they do disagree about the proper way to represent the mortality. The following statement on the Iraq Mortality Count Web site makes this clear: "All that has been firmly documented as a result of the Lancet study is that some 300 post-invasion violent

deaths occurred among the members of the households interviewed...
These 300 may be added to the roster of some 50,000 others for whom
this level of detailed knowledge is available" (Dardagan, Sloboda, and
Dougherty 2006). This conclusion dismisses the utility of statistical
inference, but in refusing to cede value to inference, the authors miss
a critical point. If a random sample of 1,849 households yielded 300
violent deaths not yet in their database, then *how many other deaths
remained uncounted?*

States and Silence

For politicians, the debate should be about whether the level of civilian
mortality in Iraq is preventable, warranted, or defensible. Yet rather than
arguing that point, the US government has chosen to state that it cannot
make conclusive statements one way or the other because it does not
collect the needed data. This is a common strategy on the part of policy
makers, but it has become especially common in the United States since
2000. Gaps in federal efforts to collect data on health disparities (Perrin
and Ver Ploeg 2004) constitute another contemporary example of state
resistance to quantification. Groups such as the Union of Concerned
Scientists (www.ucsusa.org) and congressional committees such as those
headed by Congressman Henry Waxman have documented levels of
political manipulation and suppression of science—in areas ranging
from abstinence education to global warming and missile defense
systems—that they call unprecedented.[5] This represents a strategy of
intentional and highly politicized ignorance.

The strategy of "denial through intentional ignorance" has also been
used to silence the authors of some of the Iraq mortality studies. Roberts
and colleagues' first article asked simply that their results be confirmed
through further study; after all, their data had been obtained with
only "modest funds, 4 weeks, and seven Iraqi team members" (Roberts
et al. 2004: 1863). In 2007, one of the Iraqi coauthors, Riyadh Lafta,
was denied a US visa to visit the University of Washington and make
a presentation about Iraqi mortality at a medical conference there.
His hosts invited him instead to present over the border in Canada at
Simon Fraser University, but then the British government denied him
a transit visa to stop for four hours in the United Kingdom on a flight
from Baghdad to Vancouver (Wong 2007). The famous post-Vietnam
dictum that "we don't do body counts" was thus extended to prohibit
others from doing them as well.

The Status of Measurement as a State Function

Sociologists and philosophers of science—especially Latour and Woolgar (1979), but Fleck (1935) and Kuhn (1962) before them—established a precedent for talking about scientific knowledge as created by communities of scientists. Fleck's 1935 book on this topic was titled *Genesis and Development of a Scientific Fact*. But thinking about contested epidemics is a bit like thinking about the "development of non-facts" or the "non-genesis of a scientific fact." To find an appropriate theoretical framing, one needs also to refer to levels above the laboratory and above groups of scientists, to analyses of the functioning of state-level bureaucracies. Scott's *Seeing Like a State* provides a useful framework for this analysis, in its attention to differences between the types of knowledge created and valued in state-level bureaucracies and those created and valued by local communities. The dispute over counting real bodies versus doing statistical analyses to estimate the number of such bodies is a dispute not so much between scientists as between two different communities interested in the same war. It could therefore be compared to the difference between *mētis* (local knowledge based on practice and experience) and *techne* (systematic and technical knowledge) (Scott 1998: 319–323). But state-level resistance to quantification is less often treated by theorists. There are many analyses of the growth of state interest in quantifying health, population, and production—that is, the growth of vital statistics (e.g., Anderson 1988; Poovey 1998)—yet it is more difficult to find theoretical precedents for the nonproduction or erasure of such data. Literature on how states remember and make things (and people) disappear would be one possible resource (e.g., Briggs with Mantini-Briggs 2003; Hayner 2001; Scheper-Hughes 1992).

On Research Needs, Counting, and Accounting

Looking at wartime civilian mortality as a "contested epidemic" raises a series of important research challenges. These range from the difficulty of analyzing "epidemic might-have-beens" to measuring differences between what is new disease or suffering versus what might normally be expected. Conflicts between processes of enumerating and of estimating deaths deserve more research and analysis, as does the role of state-sponsored silence in policy making (see also Briggs, this volume). Underneath all this, of course, is the discomfiting and uncontestable fact that the deaths were continuing, with no end in sight, as this chapter went to press.

What are we to make of the politics of counting civilian deaths in Iraq? Two aspects are troubling. First, the difficulties of either counting *or* estimating civilian deaths are overwhelming and unavoidable in a site where warfare is continuing and a significant portion of the populace is displaced. All those who collect data on civilian mortality in Iraq make this point, whether they champion surveillance methods or population surveys. The debate over whether one or another method of counting the dead is most appropriate masks, and perhaps substitutes for, a sense of disbelief or outrage or protest about avoidable, senseless deaths. The second troubling part is the apparent apathy on the part of the United States populace toward this problem. What would it take for counting to result in accountability? Neither well-enumerated combat deaths in the thousands nor poorly enumerated civilian deaths in the hundreds of thousands have yet led to any significant political response that would signify that the state had decided to intervene to halt this epidemic. Only after that intervention could the last stage in social response to an epidemic begin: a popular movement toward assessing the conduct of its leaders.

Notes

I am grateful to Christina Wheeler-Castillo and Max Zevin for their able research assistance, to Lynn Morgan for her trenchant comments and questions, and to my fellow participants in the Wenner-Gren symposium for their constructive suggestions.

1. I pay less attention than some other contributors to the threshold at which disease becomes plague and engenders human emotions of fear and dread or perceptions of virulence and pervasiveness. Civilian mortality in Iraq is taking place as I write and shows no signs of abating, so I also do not examine how a plague disappears or how it changes other diseases.

2. The US military updates a Web page daily at www.defenselink.mil/news/casualty.pdf.

3. The database can be accessed at www.nytimes.com/ref/us/20061228_3000FACES_TAB1.html.

4. Questions might include the following: Was a sampling strategy not truly random? Were insufficient numbers of clusters chosen? Were interviewers

likely to bias their respondents? Were respondents likely to mislead their interviewers? Were analytical procedures used improperly or interpreted inappropriately? And, should any of these have come to pass, would their effects have been strong enough to change results? If so, by how much?

5. Waxman's reports now come from his chairmanship of the House Committee on Oversight and Government Reform; previously they were from the minority (Democratic) staff of the Government Reform Committee. See, for example, www.ucsusa.org/scientific_integrity/ and US House of Representatives, Committee on Government Reform, Minority Staff, 2003, Politics and science in the Bush administration, http://oversight.house.gov/features/politics_and_science/report.htm.

Avian Influenza and the Third Epidemiological Transition

Ron Barrett

At what point does an epidemic become a plague? Despite minor differences in the ways in which this volume's authors define plague, most agree that the term denotes a certain sense of urgency, anxiety, and alarm. Indeed, it could be safely argued that definitions of plague have more to do with human perceptions of diseases than with their biological characteristics. That said, certain disease characteristics are more likely to trigger public and professional alarm than others. A series of risk perception studies finds that people are more concerned with threats that are novel, highly fatal, or personally uncontrollable, independent of their actual probability of occurring (Gray and Ropeik 2002). Extending these attributes to disease threats more specifically, it could be argued that they are defining characteristics of human plagues.

H5N1 avian influenza exemplifies these plaguelike attributes of novelty, fatality, and resistance to human agency. It appears to be a new strain with characteristic adaptations for virulence and possible transmission in human populations. It has the potential for rapid resistance to antimicrobial technologies—an inevitable evasion from long-term vaccination coverage and possibly from antiviral therapies as well. H5N1 also shares certain characteristics with the H1N1 virus associated with the 1918 "Spanish flu" pandemic (Reid et al. 1999). It therefore threatens to become the prototypical reemerging infection: the terrifying new face of an old problem that never went away. In short, "avian flu" signifies a major human plague.

Although the H5N1 pathogen is a fairly recent discovery, the circumstances surrounding its emergence are ancient and recurring. Historically, these kinds of infections have arisen in response to anthropogenic conditions such as disrupted environments, socioeconomic inequalities, and changing patterns of human subsistence, fertility, and migration. An expanded framework of epidemiological transitions explains how these conditions have shaped human disease patterns from the Paleolithic to the present day (Barrett et al. 1998). Beginning about ten thousand years ago, the first epidemiological transition brought a marked increase in acute infections as human societies developed sedentary and agricultural modes of living. Between the late eighteenth and the early twentieth centuries, the second (classic) epidemiological transition involved a shift from infectious to chronic diseases with the rise and spread of industrial economies in Europe and North America. It is important to note that these two transitions were not unilinear developments, nor were they completed stages. The globalization of human disease ecologies has since brought these complex and incomplete trends into collision, resulting in a third epidemiological transition that began in the last decades of the twentieth century and persists in the present day. This third transition is characterized by the evolution of human transmissibility in new pathogens and the evolution of virulence and antimicrobial resistance in long-standing diseases, avian influenza among them.

This chapter examines the role of these events in the emergence of avian influenza. The convergence of acute and chronic disease patterns from the first and second transitions is shaping the susceptibility of human populations to new influenza strains. Meanwhile, social responses to rapidly aging societies are producing additional reservoirs of susceptible hosts. Finally, the concentration and convergence of human and avian host environments creates unprecedented opportunities for interspecies transmission. As in ancient times, all three of these processes are strongly mediated by social and economic inequalities.

An Expanded Theory of Epidemiological Transitions

Omran's (1971) classic model of epidemiological transition explains how changing disease patterns affected the demography of affluent societies in the years leading up to and during the Industrial Revolution. From a baseline of high mortality and fertility, the stabilization and subsequent decline of infectious disease mortality brought about a major population increase despite declining fertility rates. Much like McKeown (1978), Omran attributed this population increase to the decline of infectious disease mortality, particularly among young women and children. Yet there were also important tradeoffs to this epidemiological transition, particularly with respect to increasing rates of chronic degenerative diseases at later ages.

Although this classic epidemiological transition helps explain complex interactions between economy, demography, and disease, the model has two important shortcomings. The first is historical: the notion of a single transition suggests that preindustrial populations always suffered from high rates of infectious diseases, which was not the case. During the majority of our evolutionary history, human beings mainly lived as nomadic foragers in small, dispersed bands that were too small to have sustained highly acute and virulent infections. This form of social organization selected for diseases having low virulence or longer latency periods, as is the case for many of the "heirloom" parasites that are common to higher primates (Cockburn 1971; Kliks 1983).

Long before the classic transition, the first major epidemiological transition began with the Neolithic shift from nomadic foraging (hunting and gathering) to sedentism and agriculture. Skeletal analyses show increased infection-associated lesions and indications of malnutrition and stress in populations undergoing these cultural changes (Cohen and Armelagos 1984). In these cases the rise of infectious diseases can be explained by factors commonly associated with the agricultural revolution: increased population density, decreased dietary diversity, and greater proximity to zoonotic pathogens. These factors are also likely to have had differential effects on people in and between first transition populations. Bioarchaeological evidence suggests that individual disease burdens were inversely related to social status and that life expectancies declined in societies having greater degrees of social hierarchy (Buikstra 1984; Van Gerven 1990). Far from being a natural state of affairs, high infectious disease mortality was the unintended consequence of intentional human practices, many of which have continued to the present day.

The second shortcoming of the classic transition is that it mainly addresses changes in affluent societies, implying that developing societies will experience similar changes once they have become sufficiently modernized. Although many developing societies underwent some form of epidemiological transition in the decades following World War II, their declines in infectious mortality were more modest than those in the affluent world (Ahmad, Lopez, and Inoue 2000; Riley 2005). Simultaneously, they have experienced increased rates of chronic degenerative diseases in increasingly aging populations, a "worst of both worlds" situation (Bradley 1993). Furthermore, unlike the major infectious disease declines in the pre-antibiotic era of the developed world, declines in developing countries have been much more dependent on the distribution of antimicrobial technologies, a troubling situation given the inevitable evolution of antibiotic and vaccine resistance (Hill and Pebley 1989; Ruzicka and Kane 1990). Globalization has brought these worlds into closer contact than ever before, leading some to question whether there was ever a classic transition in the first place.[1]

Considering the aforementioned issues, it is not surprising that new and resistant pathogens would eventually be discovered in affluent populations. Humankind is rapidly developing a global disease ecology, one that involves a convergence of disease patterns as well as the diffusion of pathogens across populations and national boundaries. This convergence represents a third epidemiological transition, characterized by the evolution of human transmissibility and antimicrobial resistance in infectious pathogens. This third transition is the result of syndemic interactions between acute and chronic diseases, aging populations, environmental disruptions, and global poverty. Each has played a role in the emergence of avian influenza.

Converging the Chronic and the Acute

Only a few of the human cases of highly pathogenic avian influenzas (HPAIs) detected since 1997 can reasonably be attributed to human-to-human transmission (Wong and Yuen 2006). Nearly all confirmed human cases of H5N1 avian influenza have so far occurred as a result of bird-to-human transmission, with the highest risk for infection among poultry handlers (Dinh et al. 2006; Mounts et al. 1999). As such, these HPAIs are currently exhibiting what is known as "viral chatter," a situation in which a zoonotic pathogen genetically adapts the ability to "jump" into human hosts, but not yet to the degree that it can sustain further transmission in human populations. This "chatter" consists of multiple, limited outbreaks among people in close contact with primary animal reservoirs. Viral chatter has been observed in the transmission of simian retroviruses to bushmeat hunters in central Africa (Wolfe et al. 2004). It has also been hypothesized as the source of the multiple early appearances of HIV in human populations (Hahn et al. 2000; Wolfe et al. 2005).

The viral chatter of avian influenza in human populations is especially troubling given the mutability of the virus's RNA genome, the promiscuity of its replication machinery, and the fact that a single amino acid change on a single protein could alter its choice of host

(Gambaryan et al. 2006). But even with mutations and new traits, the virus could not sustain human-to-human transmission without the proper host and environmental conditions. Such conditions probably played key roles in the differential experience of the 1918 influenza pandemic. Despite having the highest mortality in human history, the 1918 pandemic was differentially experienced within and between countries (Barrett and Brown 2008). In affluent countries such as the United States, some cities and towns were devastated while others were hardly affected (Markel et al. 2007). Similarly, while some countries were hardly affected, colonial India suffered an estimated 18 million deaths, possibly more than all other countries combined (Mills 1986).

The 1918 influenza was experienced differentially within populations as well. One of the differences was reflected in the oft-cited W-shaped age distribution of influenza/pneumonia–related mortality (fig. 5.1). In contrast to the U-shaped age distributions of most influenza epidemics, reflecting high mortality among the very young and the elderly, the 1918 flu resulted in an unusually large proportion of deaths among young adults, especially males (Noymer and Garenne 2000; see also Noymer, this volume; Swedlund, this volume). Although there is evidence to suggest that an age-mediated hyperinflammatory response (sometimes referred to as a "cytokine storm") may have played a role, co-morbidity

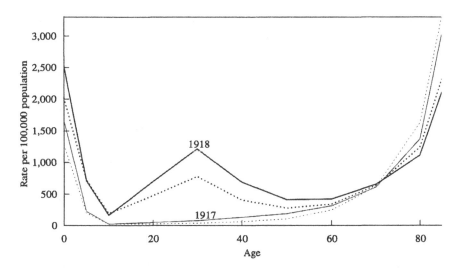

Figure 5.1 Age-specific death rates for influenza and pneumonia in the United States, 1917 and 1918. Males are indicated by solid lines, females by dotted lines. Source: US Department of Health, Education, and Welfare 1956, cited in Noymer and Garenne 2000.

issues need to be considered as well (Cheung et al. 2002; Kobasa et al. 2004; Lloberas and Celada 2002). One hypothesis is that co-infection with *M. tuberculosis* contributed to these unusual age and sex differences. TB infection was highest among young males at that time, and logistic regression for one 1919 data set shows that TB was a significant risk factor for contracting influenza. Moreover, TB death rates experienced an unusually steep decline in 1919, which proportionately accounts for the faster recovery of adult male over adult female life expectancy in the next several years, despite higher influenza mortality among males (Noymer, this volume; Noymer and Garenne 2000). These data suggest that TB played a significant role in the development of H1N1 infections into a major pandemic.

It is estimated that 30 percent of the world's population has been exposed to *M. tuberculosis*. It is therefore worth considering the potential role of TB in the emergence of future influenza pandemics. Tuberculosis has, in turn, been shaped by interactions with other diseases. For instance, the role of HIV/AIDS in the emergence of multidrug-resistant and extensively resistant tuberculosis is well documented (Castro and Farmer 2005; Corbett et al. 2003; Gandhi et al. 2006). Less known is the role of chronic degenerative diseases such as diabetes in TB susceptibility and mortality, despite its recognition early in the last century (Root 1934). One study in Tanzania found that subjects with an impaired glucose test were four times more likely to contract tuberculosis than those with normal glucose levels (Mugusi et al. 1990). The increased risk of TB infection among type II diabetes patients in southern Mexico is comparable to that of HIV patients in the same area (Ponce-De-Leon et al. 2004).

It is notable that tuberculosis and diabetes are among the most prevalent diseases of the first and second transitions, respectively. Like many other developing societies, Mexico and Tanzania have had to contend with the convergence of these two disease patterns, an intersection of flattening declines in acute infections with increasing rates of chronic degenerative diseases (Bradley 1993). Similar dynamics can be found in China, where diabetes and heart disease were significant risk factors for mortality during the SARS epidemic, an oft-cited analogy for pandemic influenza in Asia (Chan et al. 2003). The concept of syndemics best captures these broader issues of co-morbidity. A syndemic is defined as the synergistic contribution of two or more afflictions to the excess burden of disease in a population (see Singer, this volume). These afflictions, however, need not be restricted to biomedical conditions, as is the case for co-morbidity. Syndemics can include the afflictions of unsupported dependency, socioeconomic inequality, and environmental disruption, important partners in the emergence of third transition diseases.

Aging Societies

Although death rates for young adults were unusually high during the 1918 pandemic, it is notable that they were still higher among the elderly. The number and proportion of elderly people are much higher today than they were in 1918, and they are growing ever larger in most societies around the world. In the United States, for example, the percentage of elderly (defined as people aged sixty-five and over) rose more than threefold, from 5 percent in 1901 to more than 15 percent in 2000 (Kinsella and Velkoff 2001; fig. 5.2). This demographic transition is especially challenging for developing societies, which comprise more than half the world's elderly and are projected to account for most of the increase from 460 million elderly worldwide in 1990 to 1.4 billion in 2030 (World Bank 1994).

A combination of changing fertility and mortality patterns has con-tributed to this situation. The first epidemiological transition brought high mortality and fertility rates, with expansions in overall population size but without significant changes in the proportions of the elderly. The second transition brought declining mortality and fertility rates, leading to even greater population expansion due to declining childhood infectious diseases. Improved child survival initially produced broad bases at the lower end of the population age distribution. But once child mortality improvements leveled off, declining fertility drove an increasing wave of elderly into third transition populations, both rich and poor. Although total mortality and fertility declines have been relatively modest in developing societies, the more rapid rate of these changes has produced dramatic shifts in population age structure (Grigsby 1991). Such changes are already deeply felt in impoverished societies because of a lack of material resources, the dissolution of extended families, and the coexistence of infectious and chronic degenerative diseases, influenza among them (Heymann 2005; Treas and Logue 1986).

So far, HPAI has presented an even younger age pattern than the 1918 pandemic. In a sample of 172 H5N1-related deaths before June 2006, more than 95 percent occurred in persons under forty-five years of age, with slightly more in women than men overall (Chen et al. 2007). In addition to the possibility of hyper-reactions in young adults, mentioned previously, it is hypothesized that older people are protected from H5N1 infection by cross-immunity to viruses from prior seasonal

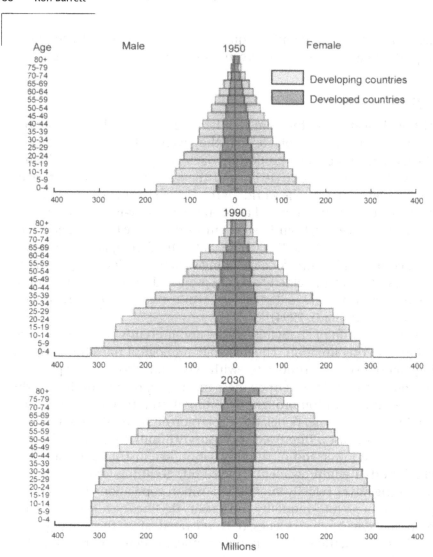

Figure 5.2 World population by age and sex, 1950, 1990, and 2030. Source: United Nations and US Bureau of the Census, cited in Kinsella and Velkoff 2001: 26.

epidemics (Chen et al. 2007). If the same factors account for the overall age distribution of H5N1, then one could expect a very different picture in the event that the virus evolves human-to-human transmissibility.

It is important to remember that the age distributions for mortality during the 1957 and 1968 influenza pandemics were relatively U shaped, with more than half the deaths in persons over sixty years of age, even though infection rates were highest among children (Cox and Subbarao 2000; Luk, Gross, and Thompson 2001; Simonsen et al. 1998). Moreover, the two strains that caused these pandemics (H2N2 and H3N2, respectively) were variants of seasonal influenzas that kill a disproportionate number of elderly every year and do so increasingly as populations continue to age (Thompson, Comanor, and Shay 2006; Thompson et al. 2003). It has been shown that the sizes of seasonal influenza epidemics contribute to the yearly antigenic variation of the virus and hence to the probability of emerging pathogenic strains (Boni et al. 2004). Consequently, the reduction of seasonal influenza among the elderly has the potential to reduce the probability of pandemic influenza in people of all ages.

In addition to seasonal influenza, there are other precedents for the susceptibility of older people to new varieties of pathogens. Dependent elderly have been unwilling reservoirs for the emergence of antibiotic resistance in bacterial pathogens such as *Staphylococcus aureus, Pseudomonas auregenosa,* and *Klebsiella pneumoniae,* which are now endemic to long-term care facilities in the United Kingdom and North America (Nicolle, Strausbaugh, and Garibaldi 1996; P. W. Smith 2000). These trends are especially relevant because secondary bacterial infections, rather than influenza itself, are the major cause of influenza-related pneumonias (Sethi 2002).

Although it is difficult to separate large-scale influenza mortality from that of other pneumonias, some argue that primary influenza pneumonias accounted for more deaths in 1918 than in subsequent influenza epidemics (Kobasa et al. 2004; Osterholm 2005). Even if this was the case, however, bacterial pneumonias were more prevalent in US Army bases before and during the early stages of the pandemic; they may have paved the way for multiple, simultaneous outbreaks during the first major wave of infections (Brundage 2006; Oxford et al. 2002). Furthermore, there is experimental evidence that persons with preexisting respiratory infections can become superspreaders for secondary infections—the so-called "cloud effect," which has been observed in the dissemination of methicillin-resistant *Staphylococcus aureus* (Sherertz et al. 1996) as well as of the coronavirus associated with severe acute respiratory syndrome (SARS), a recently discovered infection from which the elderly were more likely to die (Chan et al. 2003; Wong et al. 2004).

Human-Bird Ecologies

Most of our acute infections can be traced to zoonotic (animal-borne) diseases that crossed the species barrier as a result of ecological changes related to human subsistence (Weiss 2001). The most profound of these changes probably occurred during the ancient transitions from nomadic foraging to sedentism and agriculture, which brought humans into close and prolonged contact with domesticated animals and pests and presented greater opportunities for animal-to-human infection (Armelagos 1990; Armelagos and Harper 2005). Since then, new opportunities for interspecies contact have arisen as human populations have encroached on new environments, disrupted animal-host equilibriums, or pressured wild species to move into areas of human settlement. Avian influenza is no exception in this regard.

All influenzas have avian origins. Although only a minority of known influenza A subtypes are capable of human infection, all have been detected in birds, and the highest viral titers are found in the intestinal mucosa of waterfowl (Alexander 2000; Olsen et al. 2006). Because of its avian connections, influenza has been more closely associated with ecological issues than many other infectious diseases, with the possible exception of malaria. Several of these ecological issues, such as the interspecies role of domestic swine in the evolution of the virus, are in need of resolution and further clarification. For many years, a hypothesis of swine origin for the 1918 influenza circulated, which contributed to public alarm during the 1977 swine flu "epidemic that never was" (Neustadt and Fineberg 1983; Shope 1936). Furthermore, because pig epithelia contain receptors for both mammalian and avian influenza viruses, swine were considered potential "mixing vessels" for the reassortment of influenza's eight gene segments between two or more co-infecting strains (antigenic shift), thereby contributing to the evolution of new pathogenic influenza strains (Ito, Kida, and Kawaoka 1996; Kilbourne 1987). But although this mechanism has been demonstrated experimentally, swine-to-human infections have so far occurred only sporadically, despite a few high-profile epidemics (Cox and Subbarao 2000; Morgan 2006).

A more recent question concerns the relative contributions of wild birds and domestic poultry to the spread of avian influenza. With high titers of virions in their intestinal tracts, wild bird species such as mallards and other waterfowl are known to disseminate influenza globally along migration routes (Olsen et al. 2006). With respect to HPAI H5N1, however, the location and timing of these migrations correlate incompletely with human outbreaks since 1996, which remained bounded within China and Southeast Asia until 2004 (Gauthier-Clerc, Lebarbenchon, and Thomas 2007). This same study found that many outbreaks correlate more closely with transportation routes for the distribution of commercial poultry and fertilizer by-products.

A combined temporo-spatial and phylogenetic analysis for fifty-two human H5N1 outbreaks reveals a more complex scenario involving the introduction and spread of the virus by both wild birds and poultry in Asia and Africa, but with wild birds alone responsible for its European spread (Kilpatrick et al. 2006). This study also predicted that, without adequate biosecurity measures, commercial poultry would pose the greatest risk for the introduction of H5N1 to the Americas in the near future. Considering that the majority of human H5N1 cases have occurred among poultry handlers, and that the poultry industry accounts for more than several billion birds a year, more studies are needed concerning the political-economic and social contexts of human-poultry interactions.

Davis (2005) argues that the superurbanization of the human species has resulted in a superurbanization of its meat supply. Human densities now surpass 100,000 per square kilometer (stacked) in Amoy Gardens, Hong Kong, where the highest concentrations of SARS cases were found in 2004 (Leung et al. 2004). High-density commercial poultry cages are about 300 square centimeters per bird, comprising about 70 percent of the 12 billion chickens in East Asia (Davis 2005; see also www1.agric. gov.ab.ca/$department/deptdocs.nsf/all/pou3569 [accessed 9 August 2007]). Both humans and chickens have been squeezed into crowded conditions, subjected to nutritional and psychological stressors, and buffered with an abundance of antimicrobial drugs. With the partial exception of the latter technologies, this situation is not qualitatively different from that of the first epidemiological transition. But with the condensation and convergence of human and avian habitats, the scale is much larger than in previous transitions, and the consequences more extensive than the migration of any bird.

Conclusion: The Soil of Social Inequality

From the Neolithic to the present day, human inequalities have mediated all three epidemiological transitions. The social organization of first transition societies was hierarchical, with the upper strata living relatively longer and healthier than the lower strata (Buikstra 1984; Van Gerven 1990). The mortality benefits of the second transition were delayed and diminished among poorer societies as well as the poorest among the affluent, and they were altogether absent in some parts of the world (Ahmad, Lopez, and Inoue 2000; Riley 2005). Now, in the third epidemiological transition, the affluent and the poor are more closely connected than ever before, and the epidemic consequences of their social differences are converging within an increasingly globalized disease ecology.

Human inequalities of the third transition have important implications for the evolution and epidemiology of avian influenza. Tuberculosis has long been a disease of poverty, and acute respiratory infections are the leading cause of mortality among the impoverished majority of children under five years of age around the world (DiLiberti and Jackson 1999). Pneumonias that were once inappropriately called "the old man's friend" can now appropriately be called "the poor child's enemy," as well as a potential partner for new influenza viruses. Chronic co-morbid health conditions such as diabetes are increasingly prevalent among recently acculturated and newly developing societies (Neel 1982; Ponce-De-Leon et al. 2004; Swedlund 1997). Poverty combines with urbanization and the dissolution of traditional family structures to intensify the challenges of aging societies in the developing world and the susceptibility of the elderly to new and resistant infections (Heymann 2005; Treas and Logue 1986). Finally, large concentrations of financial capital are squeezing human and poultry environments and connecting them to one another through global trade networks and new forms of material consumption.

Given this fertile soil, the emergence of highly pathogenic influenza viruses is not surprising. Nevertheless, early studies of newly emerging human infections have focused more on the properties of pathogens than those of host and environment. An online search of the ISI Science Citation index for the fifty most cited articles from 1996 through 2007 that contained "avian influenza" in their titles revealed thirty-seven articles about the molecular and genetic properties of the virus or about the clinical diagnosis and treatment of the disease. Only ten of the remaining thirteen articles addressed issues of ecology, host susceptibility, or primary prevention (see also Herring and Lockerbie, this volume). None discussed poverty or social inequalities.

I hope this trend will change, and the number of socially and historically informed studies of avian influenza will increase. Defining a human disease as a human plague may not help to allay human anxieties. But perhaps a *little* anxiety may be a good thing if it brings attention and resources to bear on important health problems. Even then, the challenge will be to ensure that resources are well spent on addressing the core determinants of human diseases. An expanded framework of epidemiological transitions helps in this regard by identifying the socioeconomic, demographic, and environmental determinants of avian influenza in human populations. Addressing these determinants will help prevent the emergence and spread of avian influenza and many other potentially pandemic human diseases.

Note

1. Alan Swedlund (personal communication, 2006) observes that the time between the widespread use of antibiotics in the Western world and the appearance of antibiotic resistance in some microbes and of some of the newly emerging diseases (e.g., HIV/AIDS) was roughly thirty-five years. On the scale of time from the Paleolithic to the present day, this transition appears very short, even if one pushes the classic transition back to the late nineteenth century.

Deconstructing an Epidemic
Cholera in Gibraltar

Lawrence A. Sawchuk

A recurring theme in research on infectious diseases has been to empirically describe and capture the epidemic experience. This task has proved daunting, for it is not always easy to resolve the most fundamental question: When is an epidemic an epidemic? (Green et al. 2002). Frequently, the researcher is confronted with variations of the use of the term, with seemingly interchangeable expressions employed to describe epidemics such as plagues and outbreaks. To obfuscate the matter further, these emotionally charged terms are mutable over time and space. Clearly, the need for an unambiguous lexicon for the term *epidemic* is paramount for effective communication within and across discipline boundaries (Green et al. 2002: 5).

I define an epidemic simply as a marked rise in the frequency of a specific infectious disease in a community over a limited period, beyond the frequency considered normal for the population under investigation. I readily acknowledge that this definition is insufficient in scope and detail, for as Green and co-workers (2002) pointed out, each epidemic, by its very nature, is context specific. Accordingly, steps must be taken to situate the epidemic in space, place, and time. If the goal of the investigator is to empirically assess the effects of an epidemic, then contextualization is essential.

The first step in contextualizing the epidemic is to describe its fundamental epidemiological characteristics, using traditional methods. The second step is to define the prevailing state of mortality before and after the epidemic, ideally in empirical terms. The normal state of mortality then serves as the control period by which to gauge the effects of an exogenously derived epidemic on a population, as well as its short- and long-term consequences. This conceptual model divides the state of community well-being into four phases: the steady state of equilibrium, or the normal level of mortality; the stress period that disrupts equilibrium through an epidemic; the immediate aftermath of the epidemic; and the return to the steady state of mortality equilibrium. The third step in contextualizing an epidemic involves identifying, sourcing, and assessing the emergence of health inequalities. Collectively, these phases serve to contextualize the event, the ecosocial landscape, the processes at work, and the consequences. Such a scheme allows other researchers to frame their analytical work spaces in a way that will yield results that can be used to compare epidemics across space and time.

Cholera

Spreading misery and death in its wake, cholera has long drawn the attention of scholars from various disciplines (see, for example, Barua 1992; Evans 1987; Longmate 1966; McGrew 1965; Patterson 1994; Pollitzer 1959; Rabbani and Greenough 1992; Raufman 1998; Snowden 1995). Cholera is an ideal candidate for assessing the effects of an epidemic, because it can offer a classic example of crisis mortality. Outbreaks of cholera in Gibraltar in 1860 and 1865 illustrate two extremes. The former was a "slight visitation" of cholera, producing principally a shock effect that caused economic disruption and widespread community anxiety but little increase in mortality beyond the norm. The latter event was a "severe visitation" that caused not only socioeconomic shock but also extensive morbidity and mortality (table 6.1).

Cholera has retained the notoriety of being one of the most fatal of infectious diseases. It is capable of killing a patient within hours through rapid dehydration by violent vomiting and diarrhea (Watts 1997). Caused by the bacillus *Vibrio cholerae*, cholera was not endemic to Gibraltar but was a disease of importation. Despite the imposition of a wide range of quarantine measures, it was impossible to filter out everyone who carried the threat of an epidemic disease, such as cholera carriers and those with subclinical infections, who could easily slip through guarded land gates. Cholera could also have been introduced "silently" as a by-product of ships arriving from cholera epidemic regions and discharging their ballast water in the surrounding bay (see, e.g., Colwell 1996).

The carrier state for classic Asiatic cholera is thought to last from three to six days, but convalescent carriers may shed the *C. vibrio* bacillus for

Table 6.1 Nineteenth-century Cholera Pandemics in Gibraltar

Pandemic	Years	Gibraltar Outbreak	Number of Cholera Deaths			
			Civilians	Military	Convict Station[1]	Total
First	1817–1824	No appearance	—	—	—	—
Second	1829–1837	1831, rumor only				None
		1834	252	162	—	412
Third	1840–1860	1855	—	—	—	A few[2]
		1860	36	41	13	90
Fourth	1863–1875	1865	421	98	57	576
Fifth	1881–1896	1885	24	2	—	26

[1] The convict station at Gibraltar was established in 1842 and closed in 1874.
[2] Governor Gardener was reluctant to disclose the number of cases and deaths from cholera, believing that fear would aggravate the epidemic.

up to two or three weeks. Cholera transmission is further facilitated by the fact that *C. vibrio* can survive in water for extended periods of time. Smallman-Raynor and Cliff (1998) estimated that *C. vibrio* is capable of persisting for upward of three weeks in well water, given the right local conditions. Cholera epidemics have been positively correlated with climatic variables such as increases in sea temperature and air temperature and El Niño events. Kuhn and co-workers (2005: 21) wrote that sanitation and human behavior were probably more important risk factors than climatic variables.

The recurrence of cholera infection in an individual is rare, because natural infection typically confers effective, life-long immunity. Although the course of the disease is now generally understood, the issue of why some individuals suffer only mild discomfort while others die remains a mystery. Known factors that increase host susceptibility include reduced stomach acidity, the immunological burdens of other, coexistent gastrointestinal diseases, and undernourishment (Richardson 1994). Although research does not support the contention that chronic malnourishment increases the risk of contracting cholera, it can increase the risk of complications after infection, especially among children (see, e.g., Glass and Black 1992; Rabbani and Greenough 1992). Historically, cholera was linked to destitution and squalor, overcrowding, the recycling of infected clothing, defective sewage treatment, unwashed hands, contaminated produce, and impure water (Snowden 1995).

Epidemics, Colonialism, and Vulnerabilities

Cholera in Gibraltar was an imported disease that was facilitated by Gibraltar's position as a commercial center, naval port, garrison town, and British colony. Since 1804 Gibraltar has been subjected to the arrival of numerous deadly, novel pathogens that have had a profound impact on the biodemographic profile of the community. The hegemony of colonialism has always had the potential to affect the health of the colonized through a variety of possible pathways, including (1) exposure to new pathogens because of direct contact with non-indigenous peoples, (2) disruption of the local ecology through the forced adoption of new subsistence strategies, (3) alterations in the settlement pattern, frequently leading to unhealthy environs with overcrowding and poor sanitation, (4) the establishment of transportation systems that aided in the rapid and widespread diffusion of microbes, (5) the introduction of Westernized foods that promoted malnutrition and in turn greater susceptibility to infectious disease, and (6) ineffective quarantine measures that forced the local population into unemployment, a state of high anxiety, and an inability to flee from the infection site.

A number of unusual qualities of mid-nineteenth-century Gibraltar, a British colony since 1704, afford researchers the opportunity to explore deep-seated and often hidden features of a society as the result of an epidemic. These qualities included the following:

1. A small population of sufficient socioeconomic heterogeneity to permit fine-grained analysis of background mortality as well as crisis events
2. A police death registry that documents deaths according to name, age, sex, residence, birthplace, cause, and attending physician
3. A reconstituted census of 1868, as well as published yearly births, which provides information on the population at risk
4. An extremely limited habitable territory where ingress and egress were tightly controlled
5. An infrastructure in which the crucial water supply system was highly decentralized and well documented by colonial authorities at the household level
6. Copious memorials from local merchants, who were keen to minimize the economic repercussions of exaggerated reports on the number of cases of cholera
7. Numerous inquiries commissioned by the colonial Home Office (e.g., Sutherland 1867) to safeguard its troops, with the implicit

recognition that the health of the military was inseparable from that of the civilian community

An Omnipresent Ecological Stressor

Identifying the key ecological factor or factors that shaped the overall health of a community is a primary element in contextualizing an epidemic. Accordingly, attention must be given to Gibraltar's unusual water sources, its water distribution system, and the care and storage of water at the household level.

The acquisition and storage of potable water occupied a primary place in daily life in Gibraltar, because rainwater was the most important resource. The capriciousness of annual rainfall served as a constant, ecologically based psychological stressor for residents, who knew that the average cumulative rainfall for the months of June through August was less than two inches. The water distribution system was primitive and wholly inadequate (table 6.2); the garrison's quartermaster wrote in 1862 that "the inhabitants owe nothing to the British Government for the small supply of water they have had for 150 years" (Garrison Quartermaster's Office 1862). Like other essential resources, the water supply was dispersed among the hands of the military, naval, and civilian communities, each group controlling its own catchment area and storage and distribution system. Among civilians in this highly decentralized system, each housing or patio unit held individual responsibility for supplying its residents with water. Moreover, the absence of local government ordinances regarding the sanitary condition of private water tanks and of barrels used in transporting water meant that the purity of potable water was highly suspect.

Wealth was a critical determinant of household water availability, sufficiency, and quality. In Gibraltar, the wealthy more likely had access to water drawn from both a private cistern and a well, whereas the poor most likely had neither (Sawchuk 2001). Even in cases in which holding tanks were available, it was critical that residents take steps to ensure that the cisterns were filled and maintained to keep the water safe from contamination. For example, in one patio unit in the upper portion of Gibraltar, where seventy inhabitants resided in twenty households, "there is one large tank upon the premises, apparently in good condition, capable of holding 41,000 gallons of water, but it is never filled" (Roberts 1866: 20).

Any advantage the wealthy had in terms of water storage disappeared in times of protracted drought. In 1878, for example, residents were

Table 6.2 Water Supply for Gibraltar, about 1852

	Number of Houses	Water Source	Number of People	Water Consumed (Gallons per Day)	Description
Civilians	179	No wells	2,775	1.5	Conveyed on donkeys from center of town when water was available; otherwise from the North Front, water that was "sweet but hard and brackish"[1]
	133	Wells	2,330	1.0	Bad, brackish water
	136	Cisterns	4,497	1.5	Cisterns for the most part dry from 1 August to 30 September
Military	—	—	—	2.5	Garrison's quartermaster reported that even on stinted allowance, every man received 2.5 gallons a day

Source: Compiled by the military quartermaster, Gibraltar (Garrison Quartermaster's Office 1862).
[1] The North Front is the land mass outside the town of Gibraltar that extends to the Spanish border.

forced to purchase water from vendors, or *borricos*, who supplied water priced according to its scarcity, transportation distance, and difficulty of delivery. Inevitably, the poor suffered most in times of drought, because of the high cost of water when it was conveyed from the isthmus or from Spain. Sutherland's observation on the water supply for the working poor (1867: 20) bears repeating: "In the upper portions of the Rock [Gibraltar], where water is carried up the steep ramps to the highest levels, the water is sold to the poor at the rate of 7 gallons for a penny. One consequence of this condition of the water supply is that the poor used the same water for several purposes in succession." Drinking water available for civilians ranged from 1.0 to 1.5 gallons per day, an amount the inadequacy of which becomes apparent when one considers that the World Health Organization today recommends that refugees receive 3.2 to 4.4 gallons of clean water during outbreaks of cholera. In contrast, water for the military population was uniformly available and greater in quantity.

Another consequence of water shortages was felt in the production of the Gibraltarians' staple food, bread. Local medical officers were keenly aware that during the summer months sanitary water was being used by bakers: "Except in the case of actual difficulty of obtaining sufficient quantity of fresh water, I consider that sanitary water should not be used for this purpose. Although organic matter of a dangerous character is likely to be destroyed during the process of baking, a quantity of salts liable to cause dyspepsia and diarrhea remain in the bread" (MacPherson 1892: 48). Under normal circumstances, liquid nourishment from the abundance of fresh fruit available in the late summer might provide relief during the annual dry period. Yet even if the poor could afford to purchase fruit, the consumption of fresh produce posed a health risk, because crops were traditionally fertilized with human and animal waste. Not washing fresh fruit before consumption because of a lack of water could produce health consequences ranging from mild gastric distress to more serious illnesses.

The need to flush water for sanitary purposes posed a problem in Gibraltar, particularly during the hot, dry summer months, when drains were converted into nothing more than noxious cesspits. A primitive sanitary infrastructure posed further risk, as Gibraltar's health inspector observed in 1865: "The surface drainage, paving, and occasionally the cleansing of the courts or patios are little attended to. Filth is found inside houses in considerable quantities. No proper soil-pans, or other suitable domestic conveniences [exist], presenting arrangements most offensive and dangerous to the public health of the town and garrison ...

Under these circumstances, it is not to be wondered at that epidemics originate and prevail to a very serious and destructive extent at certain intervals" (Rutherford 1866).

Competing Interests and the Poverty Complex

Lack of access to potable water was just one among the myriad determinants that shaped the health of the underprivileged in nineteenth-century Gibraltar. The bulk of the civilian community was at the mercy of competing interests that directly affected Gibraltar's health infrastructure. A correspondent to the *Lancet* wrote on 23 July 1898 that the general state of sanitary affairs in Gibraltar was far from satisfactory, owing partly to the interests of the military and commercial sectors:

> First, there is the military interest, which would make Gibraltar simply a fortress with scarcely any civil population. Secondly, there is the trading interest, which finds that Gibraltar is a most convenient commercial centre and would convert the place into a vast emporium for trade with Spain and the Mediterranean... The trading element is cramped, impeded and checked by the military element; but on the other hand, the military authorities have not succeeded in preventing Gibraltar from becoming an important commercial centre. They have mainly succeeded in producing the excessive overcrowding which is the principal cause of the high death [rate].

The result was that the vast majority of Gibraltar's inhabitants were trapped in the lifestyle known as that of the working poor. Their poverty was not a singular quality but rather the sum of interconnected vulnerabilities that permeated every aspect of life. Indeed, poverty in Gibraltar is best described as a complex that included overcrowding, high unemployment, low wages, inadequate nutrition, poor personal and household hygiene, substandard household living conditions (e.g., damp living quarters, lack of amenities), and poor education about health care and treatment. Often this poverty persisted over generations. Mired in the "poverty trap," the poor eked out livings that left no financial or emotional cushion in the face of lengthy periods of unemployment and that gave them no hope of escaping their difficult lives.

For those living on the political and economic margins, housing was abysmal. The cost of accommodation in Gibraltar was unusually high, owing to the limited habitable space available for civilians as laid out by stringent military laws that restricted the height and locations of civilian housing throughout the territory of Gibraltar. To exacerbate these conditions, the habitable property that was available for civilians lay in the hands of a small number of wealthy landed owners whose only interests were pecuniary. Because wealth was concentrated among the few landlords, they could and did exploit the shortage of housing by charging exorbitant rents for crowded quarters, and they allowed unsanitary living conditions to persist. In the absence of any sanitary bylaws, minimal living standards were seldom met, subletting was rampant, and the care of common courtyards, privies, and other amenities was typically nonexistent. As an illustration of the state of affairs, during the 1865 epidemic a total of ten cholera deaths was recorded in House 23, District 27, where the government sanitary engineer recorded the following conditions:

> This house ... is a long building of two stories, each divided into eleven separate rooms, all being occupied by separate families consisting of 5 to 12 families in each... It is one of three parallel ranges of buildings erected at different slopes of the Rock ... and so close to each other as to leave only very narrow passages for access to them, and so as to exclude almost all ventilation... One of these obstructive cross buildings ... is a large privy used in common by nearly 200 persons of both sexes, and is in such a filthy condition as to be most dangerous to health, it is a large hole over an open drain which is separated by a long open iron grating; the smell from this privy is distinctly perceptible 30 to 40 yards off... The lower rooms of the house ... are about 12 ft by 11 ft and 8 ft high, containing 1056 cubic feet or about 120 ft for each person on an average; the floors are brick, apparently laid on the earth, and the ceilings of thin deal boards laid on open unceiled joists, so that [there is] only one inch of wood as a division between one dwelling and another... The door and window are both on one side, the back wall being as stated for retaining the earth behind, and very wet... The upper rooms have wooden floors (which form the ceilings of the lower rooms).... The walls of nearly all of these rooms are very damp owing chiefly to badly constructed roofs... There are no kitchens to this house, so that cooking is carried on almost entirely in small portable charcoal stoves. (Roberts 1866)

Another dimension of the health disparity in the population manifested itself during epidemics, when traditional policing measures were imposed to stop the spread of cholera through *cordons sanitaires*, quarantines, fumigation, disinfection, and isolation. The imposition of

Table 6.3 Imposition of Sanitary Cordons along the Border between Gibraltar and Spain during Cholera Epidemics in Gibraltar

Year	Cordon Closed	Cordon Reopened	Epidemic Status
1834	26 June	3 September	Cholera epidemic
1849	October	January	Cholera in England
1854	2 November	7 February	Cholera in England
1860	Remains open	—	Slight visitation of cholera
1865	24 August	23 November	Severe visitation of cholera
1884	12 August	17 October	Sporadic cases?
1885	Remains open	—	Very limited cases in Gibraltar

sanitary cordons was a well-established action implemented by Spanish authorities against Gibraltarians that began with outbreaks of yellow fever and continued with the occurrence of sporadic and epidemic cholera. The politically motivated action of isolating Gibraltar was somewhat capricious in its implementation, for it was not a universal response during cholera outbreaks (table 6.3), and paradoxically, the Spanish government itself denounced the efficacy of cordons in 1844.

By 1865 Gibraltarians had become all too accustomed to the imposition of the dreaded sanitary cordon during times of epidemic. As the local press put it, "although Spain has decided that Gibraltar is a sick man, it has recommended to him, if not to take to his bed, at least to keep to his room and enforced the recommendation by unceremoniously locking the door upon him" (*Gibraltar Chronicle*, 25 August 1865). Dependent on Spain for food, water, and other supplies, Gibraltarians found that any break in free communication with that country had a considerable effect on the well-being of the inhabitants, particularly that of the working poor.

Within days of the imposition of a sanitary cordon, an increase took place in the number of Gibraltar's poor who followed the tradition of applying for alms from the houses of the middle and upper classes on Saturdays at an appointed time. The effects of the quarantine were also felt by those dependent on the mercantile and shipping trade, such as clerks, journeymen, porters, carters, boatmen, and lightermen.

Previous outbreaks accompanied by protracted quarantines had left a permanent mark on Gibraltarians' worldview, well beyond that stemming from the risk of contracting the disease, because the economic and sociopolitical isolation meant that the economy suffered as trade came to a standstill. Under quarantine, many Gibraltarians experienced lengthy periods of unemployment. The population at large endured shortages of food and essential supplies, as well as an overall increase in the cost of living.

News of the impending imposition of a quarantine was met by heightened public anxiety, widespread fear, and, for those who could afford it, flight out of the garrison town into the surrounding countryside. Authorities readily acknowledged that this last action contributed directly to the spread and development of the epidemic (Sawchuk 2001).

Chronicling an Epidemic: Qualitative Remarks

During the study periods, 1860 and 1865, Gibraltar was struck by visitations of cholera. The first epidemic, in 1860, was characterized as a "slight visitation." A local physician described it this way:

> It could scarcely in a population of 25,000 in which less than 100 deaths occurred be strictly called an epidemic; the less so when the facilities afforded by this garrison of engendering and fostering malignant forms of disease are taken into consideration, and when it is remembered that it occurred at the end of the warm summer, when from the absence of rain, not a sewer had been flushed for 5 to 6 months in one of the worst drained and ... most densely populated towns under British rule. (Prison Report 1861)

The second visitation was most likely introduced through troop movement, a common event in Gibraltar, where troops were rotated in and out of the fortress garrison. In 1865 it is likely that cholera entered Gibraltar with the 22nd Regiment, which was restationing from Malta. Between 18 July and 27 October 1865, it was estimated that three quarters of the civil population suffered from cholera or choleriac diarrhea, which at one period was very severe (fig. 6.1).

The disease burden on Gibraltar's population in 1865 was increased by the concurrent, or syndemic, outbreak of smallpox. By the latter part of August, fifty-six people had died of the dreaded pox. The death rate during the smallpox epidemic was exacerbated by social disarray, higher food prices, and increased stress from the cholera epidemic, as well as by deep-seated cultural factors among the marginalized poor such as concealment and unwillingness to participate in vaccination (Sawchuk 2001). Although smallpox vaccination had been endorsed by the administration in 1814, the poor remained reluctant to participate because of cost and a general distrust of hospitals. For the illegally settled

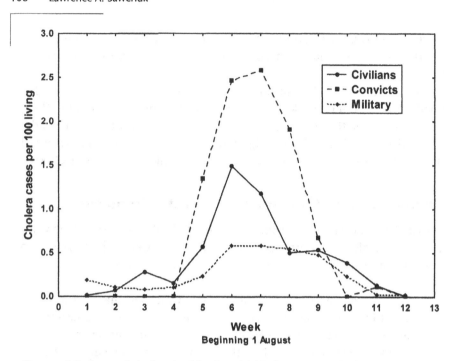

Figure 6.1 Cases of cholera in Gibraltar, 1865. Source: Sawchuk 2001.

foreign-born poor, an additional issue was possible expulsion from the fortress. Marginalized illegal residents would conceal their families from the authorities, avoiding vaccination and thereby risking death, rather than suffer removal from the garrison and secure employment.

In 1865, more than eight thousand prescriptions were made up and dispensed gratis to upward of two thousand of the unemployed poorer classes (*Gibraltar Chronicle*, 9 November 1865). Even an experienced physician remarked on the singularity of this outbreak:

> The epidemic seemed to me to be somewhat different from similar outbreaks which I had witnessed in India and in other places; firstly, the length of time of its continuance; secondly, the circumstance of its having attacked a large number of children of tender age, some mere infants, in whom the symptoms were well marked; and thirdly, the severity of many of the last cases, some of the patients seized towards the termination of the epidemic dying in a very few hours. (Rutherford 1866)

These few descriptive remarks attest to the protean nature of cholera and to the fact that local circumstances could alter the weight of the epidemic's effect.

By mid-October, cholera was on the wane (table 6.4). The government-run newspaper, the *Chronicle*, spoke metaphorically about the cessation of the epidemic: "[We] may fairly consider the epidemic visitation past and ... may reasonably hope that our 'terrible Asiatic guest' ... will take his final departure in a few days" (19 October, 1865). Further details on the 1865 cholera epidemic can be found elsewhere (see, e.g., Gross 1867; Sawchuk 2001; Sawchuk and Burke 2003; Sutherland 1867).

The Effects of Cholera on Life Expectancy

At the core of my research into the effects of cholera on life expectancy in Gibraltar is the use of life table methodology to investigate changes in mortality under epidemic and non-epidemic conditions. The life table "provides a convenient, comprehensive and self-contained summary of mortality conditions prevailing in an actual or hypothetical population" (Carlson 2006: 218). I use the period life table, which provides a snapshot of the prevailing mortality pattern summarized in a single value.

Traditionally, life tables have been used as indicators of the health of large population aggregates such as nation-states. Recently, researchers have applied the life table approach to smaller units such as local communities, and necessarily there is growing concern over the degree of confidence one can place in life table function estimates under those circumstances. Without an appreciation of the upper and lower levels of a fixed confidence level (e.g., 95 percent), it is difficult to compare small-scale communities across time and or space with statistical confidence.

The method I use here follows the Chiang approach for estimating life table parameters. The Chiang method is well entrenched in the demographic literature and dates to his seminal text, published in 1984. After comparing a number of approaches in life table methodology, Manuel and co-workers (1998: 5) recommended the Chiang method because (1) it produces the most conservative estimates for comparison between local areas; (2) it is easy to calculate (including statistical variance); (3) sensitivity analysis can be performed on the major assumptions; and (4) it is frequently used, such as by the World Health Organization, allowing for comparability. Of particular anthropological merit is that statistical comparisons can be made directly between two samples. This is extremely important in dealing with small-scale communities, which may be subject to considerable sampling error. The standard error computation of various life table functions can be found in chapter 8 of Chiang 1984. To assess the survival curve before and during the 1865

Table 6.4 Event Chronology for the 1865 Cholera Epidemic in Gibraltar

Month	Day	Description
July	18	Sporadic cases of cholera break out among military.
	31	Troops are camped outside walls of town.
August	4	Note acknowledging occurrence of cholera is attached to bills of health for ships touching Gibraltar's shores.
	10	Spain imposes five-day quarantine for any ship entering Gibraltar's port.
	11	Epidemic cholera breaks out among civilians.
	15	Principal medical officer begins issuing daily reports to governor giving number of cholera cases and deaths.
	24	Spain imposes sanitary cordon, cutting off supplies to Gibraltar. Governor issues medicine for diarrhea and cholera for the poor, at government expense.
	29	Health inspector distributes pamphlet on "simple precautions against attacks of sickness." Local paper reports "unreasonable" amount of fear among the people.
	30	Tangier Board of Health orders all vessels from Gibraltar away from Tangier and ports of Barbary.
September	6	Cholera epidemic breaks out in Gibraltar Convict Station. A relief committee opens a soup kitchen feeding about 150 families.
	7	Local merchants ask Board of Health to publish lists of cholera cases and deaths to prevent exaggeration of the epidemic.
	18	Civil practitioners are appointed to watch over poorer districts. Two physicians are put on duty at the Colonial Hospital.
October	4	Public Relief Committee established in absence of legal means of assisting economically distressed citizens.
	5	Governor contributes 1,000 pounds for public relief, in addition to private contributions by the public.

Month	Day	Description
	11	Last death due to a smallpox epidemic that began in March 1865, resulting in fifty-six recorded deaths.
	20	General holiday declared because cholera is on the wane.
	23	Special attendance of physicians at the Colonial Hospital is suspended.
	21	Bishop publishes notice to parishioners thanking "the Almighty" for ceasing his wrath in the form of cholera.
November	1	Gibraltar declared free of the epidemic. Clean bills of health can now be issued to sea vessels.
	23	Spanish authorities open border into Gibraltar nearly a month after last case of cholera is reported there.

cholera epidemic in Gibraltar, as well as the significance of cause-specific mortality attributed to cholera, I used Smith's (2004) *Survival* program.

Life table methodology reveals the variability of cholera and its effects on different age groups in Gibraltar (table 6.5). Although the 1860 epidemic produced a depression in life expectancy (LE) relative to noncholera years, the 1865 epidemic had a more marked dampening effect on LE relative to the periods representing the state of normal mortality.

The year 1866 proved interesting because of a significant rise in LE in both sexes. The subsequent period, 1867–1868, saw a significant fall in LE relative to 1866—a return of mortality to its normal background state. A comparison of the intervals 1861–1864 and 1867–1868 yielded no statistically significant difference. Consequently, the following analytical framework was constructed: (1) 1860, a period of slight visitation; (2) 1861–1864 and 1867–1868, the normal state of background mortality; (3) 1865, a period of severe visitation; (4) 1866, the year following the epidemic; and (5) a return to the "normal" state of community health.

The impact of cholera on the civilian community can be observed in the survivorship curves for the epidemic periods relative to the control periods. The survivorship curves presented in figures 6.2 and 6.3 reveal that 1865 and 1866 were both outliers in terms of survivorship. The disparity between 1865 and 1866 relative to the benchmark is particularly visible in the age intervals 5–9 years and over.

Table 6.5 Average Life Expectancy at Birth (LE) in Gibraltar, 1860–1868, in Years

Sex	Slight Cholera Outbreak, 1860		No Cholera, 1861–1864		Severe Cholera Epidemic, 1865		No Cholera, 1866		No Cholera, 1867–1868
Male	27.32 ± 1.67		31.60 ± 0.86		15.67 ± 1.15		36.22 ± 2.02		27.71 ± 1.25
		$Z = 2.28$		$Z = 8.03$		$Z = 8.86$		$Z = 3.58$	
Female	28.98 ± 1.75		36.30 ± 2.54		17.90 ± 1.25		40.46 ± 2.23		32.31 ± 1.48
		$Z = 1.09$		$Z = 8.32$		$Z = 8.68$		$Z = 3.00$	

Note: To illustrate the computation of the critical ratio of Z for a given pair, consider the difference in LE at birth by sex, $Z = e_0$ (male) $- e_0$ (female) / SE (diff), where SE (diff) $= \sqrt{}$(SE male e_0 + SE female e_0). Details on the derivation of the standard error (SE) of LE can be found in Chiang 1984: chapter 8. The computed Z scores for the period 1861–1864 versus 1867–1868 for males and females were statistically insignificant ($Z_m = 0.32$; $Z_f = 0.64$), so the two periods could be pooled as a "common phase" of normal background mortality.

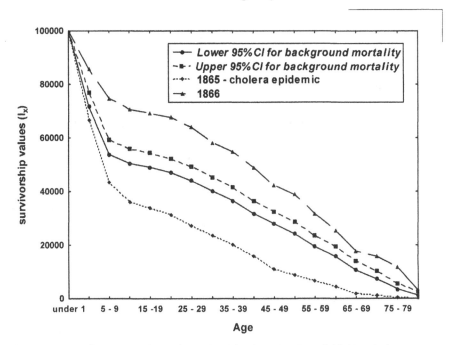

Figure 6.2 Male survivorship values (l_x), Gibraltar, 1865 and 1866, relative to the confidence interval (CI) for background mortality.

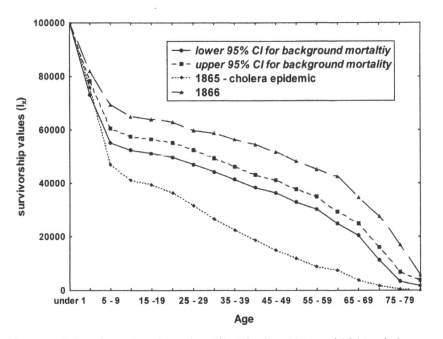

Figure 6.3 Female survivorship values (l_x), Gibraltar, 1865 and 1866, relative to the confidence interval (CI) for background mortality.

The observed gain in life expectancy is largely indirect—that is, the change in mortality produced an increase in the number of survivors who escaped the prevailing conditions at younger ages and would face the prevailing mortality pattern only later in life. A century ago, without sophisticated analytical tools, a physician in Gibraltar remarked that because cholera had "swept off a large number of the weak, the intemperate and those disposed to disease, there was therefore a more favourable condition of the population in the following year" (Stokes 1867: 47). In the aftermath of the epidemic, the removal of the frail resulted in a more robust or resilient population. Such a phenomenon is not new to epidemiologists; the concept of "harvesting" has been in the literature for decades and was most recently reintroduced in an elegant fashion in the work of Smith (2003). Dominici and co-workers (2003) use the term "short-term mortality displacement" when fewer deaths than expected occur over a period of time following a crisis. The term *harvesting* refers to an inflation, albeit temporary, in the death rate among persons of compromised health status. The harvesting effect has been used in analyzing increased mortality due to a heat wave in France (Toulemon and Barbieri 2008) and in predicting the consequences of a future influenza pandemic (Murray et al. 2006).

The results of using the cause-deleted methodology (Smith 2004), shown in table 6.6, reveal that cholera alone had no significant effect on life expectancy in 1860 relative to the period broadly defined as that of normal background mortality. In contrast, the epidemic of 1865 had a statistically significant dampening effect on LE in both sexes. A number of additional points warrant mention. In 1865, for example, the decrease in LE was felt largely in young age groups, and the majority of the effect was indirect. The loss of young persons meant that their age cohort would not follow the mortality schedule characteristic of the normal or background situation.

Origin and Destination Decomposition

Decomposition analysis is a method for pinpointing the age groups in which changes in life expectancy originate. Several popular decompositions of difference in life expectancy are available, of which Arriaga's (1984) origin-decomposition approach is probably the best known. The method employed here is an enhanced variant of this approach called the origin-decomposition and destination-decomposition approach (Carlson 2006). The method, using calculations from life table functions, was originally proposed by Andreev (1982), and the equations needed

Table 6.6 Contributions by Cholera and Other Causes of Mortality to Changes in Life Expectancy (LE), Gibraltar, 1860–1868

	Females		Males	
Cause	LE Difference	Probability	LE Difference	Probability
Slight visitation, 1860 vs. 1861–64 and 1867–68				
Cholera	−1.329	0.516	−1.463	0.434
All other causes	−1.260	0.538	−0.443	0.813
Residual (distributed among causes)	−0.004	—	0.003	—
Total	−2.589	0.205	−1.020	0.586
Severe visitation, 1865 vs. 1861–64 and 1867–68				
Cholera	−11.243	0.000	−9.607	0.000
All other causes	−1.954	0.196	−2.002	0.145
Residual (distributed among causes)	−0.001	—	0.036	—
Total	−13.197	0.000	−11.610	0.000

to implement it were provided by Carlson (2006).[1] I use it here for the first time in studying an epidemic.

Decomposition analysis has a number of useful features: (1) it requires only mortality and population data; (2) its calculations are straight-forward and can be carried out using a simple spreadsheet; (3) it identifies the age segments having the greatest influence, positive or negative, on life expectancy; (4) it provides a quantitative measure that is easily interpreted; and (5) it allows for a detailed description of the mortality patterns and the relative importance of different age intervals for life expectancy. To illustrate the value of the decomposition method for pinpointing which age groups were most affected by the 1865 cholera epidemic in Gibraltar, I look at life expectancy at birth before and during the epidemic, according to sex. During the period 1861–1864, LE at birth for females and males was 36.3 and 31.6, respectively, giving a difference of 4.7 years. For 1865, the life expectancy differential between the sexes fell to 2.2 years, with LE at birth for females and males at 17.9 and 15.7 years, respectively.

The decomposition method shown in table 6.7 reveals a number of salient points that illustrate the origin of the age mortality differentials during the 1865 cholera epidemic. For males, there was a marked decline in life expectancy at birth, of 15.98 years. The mortality burden, however, was not shared equally by all ages. In particular, infants show lower mortality rates than normal during the epidemic year. Relative to the preceding period of normal background mortality, the year 1865 showed elevated mortality, which manifested itself primarily as a "direct" effect that peaked in the age interval 15–19. This pattern of elevated mortality continued until the ages of sixty-five and older.

In comparison with men, women in 1865 showed a larger decline in life expectancy at birth, of 18.4 years. As was the case with males, there was an improvement in infant mortality during the cholera visitation. For females, however, the maximum decline of mortality is observed later than that in males, with the maximum point of decline occurring around the age interval 55–59, as shown in table 6.7.

Entropy

Another approach to assessing changes or differences in survivorship uses the concept of life table entropy. According to Romo (2003: 33), entropy of the survival function (H) is a measure of the concavity of the survival curve. Earlier research placed the bounds of H between 0 and 1. When H = 0, deaths in a population are concentrated in a

Table 6.7 Origin and Destination Decomposition of the Period 1861–1864 Compared with Life Expectancy at Birth for 1865

Age	Male		Female	
	Difference	Percent Change	Difference	Percent Change
0	0.67	–4.22	0.84	–4.56
1	–0.83	5.19	–0.55	2.98
5	–1.21	7.57	–0.99	5.37
10	–1.24	7.77	–0.96	5.24
15	–1.35	8.43	–1.11	6.03
20	–1.31	8.21	–1.10	6.00
25	–1.25	7.81	–1.11	6.03
30	–1.14	7.15	–1.11	6.03
35	–1.23	7.68	–1.33	7.23
40	–1.22	7.64	–1.37	7.47
45	–1.24	7.76	–1.51	8.22
50	–1.06	6.61	–1.46	7.96
55	–1.03	6.45	–1.64	8.93
60	–0.85	5.30	–1.46	7.93
65	–0.76	4.75	–1.42	7.73
70	–0.59	3.69	–1.09	5.92
75	–0.27	1.71	–0.54	2.96
80	–0.06	0.37	–0.29	1.59
85	–0.02	0.14	–0.17	0.94
Total	–15.98	100.00	–18.39	100.00

narrow range of age groups. If death rates are constant at all ages, then H = 1. Research suggests that H can exceed unity when life tables are characterized by extremely high death rates in the young age intervals. Individuals who survive these first few years can expect to live many more years than can newborns (Goldman and Lord 1986; Meindel and Swedlund 1977).

Entropy values obtained by using Smith's 2004 *Survival* program indicate that during times of normal background mortality in Gibraltar, death rates were fairly uniform across all age intervals. However, entropy values in the post-epidemic year, 1866, suggest a shift in mortality to a narrower range of age intervals. In contrast, during the 1865 epidemic, entropy values exceeded 1, illustrating the principle that under epidemic conditions, once children lived past the high death rates in the early age intervals, they could expect large gains in life expectancy.

Beyond the Numbers

In nineteenth-century Gibraltar, cholera was chameleon-like—in one year devastating, and in another, remaining well within the normal range of mortality. Yet there was one universal consequence of a cholera outbreak: it brought unbridled fear and shock to both individuals and the state. For the unfortunate, the personal loss brought by the deadly bacillus lingered for years as family life was irreconcilably altered. The cost of the epidemic went beyond illness or death as families diverted their limited resources from the acquisition of necessities such as food, water, and accommodation to paying for medical care and often burial expenses. For many, the loss of a lifetime of savings meant poverty, and if severe enough, the economic consequences could last for generations, forcing families into the poverty trap. At the community level there was a reduction in capital formation, a depression in spending by consumers, and a loss of productivity in local businesses. The cost of the epidemic to the state was felt immediately through an increase in the cost of hospital expenditures, care for orphans, the printing and dissemination of health-related information, the implementation of quarantine policing measures, the disinfection of households and institutions, and the cost of housing and caring for those forced to reside outside their homes in areas of quarantine.

Pelling (1978) and others have argued that sporadic epidemics such as those of cholera had no long-term biodemographic effects when viewed in the context of other prevailing diseases, falling behind many of the other common infectious diseases of the time. The evidence from Gibraltar for the epidemics of 1860 and 1865 support that proposition, but only in the narrowest of terms, for the arrival of cholera marked a rethinking of civil rights and entitlement to citizenship. It was shortly after the 1865 epidemic that civil tensions began to surface as the colonial administration implemented reforms in nationality issues, sanitation, and housing and curbs on population growth. The demographic profile of Gibraltar was altered not through the direct impact of cholera mortality but indirectly through such reforms, as political actions by the Home Office took hold and defined the very legal essence of Gibraltarian identity. The lesson from Gibraltar is that from the broad sociopolitical perspective, the effects of an epidemic cannot be measured by the toll of sick and dead alone.

Note

1. Origin and destination decompositions are calculated directly from the life table functions, where l_x = the number of survivors to age x, based on a predetermined radix; L_x = the number of person-years lived in a particular age segment; and e_x = the life expectancy in person-years to be lived by the population at age x. The result is Andreev's $_n\varepsilon_x$ age decomposition value, which assigns differences in life expectancy according to the age group in which the mortality difference first occurs (Carlson 2006).

The End of a Plague?

Tuberculosis in New Zealand

Judith Littleton, Julie Park, and *Linda Bryder*

The "white plague" label applied by Dubos and Dubos (1952) to tuberculosis (TB) has been a significant metaphor for the disease. But in what sense has TB ever been a plague, and what does appending the term *plague* to the infection achieve? After all, TB is a chronic, not an acute, condition, and it does not occur in the sort of epidemic wave and associated dramaturgical form described by Rosenberg (1992a). On the other hand, TB does connect with the ideas of affliction, pestilence, contagion, moral taint, and external threat that adhere so strongly to plagues and epidemics. Thinking of TB through the lens of plague throws these associations into high relief. For some groups, infectious disease as a category and tuberculosis are indistinguishable, linked by the recurrent image of contagion (Anderson 2008). In New Zealand, as elsewhere, TB is still a disease for which it is possible to incarcerate the uncooperative patient. When we think about plagues, therefore, TB sits in a particular position, causing mortality, but slowly, and contagious, but not like influenza. Yet because of its historical longevity, TB allows us to address two questions asked by the organizers of the symposium from which this book arose: How do plagues in the past influence the way we think about plagues today? And what happens when a plague ends?

In doing so, we draw upon the results of research into tuberculosis in New Zealand undertaken between 2002 and 2006—the "political ecology of TB" project (Littleton and King 2008). At times in New Zealand's past, TB has been a major cause of disease and death, living up to Dubos and Dubos's "white plague" label. Today New Zealand falls on the list of low-prevalence countries, those with TB disease rates of fewer than 20 cases per 100,000 persons, yet the disease persists as a real and popularly imagined entity.

In this chapter we argue that the way in which TB is conceived in contemporary New Zealand arises out of a nexus of personal experience, the distribution of the disease both historically and contemporarily, and the state's and the media's positioning of bodies. This is not a plague created de novo (see Briggs, this volume) but a disease which, although it might have faded in public consciousness, retains symbolic power (Lindenbaum 2001). The low rates of TB today simply make it easier to isolate and stigmatize those associated with the disease. In order to make this argument, we first briefly summarize the history of TB in New Zealand. Then, drawing on the historical experience, we examine the meanings that adhere to TB among patients and the broader public and the use and manipulation of these ideas by the media and politicians in the present day.

Tuberculosis in New Zealand

Although it has been hypothesized that TB existed in the Pacific before European colonization (Buckley and Tayles 2000; Butterfield 2006; contra Miles 1997), in New Zealand there is no direct evidence of its effects on Maori people until the arrival of Europeans in the eighteenth century (Finn 2006; Houghton 1980; contra Lange 1999). By 1850 the disease was endemic among New Zealanders, both indigenous and foreign born (Bryder 1991a; Pool 1991). In 1855 a Dr. A. S. Thomson, surgeon to the 58th Regiment, wrote that "in some districts twenty percent bear on their bodies the mark of the king's evil. Scrofula [a form of nonpulmonary TB] is the predisposing and remote cause of much of the sickness among New Zealanders [Maori]" (quoted in Wells 1991: 98).

The death rate from tuberculosis in New Zealand in 1872 was 126 per 100,000, significantly lower than the British death rate of around 300 per 100,000 (Bryder 1991a: 79). This figure did not include Maori deaths, of which TB was the most common cause—so much so that it was known as the "Maori disease" (Pool 1991; Wells 1991: 99). As Dr. Maui Pomare, a leading Maori doctor appointed to the Ministry of Health in 1901, who later became minister of health, put it:

Chief among the diseases I have encountered stands the dread white plague, phthisis... One is not surprised when we behold the abuse the poor bodies are subjected to through ignorance of hygiene and sanitary laws; the wonder is that there are not more who die of this disease. The Maori is generally looked down upon as an individual with weak lungs but I am sure if Pakehas [European New Zealanders] were exposed in the same way as Maoris they would disappear just as fast, and perhaps a little faster (Quoted in Wells 1991: 99).

This view of moral blame attached to the disease could easily lead to the victimization of TB patients.

Maori were not perceived as the only group in New Zealand affected by TB. Even at this early date, TB and immigration were tightly linked. With the nineteenth-century belief in the curative value of climate, the Registrar General of New Zealand, in his publications, encouraged British TB patients to consider New Zealand as a destination. However, only TB patients who could afford to support themselves and pay for their medical care in the colony were encouraged to come (Bryder 1991a: 79). Concern about immigrants becoming a drain on the social welfare and health budgets was already manifest. Once the infectiousness of the disease was more widely accepted, from the early twentieth century, more moves were made to restrict the entry of TB patients, but these were at best half-hearted, and many British TB cases continued to arrive (Bryder 1996).

Even in the early twentieth century, TB death rates were declining among New Zealand's European population, presumably as a result of improved living conditions (McKeown 1976). From 1880 to 1900 the death rate declined by 29 percent (Bryder 1991a), so the first active measures against TB in the early twentieth century took place against a declining incidence among Pakeha, although death rates among Maori remained high. Among the active measures was the establishment of a Department of Health in 1901, initially set up to deal with a bubonic plague scare.

The focus upon TB was framed in terms of the disease as "a national menace," detrimental to "national efficiency" (Bryder 1991a: 80). The annual cost of TB was calculated as "the appalling sum of £304,000" (Mason, quoted in Bryder 1991a: 80). Dealing with it was both a matter of national pride for an emerging national state and a responsibility of government: "We in New Zealand should not lag behind other countries in this matter, a matter deeply affecting the common weal of the people" (Gore Gillon 1901: 1).[1]

The early-twentieth-century antituberculosis campaign was focused on overseas models, particularly that of Britain. A sanatorium was established, with the provision of good food, fresh air, rest, and graduated labor as its major therapies. Further sanatoria and hospital annexes followed. On the public health front, compulsory TB notification was introduced in 1901, although such notifications were partial among Pakeha and Maori alike, if for different reasons (Bryder 1991a; Finn 2006; Pool 1991). Debates surrounding the introduction of compulsory notification reveal concerns over the stigma attached to the disease. The influx of immigrants with possible tuberculosis remained a fraught issue (Bryder 1991a, 1996).

Following World War I, recorded death rates due to TB continued to decline among Pakeha, apart from ex-servicemen who returned from Europe with TB. It was a matter of pride that these were some of the lowest death rates in the world (when Maori deaths were excluded), and non-Maori New Zealanders took a general attitude of complacency (Bryder 1991a). Notification records, however, were still only patchily collected.

In 1935 a Dr. H. Turbott undertook a thorough investigation into the prevalence of tuberculosis among east coast (North Island) Maori (Bryder 1991b). The death rate he recorded was 494 per 100,000. None of the ten deaths that occurred during that year had been officially reported, and the prevalence of TB had been similarly underreported (Turbott 1935). Turbott's report had a significant effect. According to Wells (1991: 100), "many white New Zealanders had regarded themselves as members of a multi-racial egalitarian society and were appalled by the racial inequities detailed in the Turbott report." A major goal of the first Labour government, 1935–1949, was to raise Maori living standards to European levels, although, as Finn (2006), Lange (1999), and Dow (1999) have reported, both formal and informal barriers to this goal remained.

The main period of action against tuberculosis among Pakeha and Maori in New Zealand was the 1940s and 1950s—ironically, as Dunsford (2008) pointed out, the decades when rates among Pakeha were reaching new lows. The shift came in response to medical interventions, particularly mass miniature radiography (in 1941), BCG vaccination (circa 1950), and effective drug treatment (after 1950). Despite a recommendation for its establishment in 1928, a Division of Tuberculosis was finally established in the Department of Health in 1943, reflecting a more proactive approach. By 1954 the Maori death rate due to TB had fallen to 77.8 per 100,000, although that was still seven times the Pakeha rate (Wells 1991). It was during this period that the first testing of dairy herds was instituted (in 1951), together with the slaughtering of all positive reactors (Bryder 1991a: 87).

Closures of sanatoriums began in the 1950s with declining preval- ence rates of tuberculosis. The last sanatorium to close was Gonville Sanatorium, for Maori children with tuberculosis (Bryder 1991a: 88).

A new link was made, however, between tuberculosis and immigration. In 1974 Pacific Islanders made up 2 percent of the New Zealand population but 20 percent of TB cases. The incidence was twenty times that of Europeans (Mackay 1991). Many were on temporary work permits issued by the Department of Labour in order to address workforce shortages. Debates over immigration and tuberculosis resurfaced. A TB officer for the Auckland Hospital Board asserted that "the arrival of active cases of tuberculosis from overseas constitutes a public health hazard and represents a financial burden to the New Zealand tax payer" (Kerr 1972: 295). In response, a Wellington doctor pointed out that rather than bringing in TB, Pacific Islanders were mainly contracting it once in New Zealand (Mackay 1972). The compromise reached in 1976 was an agreement with some Pacific Island governments that all visitors or workers staying in New Zealand for more than two months would have a chest x-ray.

From 1970 to 1987, TB notifications continued to decline, but they stalled after 1987 with, indeed, a slight increase since then (Thornley and Pikholz 2008). Current prevalence is around 10–12 per 100,000, although this masks huge gradients by ethnicity, place of birth, region of residence, and socioeconomic status (Das, Baker, and Calder 2006; Das et al. 2006; Littleton and King 2008; Thornley and Pikholz 2008). TB remains a notifiable disease, with most notifications occurring among foreign-born residents of the country. HIV and TB co-infection rates are low.

TB, however, remains a matter of government concern. The rates in New Zealand are twice as high as those in neighboring Australia, the common point of comparison for New Zealand's performance on the world stage (Harrison 2000). The increasing prevalence of tuberculosis and HIV co-infection in the western Pacific is seen as a threat at the nation's backdoor, as are the growing rates of extremely drug-resistant TB elsewhere in the world. Again, attention has been focused on the link between immigration and tuberculosis.

Relative to the prevalence of TB in the 1800s, its current prevalence represents the tail end of a plague in the sense of declining death and disease rates. Yet our analysis of patient, community, media, and pol- itical discourses and practices surrounding tuberculosis, undertaken as part of the political ecology of TB project, demonstrates the ways in which personal experience, epidemiology, and political motives coalesce to ensure that concerns and attitudes rife at the peak times of tuberculosis occurrence remain salient in today's population. TB in New Zealand is construed simultaneously as a familiar, recurrent enemy and as a new, emerging threat. In the remainder of this chapter we focus on three sources and levels of ideas about TB: the private lives of individuals, the social life of the media, and the public concerns of governmental institutions.

Disease and Personal Experience

In contemporary New Zealand, multiple understandings of TB exist. Although surveys suggest that most people understand TB as a contagious respiratory infection, more detailed work with specific communities has demonstrated how personal knowledge and experience of the disease influence not just those with TB disease but also those who surround them (Ng Shui 2006; Oh 2005; Searle 2004). In this way the epidemiological history just described has a legacy beyond the purely biological.

One salient feature is the difference between indigenous (Maori) and non-indigenous New Zealand-born (Pakeha) persons. Currently, prevalence rates of TB are five to ten times higher among Maori than Pakeha, a persistent discrepancy mirroring other contemporary health differences. For example, Maori male and female life expectancies are more than eight years less than those of non-Maori (Ministry of Social Development 2004). For TB, as for life expectancy, part of the difference is the residue of historical disparities.

TB rates among Pakeha began decreasing by 1900. Currently most TB in Pakeha occurs among the elderly, in the form of reactivation of latent TB infection or secondary reactivation of previously "cured" TB disease. In 2003 in Auckland there were thirteen Pakeha with TB disease. Of the nine who were interviewed by Searle as part of the project, four had a reactivation of old, previously treated TB disease (Searle 2004).

Of the TB patients Searle interviewed, many had had experience of the disease soon after World War II, and that experience related directly to their current attitudes toward TB. Dianne, for instance, recognizing the symptoms of TB and their significance while visiting her sick daughter in Canada, got on a plane and returned to New Zealand. Dennis challenged people in a pub—"Don't come and drink with me or I'll give you TB"—trying to deflect any potential stigma attaching to the disease. This robust attitude toward TB was not held by all participants and their families. Debbie, when asked about her illness, would talk of a nonspecific "bone infection." Dick, in fear of his fellow boarding house residents, used communal areas only at night: "That's the only way to go about it, you know, you sort of keep your distance" (Searle 2008).

In an effort to gauge other Pakeha attitudes, Searle talked to people without TB but of the same age, gender, and income level as her participants with TB (Searle 2004). She found, in general, a lack of awareness of TB as a health problem among younger people. Those with personal experience of TB remembered the stigma attached to it, whereas those without personal experience (the majority of Pakeha in New Zealand) remained relatively oblivious to the infection. Dianne's experience, however, suggests that direct confrontation with TB could provoke some long-lasting stigmatizing attitudes: "They freak, most people freak about it. They still feel very frightened of it and yet it's not the fear, you know. I thought that it's a long time since there's been any serious TB, that people would be, they'd think, oh you know, it's something they did in the dark ages, but they're not, they're still very conscious of TB" (Searle 2008:190).

In contrast, TB among Maori occurred at much higher rates and was much slower to decline, so the number of people with personal experience alive today is much greater. This means that the effects of stigma for those with TB are also much greater, particularly among older Maori (Oh 2005; van der Oest, Kelly, and Hood 2004):

> A suspected TB diagnosis has considerable impact on older Maori with previous experience of the disease. For example, the elderly mother of a PHN [public health nurse] was isolated after the doctor suspected her respiratory condition could be TB. Apparently no tests were conducted to confirm the doctor's assumptions and the patient claimed no explanation was given for her isolation. The woman spent a sleepless night worrying about whether she had infected her mokopuna [grandchildren], other whanau [family members] and people with whom she had recent contact at her local marae [meeting house]. (Oh 2005: 77)

Among participants, one effect of such stigma, regardless of ethnicity, is a lack of disclosure. Oh (2005: 45) described one person whom public health nurses treated at a "central city fast-food outlet store" by surreptitiously slipping drugs to the person "under a napkin on a plate or with a coffee or juice, ensuring other diners were unaware of the transaction."

The stigma fractured some family relationships as circles of blame were drawn. Oh's participants were concerned with being identified as TB carriers. She quoted Rau: "My own brother ... I went back one time and he said to me don't touch my kids, you know, you might have TB. I said but I've been tested, you know, and then he started saying to me, oh, well, Kowhai's got TB. So you must have TB, don't touch my kids. And that really bummed me out" (Oh 2005: 74).

In the circles of blame, TB carriers were seen as "other," and in a reversion of the tendency of dominant, less-infected groups to blame marginalized groups, some Maori sufferers directed moral responsibility back at Pakeha. They called TB "a dirty disease you Pakeha brought," and a possible carrier was described as "looking more like a Pakeha" (Oh 2005: 74).

Yet strong memories within communities could also be a help. Oh (2005: 87) quoted a public health nurse:

> When I have called the hui [meeting] of the family it's very interesting, because when you get, um, the older family members in the room or in a bigger hui, like kaumatua and kuia, they, they always remember TB from the '50s and what it did to their families. And so I find my job is, is a lot easier. Because they get up and they talk about it. And um, and then the young people that are there and it's usually them that are either the case or the contact. They start to see it from a different light... I just think that it helps, a lot.

Generational differences are observed among Pacific people, but unlike for Maori or Pakeha, for some older Pacific Islanders knowledge of TB is not a resource but a source of anxiety. As Ng Shui (2006) described, older Pacific people (those over forty, she suggests) often have heard stories of TB, and the disease for them is surrounded by fear and stigma. The treatment of TB patients through isolation (at home), the lack of a cure for the disease, and the close association of TB with leprosy (both are housed in the same clinic in Apia, Samoa) are all factors that contribute to the dismay of patients when hearing a diagnosis of TB, and the wish of some for a diagnosis of cancer rather than TB. "There were two things they were trying to find out, if it's TB or cancer... So he said to me, 'They said that they hope that I got TB' [and I said] 'Why, why?'" (Makelita, quoted in Ng Shui 2006: 89).

Younger Pacific Islanders who had some experience of TB were not so dismayed by a diagnosis, because of their limited knowledge of the disease. This generational split, based on prior knowledge of TB, affected levels of disclosure about the illness. Ng Shui's older participants often kept their diagnoses quiet and within the family; those who had no prior awareness of TB and its associated stigma continued to freely access their social networks and gain support from them.

Among newer arrivals to New Zealand, many of whom come from high-incidence countries, knowledge of TB and fear of the disease are both much more widespread. Anderson, who worked with Korean, Chinese, and Indian people, found that the fear had to do not simply with the assumed severity and contagiousness of the disease but also with the possibility of rejection and isolation from family, friends, and community, not only during the course of the disease but beyond it (Anderson 2008). One patient had not told family and friends despite a three-month hospitalization. Another, fearing divorce and rejection, hid from her husband's family the fact that she was coughing up blood. For many of Anderson's research participants, TB was associated with moral transgressions such as sexual promiscuity and failing to care for parents. In common with many TB patients from other communities, Anderson's participants coped with stigma by concealing their diagnoses and controlling information, as well as by using some of the same strategies observed by Searle (2004)—that is, humor or deflecting comments with biomedical explanations.

For each of these groups comprising part of New Zealand's population, personal experience, expectations, and knowledge of the disease reflect the historical pattern of occurrence and demonstrate the link between the broad population statistics of epidemiology and the lingering, embodied experience that colors the understandings and expectations of those faced with tuberculosis. But it also highlights the large number of people for whom there is no personal experience or family knowledge of the disease.

Broader Conceptions of Tuberculosis

As part of the political ecology of TB project, an analysis was undertaken of newspaper texts from 2001 through 2004 pertaining to TB (Lawrence et al. 2008). As demonstrated in the foregoing discussion, many New Zealanders have no personal experience of tuberculosis, and a key source of their knowledge about TB is the print media. TB is a "potent signifier" through its link with tropes such as "third world diseases" (Lawrence et al. 2008). In this instance we argue (as do Lawrence and co-workers) that the media produce effects in individuals and social bodies that, in the case of tuberculosis, are largely unchallenged by personal experience.

The majority of media coverage of TB among humans in New Zealand has been focused on reportage of particular cases or has linked TB to immigration. Such articles stress the potential of TB to affect all New Zealanders, using words such as "alert" and "scare." In doing this they accentuate the infectiousness of TB and serve to intensify its stigma by emphasizing its contagiousness and potential spread, placing TB in the position of a plague threat. This is despite press releases from district health boards that are calming in tone (*Dominion Post*, 20 December 2004).

In the survey by Lawrence and colleagues (2008) it was observed that comments by health officials tended to minimize the infectiousness of the disease. For example: "Early … TB, which I gather this is, is not very infectious at all. It's only in the later stages it is, so in the early stages it's not an issue for other people" (*New Zealand Herald*, 4 July 2002). Such calming messages contrast with Ministry of Health comments exhorting vigilance and warning against complacency in the face of TB: "Dreaded TB on rise again" (*New Zealand Herald*, 28 June 2004); "Rise in TB cases alarms health officials" (*New Zealand Herald*, 23 March 2004). These messages focus on individual responsibility for stopping the spread of the disease, an exhortation to "good citizens" (W. Anderson, personal communication, 2007).

Two sources were identified as threatening to spread TB: people in particular occupations and immigrants. The former resonates with the concern expressed by Maori in Oh's study over the notion of the TB carrier (Oh 2005: 74), the person who wittingly or unwittingly spreads the disease to the "innocent." Media coverage was greatest when a person with TB was in an occupation that held the possibility for bodily contact with others. Health workers in particular (for example, a school dental therapist, a hospital worker, and a nurse) were focused upon. In the coverage of the school dental therapist, attention was given to the number of contacts with schoolchildren the dental worker had. Health officials and the school principal both emphasized the lack of any need for panic and the fact that following up the case was a matter of controlled routine, using skin tests and so forth (Lawrence et al. 2008). Subsequent articles dealt with stories headlined "TB fear spurs dad to bar dental care for son (*Dominion Post*, 7 August 2003)" and "TB tests on school children allay fears" (*Dominion Post*, 21 October 2003).

Apart from these individualized cases, a significant number of newspaper articles linked TB to immigrants. Such articles emphasized the idea of borders: "hardening the borders" and increasing the testing and policing of migrants. Immigrants were construed as a unregulated threat to New Zealanders, as expressed in headlines such as "Immigration hunting TB man for overstaying visa" (*New Zealand Herald*, 20 November 2003) and, quoting the president of a local university students association in relation to foreign students, "It's a time bomb waiting to happen— what other illnesses and diseases are they bringing in?" (*The Press*, 10 December 2003).

Such linkage of TB to a single external cause and to a particular group serves to establish TB in people's minds as a disease of others, as a non-native threat. The link was accepted even by David, a Pakeha with TB in Searle's study, who thought his TB was the result of a recent trip to India rather than of the close contact he had as a child with his grandfather, who had TB. He described the diagnosis as a "shock, because it's sort of not a disease we think of in this country so much, or if you do, you associate it with new immigrants or asylum seekers or people from third world countries" (Searle 2008: 192).

This unthinking association of an infectious disease with particular sorts of immigrants is confirmed even in newspaper articles about particular Pakeha with TB. An informative piece in the *Dominion Post* (31 March 2003) about a Wellington solicitor's experience of TB was accompanied by a photograph of a Vietnamese man undergoing TB treatment in Hanoi, reinforcing the proximity of TB and Asians, despite the article's written content.

Such links are consequential: they contribute not only to the burden of prejudice borne by immigrants but also to the treatment of TB. The assumption that only particular people get TB appears to have contributed to delayed diagnoses among some Pakeha whom Searle (2004) interviewed. Similarly, interviews by Miller (2007) with health workers revealed an unquestioned link between TB and outsiders. An ambulance driver in Auckland described to Littleton the common practice of placing a mask on an Asian patient with respiratory symptoms but not on people of other ethnicities.

Such links, however, are also resisted by those implicated as TB carriers. Anderson (2008) found that many of her Korean, Chinese, and Indian participants, with and without TB, did not internalize this stigma. Some did not believe they could develop TB in New Zealand because of the health screening they received prior to arrival. Others attributed TB to Maori and Pacific people. Trajectories of blame move in different directions, but always outward, away from "us."

Tuberculosis and the Nation

Pervading the media construction of TB and the historical experience of people with TB is the politics of TB. In all the discussions of TB that we and team members have had, whether among patients, among health workers, or in the media, the disease reveals and confirms the particular positioning of people and animals vis-à-vis the nation. Briggs and Mantini-Briggs (2003), in their study of cholera in Venezuela, described such positioning in relation to the construction of indigenous people as unsanitary subjects, as opposed to sanitary citizens. A similar dividing line, based on supposed hygiene, has been invoked in New Zealand in relation to Maori. In the twentieth and twenty-first centuries, however, it is not easy to make such a clear division. TB reveals greater levels of complexity, the way the "modality of inclusion" (Hage 1998: 132) is regulated, and the way particular positions, especially that of the diseased other, circulate.

In common with other colonial endeavors (Anderson 2004a; Bashford 2004; Comaroff and Comaroff 1991), one of the major goals of New Zealand public health from the early twentieth century was to make hygienic citizens of the indigenous population. A 1950s film by the Department of Health explicitly compared Maori living in older settlements with Maori in a recently built house, eating three good meals a day like Europeans (Brookes 2006; Department of Health 1952).

Implicitly and explicitly the film—and much writing in the first half of the twentieth century—suggests that Maori were unsanitary subjects responsible for their own ill health because of their bad attitudes and habits. These ideas still hold some currency today. Yet commentators of the time did not situate Maori in an unambiguous category of "diseased other." The simple politics of exclusion cannot be applied. Even in the nineteenth century, when the suggested solution to TB among the Maori was "to smooth the pillow of the dying Maori race" (Featherstone 1866, quoted in Lange 1999: 65) as it succumbed to a "superior race" (Newman 1882, quoted in Lange 1999: 65) or to impersonal nature, Maori were seldom portrayed as inhuman or as a savage race: "The average colonist regards a Mongolian with repulsion, a Negro with contempt, and looks on an Australian black as very near to a wild beast; but he likes the Maori and treats them in many respects as his equal" (Reeves, cited in Lange 1999: 60).

Media coverage of TB in the first half of the twentieth century expressed a sense that, in contrast to various categories of immigrant menace, Maori were the state's responsibility, "a moral obligation which we cannot honourably ignore" (editor, *Provincial*, quoted in Lange 1999: 62)—another white man's burden.

In reality, little was done for the Maori before the mid-1930s. Government programs aimed at Maori health and the improvement of living conditions were frequently underfunded or subject to other imperatives (Dow 1999). For example, money aimed at improving Maori housing was directed toward areas visited by tourists rather than toward those off the tourist track (Finn 2006).

Historians of European colonization remain divided over the interpretation of attitudes toward Maori—whether they were explicitly racist or more complexly both racist and humanitarian (Lange 1999). Certainly, the superiority of European New Zealanders was never in question; even now, in much political rhetoric, Maori occupy a subject position. But in the twentieth century the state's responsibility, too, was rarely questioned. Maori were explicitly "our problem," even, or especially, when diseased. Both reports of Maori deaths, unattended by any effective outside assistance, after the 1918 influenza epidemic and Turbott's report on TB on the east coast of North Island in 1935 were followed by public outcry.

Maori were uneasily but surely incorporated into the nation. Disease renders them problematic but not excluded. Immigrants, on the other hand, are much more easily placed outside the borders. This is more complex than the simple exclusion of polluted others and is seen in the uneasy tension between the goals of biculturalism (Maori and Pakeha) and those of emerging multiculturalism in New Zealand. Hage (1998: 133) pointed out in relation to white multiculturalism in Australia that migrants can be seen as "an enriching/tolerable presence" and therefore something exploitable that has to be included in national space. In this respect, public health is an arena in which inclusion is regulated and debated.

The complexity is threaded throughout the history of TB in New Zealand. Physicians in the early 1900s were concerned about the number of British immigrants arriving with TB disease. Yet at a 1912 TB conference, delegates were split. Some called for stricter admission policies, particularly enforcement of the Undesirable Immigrants Restriction Act. Others argued that as British subjects, persons with early cases of TB should not be "denied the advantages that were available to their more robust fellow country men" (Mason 1903, quoted in Bryder 1991a: 82). British immigrants were desirable—after all, they were "one of us"—but Britons with TB occupied a contradictory position on the margins.

The issue reared its head again after World War II as immigration rates rose and politicians and medical staff on the Auckland Hospital Board mounted a public campaign to prevent people with TB from entering New Zealand (Dunsford 2008). The culprits were again identified as Britons with TB. This time around, much less ambiguity was expressed about the position of these immigrants: they had already endangered the other, healthy immigrants aboard ship from Britain, and in rhetoric that is often heard today, they were said to be taking the beds of deserving New Zealanders in the overcrowded hospital system. One speaker at an Auckland Hospital Board meeting in 1949 said, "A disgraceful state of affairs has been disclosed. [New Zealand] could become the happy hunting ground of anyone in England with illness" (quoted in Dunsford 2008). The solution proposed was more effective screening of immigrants. The stigma of disease, however, apparently did not attach itself to all British immigrants. Undiseased Britons were sufficiently incorporated to avoid the multiple stigmas experienced by other immigrant groups, and indeed their labor was needed in postwar economic development.

This modulation of inclusion and exclusion is evident today in the way particular classes of immigrants are excoriated. Ideas of "high-risk countries" for TB serve to justify the profiling of particular groups (*Dominion Post*, 29 January 2004). In line with the debates about the British after World War II, part of the argument centers on the economic costs of such groups. One immigration minister stated: "A country is entitled in determining whether people are eligible for residence or not to undertake—and I know it might sound harsh—a costs-benefit analysis ... if there are going to be significant costs" (*Dominion Post*, 20 January 2004).

Recent newspaper coverage of immigration and tuberculosis does frequently refer to Asians, but attention is focused on particular groups of immigrants: those who are from the third world, foreign students, asylum seekers, refugees, and, at times, migrant workers. In September 2002, parliamentary debate dealt with the "uncontrolled immigration and refugee system." The Honorable Winston Peters in 2003 accused the Ministries of Immigration and Health of allowing "hundreds of people with third world diseases including TB cases ... [to 'clog up wards'] and how can that be a reasonable way of defending the health of the New Zealand people" (*Hansard Weekly*, 35-2003009-09).

The majority of immigrants into New Zealand are encouraged (or at times discouraged) to migrate by the Department of Labour. When these immigrants are reported among TB cases, they are portrayed not as contributing taxpayers but as consumers of the resources of real New Zealanders. The notion of nonproductivity is stronger in relation to refugees and asylum seekers than to other immigrants. As Lawrence and co-workers (2008) pointed out, asylum seekers tend to be imagined as the least desirable and most dangerous of immigrants. Similarly, foreign students, particularly Asian students, are targeted. The same rhetoric of risk to "domestic" (local) students is evoked.

These fine lines of inclusion and exclusion are not restricted to humans. Much research in New Zealand is devoted to bovine tuberculosis, and nearly half the TB coverage in newspapers is devoted to the matter (Lawrence et al. 2008). The significance of bovine TB is its potential impact on agricultural earnings: loss of TB-free status would have devastating trade effects. Despite testing, TB threatens cattle and deer because of a reservoir of non-native possums, originally imported from Australia in the nineteenth century, which—although this seems never to be mentioned—initially caught TB from cattle. Not one of the three species is indigenous to New Zealand, but cattle are the "national herd," deer occupy a somewhat ambiguous place because some are feral and others are farmed, and opossums, those "little Aussie imports," are portrayed as diseased others that should be exterminated.[2] Hage (1998: 100) discussed the parallels between the categories of domesticated, tame, and captive animals and various forms of inclusion, and Lawrence and colleagues (2008) drew the parallel between the encroaching possums and foreign students, both of whom pose a threat to domestic products, whether cattle or other students.

Such debates over inclusion and exclusion in the face of TB focus attention on the policing of borders. Proposed health measures inevitably have to do with tighter immigration controls—"hardening the borders"— and with more screening offshore (Lawrence et al. 2008). Even with an understanding of the disease process, including the recognition that most immigrants with TB develop the active disease after their arrival and that screening therefore has limited effectiveness, a recent editorial in the *New Zealand Medical Journal* ended with hyperbole: "Beware the recent Asian immigrant with fever and chronic illness or even the recent Asian immigrant who is afebrile and has just a single persistently enlarged cervical lymph node!" (Thomas and Ellis-Pegler 2006: 3).

Whereas TB among Maori in the 1930s prompted calls to improve social conditions, TB in contemporary New Zealand promotes calls for selective exclusion. Briggs and Mantini-Briggs have written, in relation to cholera, that the "social construction of citizenship crucially shaped how people perceived the disease and what they were willing to do in preparation for a possible epidemic. The epidemic in turn reshaped categories of citizenship and how social and political exclusion affected people's lives" (Briggs with Mantini-Briggs 2003: 58). Not since the mass x-ray campaigns of the 1950s (Dunsford 2008) has TB in New Zealand prompted mass mobilization, but perceptions of it do rely on which communities it is seen to occur in. Then it was seen as affecting "our community"; now the focus is on keeping it out of "our community." That perception creates specific responses, such as the deportation of a patient with TB who was picked up while attending a TB clinic. Such responses serve to decrease people's willingness to acknowledge symptoms (Anderson 2008), to agree to contact tracing, and, in non-implicated communities, to recognize their own possibility of TB (Searle 2004). Beyond that, such responses serve as justifications for the further marginalization and stigmatization of particular groups, as well as re-inforcing the idea that TB does not exist in the domestic space. These are practical outcomes, but they overlie a complex of personal interpretations and experiences.

Conclusion

There is a conundrum here. In New Zealand's past, TB was a major cause of death. It was a pestilence and was seen as a form of moral contagion or taint (Bryder 1991a; Lange 1999). At the same time, it is a chronic disease, contrary to classic plagues (Rosenberg 1992a) and modern plagues (Lindenbaum 2001), and it is one for which the cause and process of transmission have been understood since the 1880s. In most developed parts of the world, it is now "a minor public health issue."[3] Why, then, does the aura of plague still adhere to TB? Why does the account of TB in a dental therapist or in a non–New Zealand–born schoolchild prompt such strong responses? Why does legislation still exist that can permit the incarceration of uncooperative infectious people with TB?

One explanation has to do with history: there are many people alive from earlier generations or from different places with memories of TB as a serious contagious disease. Personal experience matters. In this case the strength of those memories adheres, perhaps because the disease was a lengthy process, unlike the "forgotten" plague of 1918 influenza (see Swedlund, this volume).

Another is that TB is conflated with other infectious diseases, is indistinguishable, for some people, with HIV/AIDS (Anderson 2008) or leprosy (Ng Shui 2006), or is worse than cancer (Searle 2004). Perhaps its chronic nature—the notion of a long sentence, older ideas of a lifetime trait, the fear of a carrier—elevate anxieties. Such ideas, however, are not particularly visible in media discourse or in comments by politicians, although they do occur in some accounts by TB patients and health workers.

Beyond individuals with TB, public discourse centers on ideas of foreignness, of pollution (Douglas 1992; Sontag 2001). In the case of Maori, pollution is from within the nation or is the pollution of an originally pristine world by immigrants and colonizers, depending on who is speaking. In the case of possums and particular immigrants, the pollution is from without, regardless of the realities of New Zealand–born status or long-term New Zealand residence.

The current climate of growing inequality and the visual impact of particular sorts of migrants (Hage 1998) facilitates certain forms of scape-goating. Douglas (1992: 119) predicted in relation to AIDS that "when the poor are perceived as a distinctive subculture the centre community will be more likely to respond punitively." TB in New Zealand today is adhering to the multiple ways in which immigrants are blamed for social ills. It is yet another stick. The difficulty, given the discourses of blame and risk, is in how to raise concern about the social determinants of TB.

In the 1940s, Dr. C. Taylor, director of the TB Division of the Department of Health, wrote:

> The health services of the Dominion must not be expected to solve the problem without public encouragement and support. The Europeans of the community have long remained oblivious to the plight of the Maoris. If the apathetic European conscience cannot be stirred by some desire to prevent and alleviate Maori morbidity then perhaps some appeal to self interest may be more efficacious. Until the reservoir of TB infection existing among the Maoris has been drained to a smaller volume there is no hope of eradicating TB from the homes of New Zealand, white and Maori alike. (Taylor 1943: 110)

This is a confirmation of Douglas's comment that "the central community's attitude to expenditure on research and health and medical treatment for the sick is conditioned for each disease in the expectation of getting the disease" (Douglas 1992: 120). The construction of TB in public discourse in New Zealand today suggests a lack of will for long-term solutions to the issue.

But in relation to the themes of the Wenner-Gren symposium, can we use TB to answer the question, What happens when a plague ends?—

which was after all the beginning point of this chapter? The answer is no. For all its position as "a minor public health problem," TB as a plague is still with us in public imaginings. It is one of those diseases that are socially sedimented (Shirley Lindenbaum, personal communication, 2007) in the memories of individuals, in stories from elsewhere, and even in legislation. Thinking of TB as a plague forces us to face the conundrum that diseases that are "minor public health problems" can retain the power to afflict their sufferers. The effect of plague is the disproportionate relationship between the physical threat of a disease and its symbolic power.

Notes

1. New Zealand became a self-governing colony in 1854. It was given dominion status by Britain in 1907 but progressively gained control over its foreign policy in the following decades.

2. Possums are linked with plague in their own right, following the familiar motifs of contamination and non-nativeness.

3. At a recent workshop on TB in Canada, we were all stunned to hear Dr. Kue Young refer to TB as a "minor public health problem," which, upon reflection, it certainly is currently in New Zealand and Canada. Such a description, of course, masks its effects on particular communities while describing the national situation.

Epidemics and Time
Influenza and Tuberculosis during and after the 1918–1919 Pandemic

Andrew Noymer

In this chapter I advance the idea that diseases are interrelated and therefore that "plagues" cannot be understood in isolation. A plague of a given disease affects and is affected by the epidemiological situation in the population it strikes. The idea that context matters is unlikely to be controversial in contemporary social science. The idea that a holistic understanding will yield insights not produced by particularistic approaches, likewise, will not arouse fierce debate. What I suggest, however, is more specific than either of those notions. I argue that often, if not always, the true effect of a plague can be seen only in the long term. This is in spite of the fact that severe short-term mortality is the defining characteristic of some plagues—for example, cholera epidemics in Victorian London and yellow fever epidemics in colonial America. There are also examples of plagues that play out over decades, such as the late-twentieth- and early-twenty-first-century plague of HIV/AIDS, but this does not diminish the point.

My central tenet in this chapter is that the effects of a plague need to be judged not only by the characteristic mortality of the outbreak and the long-term trends of the disease in question but also by changes in *all* diseases in the wake of the plague. This is emphatically not to eschew the notion that disease outbreaks have specific etiologies: a plague of influenza cannot happen without influenza virus, a plague of malaria needs *Plasmodium* species, a plague of plague requires *Yersinia pestis,* and so on. Rather, the idea is that the population in the wake of a plague is not the same as the population before the plague, and this phenomenon can (and, I postulate, often does) introduce perturbations in the epidemiology of seemingly unrelated diseases.

The idea of interrelated diseases in this sense has been suggested before. McNeill (1976) speculated that the Black Death might have paved the way for the reduction of leprosy in Europe. The argument was that "the pestilence," as the Black Death was known to contemporaries, killed people with leprosy disproportionately. The Black Death came and went, wreaking havoc but also leaving behind a population—though smaller by far—that was healthier, at least as far as leprosy was concerned. One caveat is that fourteenth-century records are not always reliable. Creighton (1891) was dubious about the prevalence estimates for leprosy in medieval Britain; it is unclear whether all the patients in Europe's many leprosariums actually had leprosy (*Mycobacterium leprae* infection). Moreover, the etiology of the Black Death itself is perhaps the most historiographically contentious issue in historical epidemiology today (Noymer 2007; Theilmann and Cate 2007). Whatever caused the Black Death, recent research on skeletal remains suggests that victims were not a random sample of the population (DeWitte and Wood 2008), which seems to buttress McNeill's argument, albeit not specifically with regard to leprosy.

The dominant modi operandi in historical epidemiology are the disease-specific study of a particular plague and a chronological approach that documents individual plagues in a given national or regional setting. I maintain that we need to think of a plague as a disturbance of a pre-plague (dis-)equilibrium that leads to a new post-plague (dis-) equilibrium and thus to look at all diseases, not just the plague itself. In this chapter I argue from an example for which much better data are available than for fourteenth-century leprosy. The case is the 1918–1919 influenza pandemic, which killed about 50 million people worldwide, or 2.5 percent of the global population. Despite being six hundred years more recent than the Black Death, data quality is a problem for the 1918–1919 pandemic, too (see Johnson and Mueller 2002). Nonetheless, much may be said about this early-twentieth-century plague.

I offer an overview of the 1918–1919 flu pandemic and then illustrate the preceding point by discussing some findings that make the long-term effects of the flu just as noteworthy as the short-term effects. I conclude by placing these findings in the context of disease ecology and the so-called McKeown debate.

The 1918 Plague Selection Story in a Nutshell

The 1918–1919 influenza pandemic killed many tuberculous persons, at least in the United States. Tuberculosis is a chronic disease, a slow killer. By killing many tuberculous people all at once, the 1918–1919 flu removed from the population individuals who would have died of tuberculosis in later years, lowering tuberculosis death rates. Therefore, the 1918–1919 influenza pandemic was a factor in the decline of tuberculosis. Conceptually, this description follows exactly the same lines as McNeill's suggestion that the Black Death hastened the decline of leprosy (and intriguingly, the pathogens of tuberculosis and leprosy are related at the genus level, *Mycobacterium*). The available data, however, permit a much greater elaboration of the story when it comes to influenza and tuberculosis.

This detailed elaboration is noteworthy because tuberculosis was historically an important cause of death in the United States. Indeed, it has been called "the chief cause of death" (Long 1948), and its decline during the first half of the twentieth century is a key part of the story of health improvements during that time. Tuberculosis was a killer at adult ages, which gave its decline signature importance (Frost 1939). Unlike causes of death that predominated in childhood, such as measles, pertussis, and diarrheal diseases, tuberculosis stood alone as the major infectious disease killer of young adults. The decline of tuberculosis thus paved the way for much longer life among those who survived childhood. Worldwide, tuberculosis remains an important cause of death and illness today (Dye et al. 1999; Maher and Raviglione 2005).

Influenza

Influenza, or flu, is an acute respiratory tract infection caused by the influenza virus (Wright and Webster 2001). Symptoms are similar to those of the "common cold" but can be much more severe, and development of a secondary pneumonia is common. High fever also distinguishes influenza symptoms from those of some other viral infections of the respiratory tract. Influenza virus can be transmitted through droplets, aerosols, or surface contamination (see Tellier 2006, which also discusses the distinction between droplets and aerosols). Epidemics of influenza occur annually and are sometimes called the "flu season." Influenza is an important cause of death: in the United States in 2003, influenza and pneumonia, counted together, killed more than 65,000 people, 2.7 percent of all deaths, making it the seventh leading cause of death

(Heron and Smith 2007). Year-to-year fluctuations are not uncommon: in 2004, the most recent year for which data are available, flu and pneumonia killed just under 60,000 people (2.5 percent of all deaths) and was the eighth leading cause of death, just behind Alzheimer's disease (Miniño et al. 2007). Note that heart disease and cancer together account for more than half of all deaths, which leaves all other causes fighting for table scraps of percentages of the total.

The 1918–1919 Influenza Pandemic

The 1918–1919 influenza pandemic, sometimes called the "Spanish flu," was the most deadly outbreak of any disease in the twentieth century. An influenza pandemic is a global epidemic of the same new strain of influenza virus (Kilbourne 1987: 14); I use "1918–1919 epidemic" and "1918–1919 pandemic" interchangeably. Influenza virologists use the term *antigenic shift* when a major genetic change takes place in circulating viruses, resulting in a new (pandemic) strain of virus. Inter-pandemic periods are characterized by seasonal influenza (and thus asynchronous hemispheric outbreaks) with slowly changing strains; these incremental changes are termed *antigenic drift*. Shift and drift are discussed in Pereira (1980) and Steinhauer and Skehel (2002). Influenza is a zoonosis, a disease that comes to humans from an animal reservoir. The animal hosts of influenza are swine and, especially, birds. Webby and Webster (2001) discuss the particulars of avian-porcine-human influenza virus cycling.

The 1918–1919 pandemic was not Spanish in origin, but Spain's neutrality in the 1914–1918 world war meant that Spanish newspapers did not censor bad news about the pandemic, in contrast to newspapers in belligerent European countries. This led to the pandemic's being known as the "Spanish flu" (Echeverri 2003). The name was reinforced over the years in books such as Collier's *The Plague of the Spanish Lady* (1996 [1974]), but it is used less nowadays. Estimates of global mortality from the pandemic are 40 million to 100 million (Johnson and Mueller 2002). In 1918, most of the world's population lived in jurisdictions without registration of vital events, which means that any estimate of the pandemic's mortality is little more than an educated guess. The 1833 influenza pandemic was also noted for its mortality (Patterson 1985, 1986), but the nineteenth-century data are less detailed than the 1918–1919 data.

The 1918–1919 flu was also qualitatively different. The age-mortality profile (a plot with age on the horizontal axis and death rates on the vertical axis) for influenza is normally U shaped. Children and the elderly have the weakest immunity, and the U profile reflects that. Adults, who have the greatest resistance, form the base of the U. By contrast, in 1918–1919 the age-mortality profile was W shaped. Typical mortality among the youngest and oldest was accompanied by a third peak, among young adults, which was unprecedented for influenza as well as puzzling theoretically. These patterns are illustrated in figure 8.1, which shows 1917 (U) and 1918 (W) influenza and pneumonia mortality by age in the United States. The data come from the US death registration area and so include both soldiers and civilians on US soil but exclude overseas war deaths. Military recruitment may have played a role in the spread of flu in the United States, but it does not explain the high mortality among females or the lethality of the flu in other, nonbelligerent countries.

The W pattern in 1918–1919 is completely atypical, even for a pandemic. Such a pattern is unusual among biological causes of death, with tuberculosis being the closest match among the major diseases.

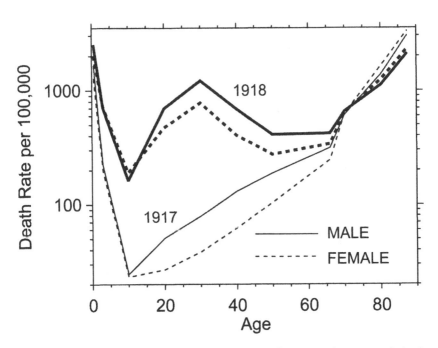

Figure 8.1 Age distribution of death rates from influenza and pneumonia in the United States death registration area, 1917 and 1918. Death rate is deaths per 100,000 person-years lived. Data from US Department of Health, Education, and Welfare 1956.

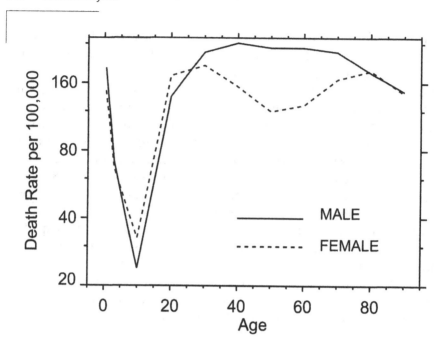

Figure 8.2 Age-mortality profile for the United States for deaths from all forms of tuberculosis, 1917. Death rate is deaths per 100,000 person-years lived. Data from US Department of Health, Education, and Welfare 1956.

This is seen in figure 8.2, which illustrates death rates for all forms of tuberculosis (TB) for the United States in the relevant time period (1917). By far the most deadly form is pulmonary tuberculosis, a graph of which would not look markedly different except that the mode among infants would be smaller, because other forms of tuberculosis are more important at the youngest ages.

What Caused the W Shape?

The entire influenza mortality curve in 1918 (fig. 8.1) lies above the 100 per 100,000 line, reflecting the severity of the epidemic. The male excess over females in death rate, in absolute terms, was also exaggerated in 1918, particularly at the middle-age mode of the W. The leading explanation for the W shape is that some flu victims experienced an unchecked immune response that flooded their lungs with fluid. This is called a "proinflammatory cytokine response," or, more colloquially, a "cytokine storm" (see Chan et al. 2005; Osterholm 2005; Wong and Yuen 2006); cytokines are a type of immune system protein. Adults, not the young or the elderly, have the strongest immune systems, and adults in 1918–1919 would have experienced this pulmonary complication most severely. Fluid-filled lungs are consistent with clinical reports from 1918–1919 (Crosby 1989; Taubenberger 2005). This adult peak, superimposed on the usual U shape, putatively accounts for the W.

The verb *superimposed* in the last sentence is noteworthy. There is evidence that the W in fact represents an inverted V (or A-frame) shape plus the typical U shape. The inverted V, or the middle mode of the W, comes from the strain-specific mortality of the 1918 influenza, while the right-most (oldest) mode of the W comes from the typical flu mortality of the preceding winter. The evidence for this was presented by Olson and colleagues (2005), who analyzed age-stratified monthly mortality data from New York City and showed that the winter 1917–1918 normal flu season exhibited the typical high mortality at old ages. The autumn 1918 (pandemic) wave of mortality preceded the timing that would have been expected for the 1918–1919 winter flu season; this is well known. Olson and coauthors go on to show that this fall wave exhibited unusual mortality at young and especially middle ages, but not at older ages. If this finding is replicated nationwide, it would mean that the right-most (oldest) mode of the W is not truly an aspect of the 1918–1919 influenza pandemic but an artifact of looking at calendar-year data (i.e., a holdover from the winter 1917–1918 normal influenza season). On the other hand, the middle and left-most (youngest) modes of the W are part of the 1918 pandemic. A prior-immunity argument suggests that the diminution of mortality among older cohorts (that is, the right-most trough of the W) was due to acquired immunity in these cohorts from the 1890 pandemic (Palese 2004; Palese, Tumpey, and Garcia-Sastre 2006); this is also consistent with the available data.

Because the present study uses annual data throughout, the portrayal of influenza and pneumonia death rates in calendar-year terms (fig. 8.1) is the correct comparison graph. The selective mortality findings, which I discuss in more detail later, rest on the middle mode and not the W shape per se and are not affected by the findings of Olson and colleagues (2005). Nonetheless, it is worth remembering that the W shape is the 1918 calendar-year age-mortality profile.

The 1918 Plague Selection Hypothesis in Greater Detail

Selection theories in demography are often highly mathematical, but selection in the 1918–1919 flu can be summarized according to the questions, Who died, who survived, and did this change the ante- versus post-epidemic population composition?

The selection hypothesis centers on the W-shaped age-mortality profile. It posits that young adults who died of the 1918–1919 influenza—the middle of the W—were on average less healthy prior to the epidemic. The surviving population, in 1919 and afterward, was therefore that much healthier on average. Tuberculosis is the nexus with the less healthy because, among other things, the lungs are attacked by both diseases. Since many influenza deaths were among tubercular people, the post-epidemic population was healthier. The hypothesis is corroborated by a variety of data, including plummeting tuberculosis death rates in 1919 and thereafter (Noymer and Garenne 2000). It is no coincidence that tuberculosis was, in that period, typically a disease of adults rather than of children or the elderly (fig. 8.2), and it was the most important cause of death among adults.

Figure 8.3 is the key to the story. It plots the age-standardized death rate for all forms of tuberculosis in the United States for each sex, from 1900 through 1940. Throughout the twentieth century, tuberculosis was in retreat. This also holds going back to the mid-nineteenth century for

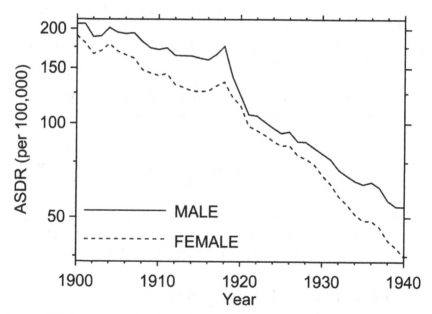

Figure 8.3 Age-standardized death rate (ASDR) in the United States for all forms of tuberculosis, 1900–1940. Data from US Department of Health, Education, and Welfare 1956.

Massachusetts, the state with the oldest available data. Yet the steepest decline clearly came after the 1918–1919 flu pandemic, and the steepness of the decline is not an artifact of the uptick in tuberculosis deaths that accompanied the flu in 1918. In short, tuberculosis death rates fell precipitously in the close wake of the influenza pandemic, more than they had been falling already. As figure 8.4 shows, the flu pandemic came and went. The strength of looking at the overall epidemiological situation becomes apparent when figures 8.3 and 8.4 are considered together. The seismic shock is in influenza (fig. 8.4), whereas the long-term reverberations are felt in the tuberculosis time series (fig. 8.3).

Note that the vertical axis in figure 8.3 is logarithmic (e.g., equal distance denotes a factor change such as doubling or halving, not absolute change). The male series falls more steeply than the female series. This is not simply because both sexes fell by a certain proportion, and the males started higher and therefore fell more. Slope in semi-log-scale plots signifies proportional change, and a proportionally equal fall for both sexes would be denoted by parallel downward-sloping lines. The distance between the male and female series in figure 8.3 is

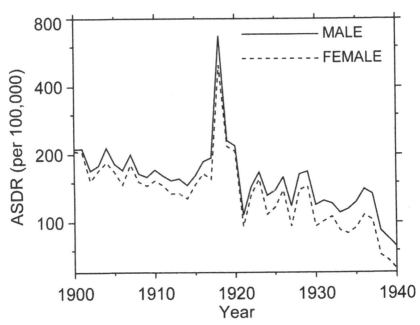

Figure 8.4 Age-standardized death rate (ASDR) in the United States for influenza and pneumonia combined, 1900–1940. Data from US Department of Health, Education, and Welfare 1956.

choked after the pandemic, so the male rates fell more steeply in both an absolute and a relative sense, which is consistent with the male excess death rate (relative to females) in the selector (the flu pandemic).

Figure 8.3 is age-standardized. Noymer and Garenne (2000) provide a breakdown of this relationship by specific age groups, which shows, as the selection hypothesis would predict, that the ages driving the changes in the age-standardized rate are at the middle mode of the W-shaped flu mortality.

It bears repeating that the most important mode of the W is the middle one. Naturally, it is the unusual mode. More directly, the middle mode of the rates (i.e., the W) coincides with the largest denominators of underlying population. The right-most (oldest) mode did not apply to a large underlying population in 1918: the population sixty-five and older constituted less than 5 percent of the 1920 census enumeration (Linder and Grove 1943). Influenza death rates declined steeply through the childhood years, so the left-most (youngest) mode in the rates likewise did not result in a huge number of deaths. The middle mode applied to a large population at risk and therefore had the greatest impact by far in terms of number of deaths. This is illustrated in figure 8.5, which shows death counts for influenza and pneumonia for the death registration area of the United States in 1918. Complete death registration did not exist in the United States at that time, so there were more deaths in the whole country than are represented in figure 8.5. Given that the W shape in the rates was seen worldwide, the overall shape of figure 8.5 is extremely unlikely to have been altered importantly by the incompleteness of the United States death registration area.

The Standard Story of the 1918 Plague

Despite the magnitude of the 1918–1919 flu and its peculiar age-mortality profile, demographers have paid relatively little attention to it. Part of the reason is that the 1918–1919 epidemic was short-lived. Although it shortened United States life expectancy by 12 years in 1918 (relative to 1917), mortality decline continued apace in 1919 as if nothing had happened. Historically, the 1918–1919 influenza has not fit well into the story of long-term expansion of life expectancy. Ironically, the selection hypothesis postulates that the 1918–1919 flu actually hastened the decline in mortality in the years following 1918, by removing sicker-than-average people from the population.

Trostle (1986: 60) noted the role of the pandemic in the development of modern notions of host-environment interactions in disease

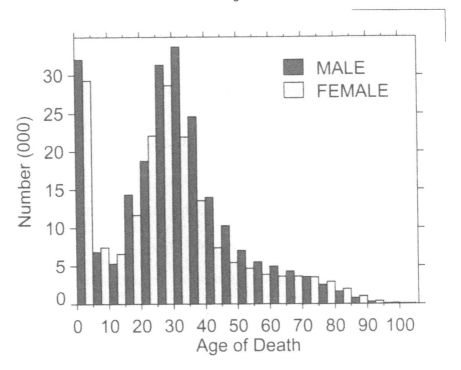

Figure 8.5 Age distribution of deaths from influenza and pneumonia in the United States death registration area, 1918. Data from US Bureau of the Census 1920.

processes, and Kunitz (1987: 383) made a similar point. But for the most part, even when the population literature includes an awareness of the 1918–1919 epidemic, it treats the event as a one-off curio. Medical historians and medical geographers over the years have published occasionally on the 1918 pandemic (see Galishoff 1969; Hildreth 1991; Katz 1974, 1977; Killingray 1994; Palmer and Rice 1992; Patterson 1983, 1986; Patterson and Pyle 1983, 1991; Pyle 1986; Tomkins 1992a, 1992b; van Hartesveldt 1992), but until lately, 1918 was not a major focus of research in the social sciences, especially outside medical history.

More recently, having recognized that the 1918 flu is under-studied, scholars have begun to devote more attention to the topic (e.g., Afkhami 2003; Almond 2006; Ammon 2001; Johnson 2006; Langford 2005; MacDougall 2007; Mamelund 2003, 2004, 2006; Reid 2005; Smallman-Raynor, Johnson, and Cliff 2002; Tognotti 2003; Tomes 2002). Epidemiologists also show a renewed interest in the pandemic (e.g., Azambuja 2004; Azambuja and Duncan 2002; Chowell et al. 2006a, 2006b; Mills, Robins, and Lipsitch 2004; Olson et al. 2005; Sattenspiel and Herring 2003). For obvious reasons, epidemiologists never forgot about 1918 to the extent that social scientists did (see, e.g., Doll 1987). Using data from Chicago for the years 1850 through 1925, Ferrie and Troesken (2008: 12) noted that "influenza and scarlet fever appear to have been killing off the weakest and most vulnerable parts of the population so that high death rates from these diseases actually reduced death rates from other causes." My sentiments exactly.

Differential Social Effects

There is a general sense in the literature that the 1918 pandemic killed in a relatively socially neutral way, unlike most diseases. This belief was perhaps borne of the fact that the middle mode of the W represents the strongest people in society. But an aggregate age-mortality profile says nothing about the social class, however defined, of the decedents.

Crosby (1989: 227) noted: "Unlike tuberculosis, typhoid fever, and venereal disease, [the 1918 pandemic] did not show a clear preference for the poor, the ill-fed, ill-housed and shabbily clothed ... by and large the rich died as easily as the poor." In fairness, socially neutral impact was not one of the major themes of Crosby's book, but to the extent to which he dealt with it, he cautiously leaned that way. Sydenstricker (1931) began his classic article on the subject with the sentence, "Perhaps no observation during the great influenza epidemic of 1918–1919 was more common than the familiar comment that 'the flu hit the rich and the poor alike.'" Although Sydenstricker did much to show that this was not the case, by and large his lesson has been ignored.

The approach I advocate also casts doubt on social neutrality, and indeed tuberculosis, which Crosby mentioned as an example of a socially mediated disease, is the nexus between social class and influenza mortality. Mamelund, in some recent papers (2003, 2006), has also looked at the 1918 flu and social status and reached similar conclusions about the non–social neutrality of the 1918 pandemic. Tuckel and colleagues (2006) concur (see also Swedlund, this volume).

Here I examine tuberculosis data that do not contain explicit social class information. However, tuberculosis is well known to be associated with poverty and crowding (Barnes 1995; Brandt 1903; Kitagawa and Hauser 1973; Lowell, Edwards, and Palmer 1969; Myers et al. 2006; Paluzzi 2004; Rothman 1994; Tiruviluamala and Reichman 2002) and with poor nutrition (Scrimshaw 2003). This knowledge is in spite of the fact that a number of books on tuberculosis devote disproportionate coverage to famous people—Chopin and the Brontë sisters, among others—who died of tuberculosis (e.g., Daniel 1997; Dormandy 1999; Dubos and Dubos 1952). If the tuberculous were affected disproportionately by the 1918–1919 plague, then the finding suggests strongly that the poor were as well.

Historical epidemiology is an endeavor that strives to be good historiography as well as good epidemiology. As such, one of its goals is to use records of past diseases as lenses into past societies. By enabling comment on the social non-neutrality of the 1918–1919 pandemic, the approach yields greater insight into social history than a more literal reading of the influenza time series data.

Discussion: The Long-term Effects of Plagues

Context matters. This has been recognized in a comparative-statistics sense for a long time. That is to say, two different populations experiencing the same plague will react differently. Nutrition is thought to play a strong role here. The death rate from the 1918–1919 pandemic in the United States is estimated at around 0.5 percent, whereas globally it is thought to have been around 2.5 percent—a fivefold difference. The level of industrialization of American society in 1918 relative to that of the rest of the world requires little elaboration. But inter- or intranational inequality of health outcomes according to resources is only one type of important context.

Context matters with respect to comparative dynamics as well. Within a given population, health is not a fixed object that is diminished by a plague, temporarily or permanently. Rather, health is a complex system that is in motion before, during, and after a plague. As Epstein (2007: 69) put it, epidemics "are embedded in the social ecology of the populations through which they spread. We may not like to think so, but we are still part of nature, and our fate is entwined in a constantly evolving system of relationships to each other, our predators, and our prey." Looking at post-plague changes throughout the system is therefore desirable.

The 1918 influenza pandemic had a longer-term impact and affected a broader swath of disease patterns than has been previously acknowledged. Using data from the United States, I have shown that in the wake of the 1918 pandemic, tuberculosis death rates tumbled. This fall was great enough to be seen even when superimposed on the secular decline of tuberculosis death rates in the twentieth century. I interpret this as selective mortality, or what in biology is sometimes called a harvesting effect. The pandemic killed many tuberculous people, affecting the tuberculosis death rate in later years by diminishing the size of the pool of tuberculous persons and interrupting transmission. Golubovsky's (1980: 146) observation that "viral infections act as potent selective agents in natural populations" holds true for humans as well.

It is worth reiterating that the selection hypothesis does *not* posit that the unusual virulence of the 1918 pandemic was due to the confluence of tuberculosis and influenza. After all, both high tuberculosis prevalence and winter flu epidemics were constants throughout the early twentieth century (and before), and only the 1918 pandemic had the unusual W-shaped age-mortality profile. Tuberculosis was not a *cause* of the unusual virulence of the 1918 influenza. Rather, according to the selection hypothesis, changes in tuberculosis epidemiology were a *consequence* of the influenza pandemic.

Tuberculosis is with us still, especially in poor countries, and it still seems to be disproportionately a male disease (Watkins and Plant 2006). The findings on the influenza pandemic reported in this chapter point clearly to the idea that the effects of the next influenza pandemic will depend in part on the way it interacts with other diseases, especially tuberculosis and HIV. Those two diseases overlap (Nunn et al. 2005), which could create two- and three-way synergies and antagonisms with an influenza pandemic. The possible outcomes, which are difficult to foresee, range from counterintuitive protective effects (e.g., reduced immune response from HIV status could be protective from a runaway immune response) to devastating enhancing effects.

The approach I have taken fits squarely within the tradition of disease ecology. This school of thought is often associated with William McNeill, whose book *Plagues and Peoples* (1976) was influential and controversial and whose postulate about leprosy and the Black Death began this chapter. Alfred Crosby, whose 1989 book on the 1918–1919 influenza was important, is also often associated with the ecological approach to disease, through his earlier book *The Columbian Exchange: Biological and Cultural Consequences of 1492* (1972), which was likewise influential and controversial.

There are, however, a number of chronologically and theoretically important strands of the disease ecology literature in addition to Crosby's and McNeill's. Mirko Grmek's (1969) concept of pathocoenosis antedates both Crosby 1972 and McNeill 1976. Pathocoenosis, or the idea that disease frequencies and distributions are jointly dependent on each other in a given population, has an obvious theoretical fit with the influenza pandemic's effects on tuberculosis. The theoretical affinities between pathocoenosis and Merrill Singer's syndemics concept (Singer, this volume; Singer and Clair 2003) are likewise salient.

René Dubos's book *Man Adapting* (1980), originally published in 1965, is another example of the disease ecology approach, and one that predates Crosby, McNeill, and Grmek. Indeed, Warwick Anderson (2004b) traced disease ecology back to Theobald Smith (1859–1934). Smith's book *Parasitism and Disease* (1934), based on lectures delivered a year before his death, bridged the gap between the then-young sciences of microbiology and epidemiology. Not surprisingly, given the contemporary importance of tuberculosis, Smith also worked extensively on that disease (Smith 1917). On Smith, see also Dolman and Wolfe 2003.

This chapter has a clearly demographic flavor, with age-standardized death rates, age-mortality profiles, and so on. Historical demography is well in step with the ecological approach to population health (Swedlund 1978). And disease ecology still brings new insights to our understanding of plagues, even such pored-over plagues as the 1918–1919 influenza pandemic and tuberculosis.

Conclusion: Tuberculosis Decline, a Reappraisal

The decline of tuberculosis has been a major component of worldwide mortality decline in general. This observation was center stage in Thomas McKeown's (1976) argument that improved socioeconomic conditions in general and nutrition in particular were more important than medicine in the decline of mortality. On the other hand, Samuel Preston (1990) gave the demographer's bill of particulars against McKeown, including the finding that life expectancy has increased over time even at constant levels of per-capita income (Preston 1975) and that the fall of tuberculosis in England and Wales (on which McKeown focused) was larger than in other populations (Preston and van de Walle 1978). These questions are still debated today (see Birchenall 2007a, 2007b for some recent contributions).

I have not spoken in this chapter to all the causes of the historical decline of tuberculosis. For example, as I noted earlier, tuberculosis was already in retreat when the pandemic struck. But the fact that tuberculosis decline was greatly abetted by the intercession of a seemingly unrelated pandemic of influenza is a caution against assigning responsibility for mortality decline to a single factor, whether nutrition, public health interventions, clinical medicine, or something else. Riley (2001) also argued against particularistic approaches. But if tuberculosis was such an important disease in history—and it was—then why have the present findings not been noted before now?

Tuberculosis in the United States was in decline before the 1918 influenza struck. Even without the pandemic, it would have declined to its historical nadir. Nonetheless, interesting and important patterns and processes are layered on top of the secular decline of tuberculosis. These patterns and processes become evident when disease is considered as a system, of which individual diseases are constituent parts. A plague is a shock in an individual disease, but its echoes may be felt through the entire system, and as such the true (i.e., long-term) impact of a plague may be seen in other diseases. The single most important thing to accelerate the decline of tuberculosis in the twentieth century in the United States was the 1918 influenza pandemic. This conclusion comes from thinking about diseases as interrelated and showing in a concrete example the value of this way of looking at plagues. It would seem that the traditional, particularistic approach of much historical epidemiology work is the reason this large effect has been overlooked.

Everyday Mortality in the Time of Plague

Ordinary People in Massachusetts before and during the 1918 Influenza Epidemic

Alan C. Swedlund

Her story begins on the eve of the cholera epidemic in Sunderland, England, in 1832. Sheri Holman, in her historical novel *The Dress Lodger*, describes a scene taking place in the working-class pub the "Labour in Vain." The flawed protagonist, Dr. Henry Chiver, wonders whether the young medical students he tutors and who have joined him at the table are paying any attention to their surroundings:

> Did they give more than a passing glance to the shy girl who came in to retrieve her father tonight? Mark her too bright eyes, notice the dainty drops of blood blooming on the handkerchief she touched to her mouth? Over by the door, did they observe the once-handsome face craterous with smallpox, or his companion, the swine-eyed old man whose nose has been eaten down to a snout by syphilis? Disease is drinking in the bar with us. For all we know, Cholera Morbus is even now thumping the bar for a gin. "I am wasting my time on these boys," Henry thinks. (Holman 2000: 20–21).[1]

My story begins in a small town in Massachusetts in 1918. In September, two young soldiers from Camp Devens are on leave for the weekend. They are due to ship out for France soon. Patrick brings his newfound buddy from Vermont home to the industrial village of Turners Falls to meet his family. The Vermonter is feeling unwell but looks forward to some home cooking and a chance to meet a local girl or two. Patrick's father welcomes the two boys at the door. As they sit down in the small front room, the soldier from Vermont watches as the father puffs his cigarette, coughs violently, and complains of his case of "cutler's lung."[2] Patrick's mother is boiling up a fine-smelling pot of something, and his younger sister is paying the visitor close attention. Patrick's older sister is there, too, but she looks pale and exhausted after the difficult birth of her son three days earlier. Five days later, two of these people are seriously ill with aches, chills, and fever, and another two, Patrick's father and older sister, are already dead.[3]

In these fictional accounts we are able to conjure up the simultaneity of compound risk factors and the ways in which class, gender, and ethnicity are connected in the emergent phase of a full-scale epidemic. They also capture, perhaps in a glancing sort of way, the kinds of everyday, underlying diseases to which communities are subject in normal times, as well as the scars of plagues past and the hazards of the workplace. Holman is especially effective in drawing attention to the manifest reality of infectious diseases in England in the 1830s. Too often, accounts of plague in the medical-historical literature omit the complexity of the disease environment, the multiple risk factors, and the everyday experiences of those in harm's way. In part this may be a function of the ways in which historical accounts of plagues reflect the limited knowledge of the "expert" observers of the time, obstructing ready access to a more nuanced account. And in part I think it is because the biomedical tradition of recounting the history of epidemics is prone to selecting at most two or three key causes and a single response variable—the named disease.[4]

Contemporary epidemiological studies are less constrained by the censoring and selectivity that characterize the historical record and have the advantage of an expanded window of simultaneous observation. As illustrated by Merrill Singer's construction of *syndemics* (e.g., Singer and Scott 2003), the concurrent appearance of multiple and interacting diseases and multifactorial risks can be rendered in sharp relief for many contemporary populations.

In this chapter I address a few of the knotty problems involved in reconstructing historical epidemiology. I also want to portray how citizens of ordinary communities, fully aware of an epidemic's approach and arrival, might have experienced what I call "plague time." These are people who were not in the eye of the storm but at its edges. What other experiences with disease and death filled their lives and occupied their attention? The reconstruction of historical experience requires multiple sources, imagination, plausibility, and a reader's trust. The result often leads to an unproven scenario, which is one reason I chose to open this chapter using fictionalized accounts.[5]

One motivation for this project was Alfred Crosby's moving and compelling afterword in *America's Forgotten Pandemic* (2003), in which he recounts how a "plague" that took probably more people than any previous plague in history—the influenza pandemic of 1918—was so quickly forgotten, even in its immediate aftermath.[6] Crosby goes on to note that this was primarily a loss of institutional memory and by no means forgetfulness by all who survived it. A second motivation was the observation made by both Crosby and John Barry (2004) that although the epidemic took a heavy toll on a particular age group, young adults, it was relatively indiscriminate with regard to class. Barry echoes others in saying that it was "not tied to race or class"; it was "too universal" (Barry 2004: 395).[7] I find these observations intriguing, given my own research experience in historical epidemiology and that of other scholars (e.g., see Herring, this volume, Noymer, this volume; Swedlund 2010).

The primary sites for this investigation are four towns and two villages in Franklin County, western Massachusetts, in the early twentieth century: Greenfield, Deerfield, and the villages of Shelburne Falls in the town of Shelburne and Turners Falls in Montague (fig. 9.1). The "plague" is the 1918 flu pandemic. This disease episode has the advantage of being recent enough to fall within the age of state medicine and within the memories of the few people still living who experienced the epidemic.[8] I deploy the "official" record of the state and local medical authorities, accounts from the popular media, and local narratives of the epidemic. For the state I looked at the annual reports of the Massachusetts Office of Vital Statistics and Board of Health to see how each captured the events of 1918. I also consulted the *Boston Globe*, the state's largest newspaper. At the most local level, I looked at the minutes of the District Medical Society for Franklin County, the town reports for four contiguous towns in the county (all in the Pocumtuck Valley Memorial Association Library, Deerfield, Massachusetts), and the local newspaper of record. I also consulted personal accounts from the time and recollections of survivors.

Anthropologists often attempt to tell big stories in small places. My aim is not just to provide another prosaic story of the flu told close up about small towns and their inhabitants. On top of that, this slice of small-town New England can add to our growing understanding of life and death in Progressive Era America. Larger generalizations regarding the 1918 influenza epidemic can be either supported or challenged.

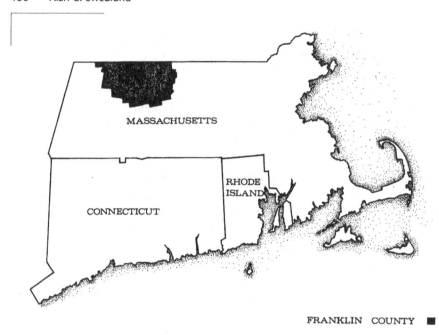

FRANKLIN COUNTY ■

Figure 9.1 Shaded area location of Franklin County, Massachusetts and the four towns. After Garmsun, 1991, with permission.

The broad outline of the 1918 influenza pandemic is now well known. Worldwide estimates of total deaths vary from 20 million to 100 million persons, and most researchers now agree that the higher numbers are the more plausible, given the underreporting in many regions of the world (Noymer, this volume).[9] At least 500,000 Americans died in the epidemic, and it is estimated that as much as 25 percent of the US population was symptomatic at some time during the active period of the flu's presence. The flu killed at least 2.5 percent of its victims, but at Camp Devens, an army base in Ayer, Massachusetts, the mortality rate was 27.9 percent—2,817 cases were reported there between 4 September and 29 October, with 787 deaths. In the month of October alone, the death rate at Camp Devens was 54.9 percent of those afflicted (Massachusetts Department of Health 1919: 199).[10]

The 1918 flu first appeared in Massachusetts at the Chelsea Naval Hospital on 10 August. This was also one of the earliest occurrences in the whole country. The first civilian cases in Chelsea were reported on 28 August. Civilian cases had hopscotched across the state, first passing over and then returning to Greenfield and Turners Falls in the middle Connecticut River valley and arriving in the western Massachusetts city of Pittsfield by 13 September (Massachusetts Department of Health 1919: 198).

When the crisis had passed and the year ended, the state reported a total of 145,262 confirmed cases of influenza, with 11,100 deaths. We know, however, that many cases went unreported, and the total number was probably closer to 400,000 (Massachusetts Department of Health 1919: 200).[11] Influenza was not even made a reportable disease until 4 October, so no cases or fatalities were counted for all of September, except at the army base (Massachusetts Department of Health 1919: 202). In addition, flu cases resulting in death were most frequently due to complications from pneumonia, so those dying from what the attending physician called influenza and those dying from lobar pneumonia, for example, are difficult to parse. Other, competing complications and causes increased the risk of death from contracting the flu as well. A further complication, as Condran (1995: 40) observed, was that "the path between the physical cause of someone's death and its appearance in a municipal summary of vital statistics is long and involves a complex set of agreements on the part of the patient, the family, the physician certifying the death, and the city government recording it." Epidemics can both magnify and narrow the field of observation, so that historical morbidity and death statistics may be relatively coherent and reliable but still entail issues of accuracy.

Massachusetts reported 13,374 cases of lobar pneumonia in 1918, with 9,787 fatalities (Massachusetts Department of Health 1919: 201).[12] Interpolating by the seat-of-the-pants method, I think it is safe to assume that at least 20,000 deaths occurred in Massachusetts as a direct result of the 1918 flu and its complications. In a table prepared by the Office of Vital Statistics of Massachusetts that included influenza deaths "in combination" with other causes, officials placed the total at 18,426 deaths. Influenza cases and deaths rose rapidly in September, peaked in October, declined rapidly in November, and then rose slightly again in December before ultimately trailing off to negligible numbers.

One characteristic of the 1918 flu that has been commented on frequently is that so many young and middle-aged adults died worldwide. The characteristic U-shaped mortality curve, reflecting death rates highest among the very young and the elderly, was transformed into a W shape, with the middle peak consisting of these adults (see Noymer, this volume). Some researchers have hypothesized that this was because of the large numbers of young men concentrated in military installations and engaged in the European theater of war, but the statistics from Massachusetts and elsewhere illustrate that in at least some cases, sex ratios in the 20–49 year age groups were actually fairly even (e.g., Office of the Secretary of State of Massachusetts 1918: table 56, 180–181). The age-mortality pattern was not just a matter of having high concentrations of susceptible males in conditions where the virus could easily spread. People in these age groups, both male and female, seem in fact to have had a greater risk of severe symptoms and death (see Barrett, this volume; Noymer, this volume).[13]

To attempt to characterize mortality in 1918 America and Massachusetts without reference to the influenza pandemic would be absurd and would neglect the most deadly pandemic in history. Yet as I mentioned earlier, writers on the epidemic point out how easily it was, until recently, forgotten. Part of my aim in the rest of this chapter is to unwrap the other epidemiological events that took place at this juncture in Progressive Era Massachusetts and to evaluate the behavior and actions of the medical establishment and public around general issues of health and disease. The epidemic occupied the last four excruciating months of 1918. What else happened in communities in Massachusetts and throughout the United States? Was it only the short duration of the epidemic and the fact that the flu story was swamped by the number of war casualties and the front-page events of World War I that explains this phenomenon? Is it our current anxiety about future pandemics that makes the apparent "letting go" of a past crisis seem so incomprehensible to many today?

Background

The United States officially declared war on Germany on 6 April 1917, but the considerable lead-up to America's participation had citizens well attuned to the imminent event. Propaganda against Germany was already prevalent in the popular media. Franklin County readers of the *Greenfield Recorder* would have seen on 25 April 1918, alongside separate stories about the evil Huns, the headline "Be Vigilant for Health." They learned that "keeping a close watch for sickness" was a role they could play in "everyday preparedness," and it was especially at times such as these that serious harm to the town and country could result from epidemic diseases.[14] The Greenfield Board of Health had noticed numerous cases of measles and scarlet fever in recent months and cautioned that scarlet fever especially "constitutes a serious menace to any community in which it gains a foothold," particularly if it was the "old fashioned" and "more active type" of the disease.[15] Monitoring infectious disease was not just a matter of public health; it was also patriotic.

In Massachusetts the reportable infectious diseases of greatest concern in 1917 and early 1918 were tuberculosis, illnesses causing infant mortality, and the traditional childhood diseases—measles, diphtheria, and scarlet fever—together with a more recent worry, poliomyelitis.[16] Although polio had been known, if not well understood, since at least the mid-1800s, a widespread epidemic of it struck the United States in 1916. Massachusetts was affected, and Franklin County was not spared. In the town of Montague, within the borders of which Turners Falls was an industrial village, the Grange suspended meetings in late summer "on account of the infantile paralysis." The Congregational church suspended its Sunday school, and the Parent Teacher Association lawn party was "indefinitely postponed" (*Greenfield Recorder*, various dates, August 1916). Cases were reported from several Franklin County towns, and the newspaper advised readers on "what to do for paralysis" (cleanliness, quarantine, etc.). Greenfield underwent quarantines in July, and other towns in August.

As the summer of 1917 approached, citizens worried about a repeat of polio, but in general they sensed that they were living in the "modern era." Infectious disease was still a threat, but they knew about germs and how to avoid them (see, e.g., Tomes 1998). And had not the rates of infectious diseases been going down for the last several years? The Massachusetts Board of Health had reported it so, and the newspaper occasionally published statistics to prove it. Sanitary engineering, quarantines, and recent developments such as vaccines and diphtheria antitoxin were marvels of this new age.[17] Massachusetts was at the forefront of states monitoring the public's health.

Indeed, a lengthy time series of data collected by state bureaucracies involved in the public's welfare was at hand for the use of experts and laypersons alike.[18] Beginning with 1870, the first full year after the founding of the Massachusetts Department of Public Health in 1869, infant mortality dropped from 162 deaths per thousand live births to 102 by 1915. Combined deaths due to measles, scarlet fever, and diphtheria-croup dropped from 147 to 34. Deaths from pulmonary consumption–tuberculosis dropped from 339 to 114. The results represented a 37 percent reduction in infant mortality, a 77 percent reduction in childhood fevers, and a 66 percent reduction in pulmonary tuberculosis (Office of the Secretary of State of Massachusetts 1915: 150, 211).[19] The trends were not entirely smooth, occasionally rising slightly or falling more abruptly, but overall each infectious cause of death declined over time.

Plague Time

The *Greenfield Recorder*, a weekly, served all of Franklin County during this period.[20] The year 1917 passed without the newspaper's reporting any serious disease episodes. The spring wave of mild influenza in 1918, too, went unremarked. On 24 August, no mention of influenza appeared in the *Recorder*, but it was noted that several local conscripts were leaving to report at Camp Devens. News of the "Grippe" was traveling fast by word of mouth, and people were hearing of cases in Boston—some would have seen or heard of reports in the *Boston Daily Globe*. On 6 September 1918 the *Globe* reported fear of a possible influenza outbreak, and it followed up with a series of articles chronicling the rising number of cases in Massachusetts and elsewhere. It dutifully repeated the claim made by the military health agent, Colonel Philip Doane, that the germs might have been deliberately "planted"—introduced from German U-boats (*Boston Daily Globe*, 19 September 1918). It tracked the increasing number of cases at Camp Devens and other military posts in the state and told people how to avoid the flu by keeping clean, taking fresh air, avoiding crowds, and so forth (*Boston Daily Globe*, 28 September 1918). It repeated US Surgeon General Rupert Blue's recommendations for taking care of oneself once infected: "rest in bed, fresh air, abundant food ... and Dover's Powders for the pain" (*Boston Daily Globe*, 14 September 1918). Local newspapers quickly picked up national reports and stories out of Boston. One trend found in the *Globe* throughout September and October was a tendency every few days to assure the public that the situation was improving—that fewer new cases were expected.

But the most important newspaper story for Massachusetts residents in early September 1918 was that the Boston Red Sox were playing in the World Series, with Babe Ruth wearing a Red Sox uniform. The Red Sox would win that series on 11 September, the same day that three civilians dropped dead on the streets of Quincy (Crosby 2003). The first local story in Franklin County to note the appearance of the epidemic came in the *Greenfield Recorder* on 25 September 1918.[21] It was not front-page news, and it was not about deaths in the county but about the death of a Turners Falls man at Camp Devens. Back on page 8 was the obituary of Richard Hastings, "a fine specimen of physical manhood," who died on 20 September after a "short illness with pneumonia."

The newspaper for 2 October was another story. The headline read "INFLUENZA WITH US," and the article recorded that 234 cases had already been reported for Greenfield, and another 100 cases for Turners Falls. The state Board of Health recommended the closing of all places of public assembly and made the closing of churches and schools mandatory until further notice. There were deaths to report in Greenfield, Turners Falls, Shelburne, and Deerfield, all having occurred within the past few days. Still, the Board of Health claimed there was "no need for the public to become panic stricken." On 9 October the front page of the *Recorder* announced there were now eight hundred cases in Greenfield, and the Board of Health required the closing of "saloons and soda fountains." Death notices were appearing from towns throughout the county. The paper published the Board of Health's "Rules for Avoidance of Influenza" ("keep clean." "don't go to crowded places," etc.). In a moment of unabashed commercial opportunism, page 9 carried an advertisement featuring images of women in "Smart Hats for Those in Mourning" (fig. 9.2).

On 16 October, Franklin County residents opened the *Recorder* to read competing front-page headlines: "Epidemic Declines: Fewer new cases" and "Many Deaths Yesterday: Rest of County beginning to feel effects." Readers were told that mobilization of health care in the community, including the arrival of additional physicians sent by state and federal health departments, was working. The Red Cross and visiting nurses were successfully getting food and assistance to families overcome by the flu. Despite the number of deaths, daily reports claimed that the incidence of cases was steadily declining. On 23 October the paper announced that the ban on assembly was to be lifted. Churches could meet on Sunday, 27 October, and on Monday morning schools could open, along with saloons and soda fountains in the afternoon and moving picture theaters in the evening. The recent cases of flu were much milder than the earlier ones, according to the paper, although 199 people had died in the county between 1 and 23 October. "Undertakers were under nearly as great a strain as the doctors" (*Greenfield Recorder*, 23 October 1918).

Although the pages of the *Recorder*, the *Greenfield Gazette and Courier*, and the *Turners Falls Reporter* continued to carry stories regarding the epidemic in the weeks that followed, increasingly their coverage was about the national epidemic or about being "careful after flu" (*Greenfield Gazette and Courier*, 4 December 1918). Short columns appeared from time to time about a fatal case here or a few mild cases there, but for all intents and purposes the local encounter was over.[22] Barely six weeks after the first knowledge of the Massachusetts epidemic in mid-September, the sense was that the crisis was passing or had passed. People who had lost family and friends were by no means beyond

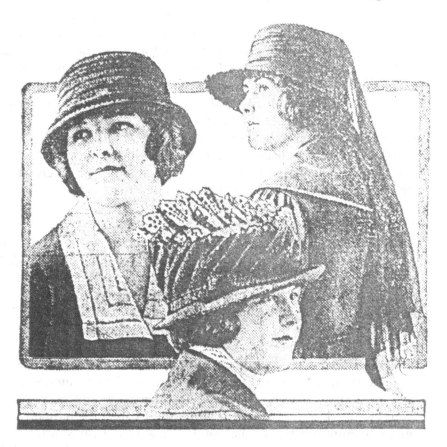

Smart Hats for Those in Mourning

Figure 9.2 Advertisement for hats for women in mourning. *Greenfield Recorder,* Greenfield, Massachusetts, 9 October 1918, page 9.

mourning, anxiety, and depression, but hope and confidence were being restored. Citizens felt renewed faith that the medical community had responded and done its job.

Throughout those six weeks, newspaper columns carrying other news competed for space with stories about the flu. The war effort received front-page attention, of course, and often superseded the epidemic. But other pages carried results from the county fair and garden competitions, stories about one town's purchase of a fire truck, and accounts of the Boston and Maine Railroad's being sued by widows. All the papers found ample room for news besides that of illness and death. Advertisements for

IMMEDIATE ACTION   NO DELAYS   NO RED TAPE

GERMIFUME The Magic Disinfectant GERMIFUME

SPANISH INFLUENZA	GERMIFUME	Influenza is widespread.
In Greenfield 1,000 cases.		How can you avoid it?
In Turners Falls 600 cases.		
In Millers Falls 300 cases.	The Magic Disinfectant	Spray your handkerchief with GERMIFUME, a magical, handy anti-
In Massachusetts 265,000 cases.		septic. Use your handkerchief over
	An Essential in Modern Sanitation	nostrils in close, public places.
Stamp It Out!		GERMIFUME fights for you; pro-
With Germifume	In proper use prevents sickness by de-	tects you, will save you.
	stroying microbes, bacteria, or bacillus in any	
It is O. K. The Board of Health	contagious or infectious malady or epidemic.	Buy it TODAY.
says so. Use lots of it; the Public	Especially efficient as a preventative in	At All Leading Druggists.
Health Service wants you to.	scarlet fever, diphtheria, La Grippe or colds.	
It is Pungent, Pleasant, Power-	It kills the germ in process of incubation.	For 35 cents
ful in effect. It meets the exacting	It affords valued after treatment of the prem-	
demands of the sick room, the home	ises, and is a real aid to medical attendants	Manufactured and Guaranteed by the
and hospital.	and nurses.	Onota Chemical Co.,
Invest 35 cents for Health	Fully recommended by Massachusetts health officials and physicians.	Pittsfield, Mass.

ANTISEPTIC LIFE INSURANCE

Figure 9.3 "Protection against influenza," Germifume. Advertisement from the *Greenfield Recorder,* Greenfield, Massachusetts, 16 October 1918, page 5.

the new Overland automobile and furnishings from the local furniture store found their way into the papers next to ads for war bonds and patent medicines: "For Spanish Influenza ... try Peruna first"; "Fruit-a-tives—The wonderful fruit medicine—greatly helps to resist this disease" (fig. 9.3). One gains the impression of both a deliberate effort by the media to keep people calm and an attempt to offer genuine reflection, reassuring people that life was going on somewhat normally despite the sudden epidemic and significant loss of life.

Personal Narratives

Letters, diaries, and other personal recollections of the epidemic in western Massachusetts do not vary significantly from those collected in other regions that were hard hit. Agnes Higginson Fuller, widow of the famous Deerfield artist George Fuller, who died in 1884, recounted in her diary the series of family members and friends who came down with the "grippe." She lived in both Deerfield and Boston and traveled back and forth regularly, although on Friday, 4 October 1918, she wrote, "Grippe epidemic spreading in Greenfield, we do not go there" (Fuller-Higginson Papers). Her brief remarks about who had become sick are interspersed with daily comments on the beautiful Indian summer and an occasional highlight from the newspaper stories on gains by the Allies in the war. The only death she reported was in a family being cared for by "Mrs. McC," presumably her housekeeper. There is no hint of extreme fear of the disease.

Several adult children corresponded with their parents living in Deerfield or other Franklin County towns from their colleges or positions of work. Gladys Brown wrote to her mother on 5 November 1918 that the cases of influenza in New York City were "dropping fast," and the "bans are off tomorrow." Her sister Mabel wrote to their mother on 6 November that the top floor of her dormitory in Keene, New Hampshire, had been taken by the Board of Health as an emergency hospital. Mabel wanted to volunteer with the nurses so she could learn "all about the care of sick people... It would be sure to come in handy some day" (Brown Family Papers). Jane Arms, of Greenfield, wrote from Smith College on 7 October 1918 that her dormitory was under quarantine but that the students were encouraged by faculty to "stay outside and breath fresh air" (Arms Family Papers).

People who were young in 1918 and who remembered the epidemic recalled people losing their minds from grief or from having endured a bout of the pneumonia. They described wearing bags of camphor around their necks and other herbal treatments, being given sips of whiskey by their parents, the schools being closed, and the extreme quiet of the streets. Some reported that the epidemic passed quickly, and people did not talk about it afterward. It was considered impolite for children to ask about a missing school chum.[23] On the part of many there must have been a desire to forget loss, but also these people were young children at the time and perhaps transitioned more easily than adults.

The Medical Community

The Franklin District Medical Society, founded in 1851, was a recognized chapter of the Massachusetts Medical Society and the American Medical Association. In the latter part of 1917, a portion of its quarterly meetings was often devoted to topics of how the war was affecting medicine and the members' practices.[24] At the May meeting there was much talk about physicians who were absent in "government service" to the war effort. A long discussion revolved around the question of what portion of an attending physician's fees should go to the family, if any, of the absent physician who normally treated that patient. (No action was recorded.)

At the May meeting of 1918, Dr. H. A. Streeter, of the state Board of Health, discussed protocols for "Reporting Specific Diseases." A recent concern was the high rate of venereal infections in prostitutes (90 percent) and its implications for contact: "One prostitute took care of 140 visitors in 10 days." It was also noted that the "Drafted Army" showed much higher rates of venereal infection than the "regular Army." Other topics included medical care for returning soldiers and maternal and infant care.

In July 1918, topics turned to the experience of one doctor "in camp," of lobbying related to medical legislation, and the state Board of Labor's invitation to participate in the upcoming "Industrial Health Conference." Then the record falls silent until 19 January 1919. The fall meeting clearly was cancelled because of the epidemic. In January 1919, the discussions all revolved around the influenza epidemic and epidemics in general. A Dr. Champion, of the state Board of Health, gave an overview of the epidemic, which came on so fast that it "near paralyzed our social forces," and described the need for improvements in efficiency and coordination of community resources. He said that estimates for Massachusetts were 300,000 cases, with 7,000 to 8,000 deaths. He was off by a factor of at least three for deaths.

In open discussion, a Dr. Upton said he would call it "a pneumonia rather than other epidemic." Dr. Leach connected "weather with severity" of the flu. Mr. Maurice Taylor of the US Public Health Service Commissioned Corps hoped the group might be able to get "a survey of all possible cases and to learn of after effects, physical as well as mental." A Dr. Goldsbury reported that between 26 September and 31 December there had been 1,664 cases of influenza in Greenfield.

Influenza was not a topic of discussion on 14 May 1919. In July 1919 the whole meeting was devoted to hearing reports from Franklin County physicians who had served as doctors in military camps or overseas in the preceding months. Of the three or four doctors who spoke, only a Dr. Mather, according to the recording secretary's notes, mentioned his experience with "the flu," during his time in Hingham and Boston. At the September 1919 meeting the main topic was treating emphysema, but on 11 November—the first anniversary of Armistice Day—Dr. Timothy Leary spoke on "acute respiratory diseases with special reference to influenza." He reported that he thought the class of "smokers and drinkers" had been least affected by the recent flu pandemic, whereas "healthy young adults [were the] most susceptible." His recommendations for prophylaxis were masks, isolation, and vaccines. On 20 January 1920 the society's topic was malignancies.

Throughout the remainder of the year, the local medical society was back to its usual rhythm of discussing topics such as tumors, puerperal septicemias, and other maladies of everyday treatment.

Municipal Accounts

Annual town reports were already a long tradition in New England in 1918, as they continue to be today. They were not standardized by any state code or mandate, so each took its own form by custom and preference. Each town had to include, however, births, marriages, and deaths for the calendar year. These records provide insights into the individual experiences of each town in Franklin County.

At the end of 1918, the health agent and milk inspector for the town of Greenfield, Massachusetts, dutifully presented the number of "reportable contagious diseases" occurring during that year. They were as follows: chicken pox, 80 cases; diphtheria, 8; German measles, 138; measles, 30; mumps, 274; scarlet fever, 31; and whooping cough, 66, for a total of 427 cases. In addition, he listed the number of houses he had "disinfected" for diseases: diphtheria, 8; scarlet fever, 31; tuberculosis, 4; cancer, 1; and pneumonia, 3 (Annual Report of the Town of Greenfield 1918). He did not report the more than 1,600 cases of influenza and the approximately 147 deaths that resulted from it. Again, influenza was not even classified as a "reportable" infectious disease, as designated by the state Board of Health, until 4 October 1918 (Massachusetts Department of Health 1919: 202). The town report did, however, reveal the effects of the epidemic on the town. A list of numbers of deaths by month, although it gave no causes, showed a total of 24 deaths in August. In September the number jumped to 34, and in October it rocketed to 132, of which 82 were deaths of persons between the ages of 20 and 46. Influenza eventually took approximately 115 Greenfield residents aged 20–46, in scarcely two months' time.

The Greenfield Board of Health inaugurated a Health Department in March 1918, prior to which time the board had no official office or headquarters. From this office it was able to mobilize doctors and nurses when the epidemic struck in the fall. Five town physicians and several nurses were already away doing war work as the epidemic struck heavily in mid-September. The town appealed to the state for aid, and four physicians were sent, but no nurses were available. The District Nurse Association provided backup support. The hospital was forced to close for about a week because too many cases were coming in. Volunteers joined the regular staff, and a roof was quickly constructed on the grounds to provide an outside "piazza" to accommodate the patient overflow. Patients, with their beds screened, were left in the open air, providing "the most satisfactory results" (Annual Report of the Town of Greenfield 1918: 120–139). As noted in the newspapers, schools and theaters were closed on 28 September, and soon afterward, so were saloons, club rooms, and soda fountains. The restrictions were maintained for a full month.

In assessing the progress of the epidemic, the Board of Health noted that it increased "gradually" during the first week and "very rapidly" during the second, reached its "highest mortality" in the third, and "dropped rapidly during the fourth week." The board's assessment of countermeasures and implications for a future epidemic held that the closing of places where people congregated was essential: "Droplet infection is an assured fact; this means that while coughing and even during ordinary conversation, fine drops of saliva are sprayed about, and it is a fact beyond contradiction that where people are gathered together, a person who carries the infection in his nose and throat can infect many others, even though he does not feel sick himself at the time" (Annual Report of the Town of Greenfield 1918: 134).

In its report, the town of Greenfield chose not to list the cause of death for each person who died in 1918, but the next town over, Montague, did so, and Montague included the manufacturing villages of Turners Falls and Millers Falls. On 16 September, sixty-year-old Mary Pavlak Hess died of "la grippe." On 17 September it was Richard Hastings, that "fine physical specimen." In the second half of September nine persons died of influenza or pneumonia. Then came October. In that month alone, eighty people died of influenza or pneumonia, and seventeen deaths from other causes were listed. At least one death, and usually two or three, took place every day until 24 October. Then, for the entire month of November, only three deaths were attributed to flu or pneumonia, and for December, seven. The Montague Board of Health concluded that the town had seen 1,069 cases of influenza and 96 deaths from influenza and pneumonia. Other "reportable" diseases that were noteworthy included measles and scarlet fever. The school physician reported two epidemics for the year, one of scarlet fever in the spring and the influenza epidemic in the autumn. The case fatality rate for measles was 8 percent, and for influenza, 11 percent (Annual Report of the Town of Montague 1918).

Deerfield, to the south of Greenfield and across the Connecticut River from Montague, passed through the epidemic relatively unscathed. Deerfield did not report causes of death in its annual town report, but by cross-referencing it is possible to pick out influenza deaths by the end of the third week of September. October saw only six deaths in town, and November, four. The school superintendent observed that students and parents were taking undue advantage of the school closings and "irregular conditions ... to detain their children for work" (Annual Report of the Town of Deerfield 1918). He reported that where families had sickness at home, the children were not allowed to attend school. The town of Shelburne's experience was similar to Deerfield's, each reporting to the state six deaths from influenza.

The State

The Massachusetts Office of Vital Statistics, in its dry, deliberate way, compiled the mortality statistics for 1918 in two reports, the first in 1919 and then a slightly expanded version in 1920. The tradition of vital statistics reporting in Massachusetts was to spare the words and lavish the numbers. The 1920 report's section on mortality is 142 pages long and contains 33 tables, most of them running for many pages. Of the 142-page section on mortality, the discussion portion makes up only 18 pages. The subsection devoted exclusively to influenza is one sentence long. The tables were the raison d'etre. In addition to numerous tables on general mortality, classified by sex, age, nativity, and so forth, there are tables on influenza by age, by frequency during months of the year, by municipality, and by coincidence with other causes. The officials reported 84 deaths for Greenfield, 50 for Montague, 6 for Deerfield, 6 for Shelburne, and a total of 201 for all of Franklin County (Office of the Secretary of State of Massachusetts 1918: table 57, 195).[25]

The Office of Vital Statistics was not constrained by the state Department of Health's regulations for submitting "reportable diseases," and it received records of all deaths in the state. This meant that it could include 4,207 influenza deaths for the month of September, when the Department of Health showed none. By choosing to investigate the coincidence of influenza with other causes, the statistics office could produce important insights into the association of influenza with types of pneumonia, with tuberculosis, with complications of pregnancy, and with other categories (fig. 9.4). The report included no epidemiological analysis and no in-depth discussion, but by presenting the data in this way, the statisticians signaled their relatively sophisticated understanding of disease associations. They provided four tables of detailed population statistics for the state, so denominators were often available for interested health officials and the general public. And the

Figure 9.4 Leading Causes of Death from Influenza Together with
Other Diseases, Massachusetts, 1918

Combined Cause	Total Cases
Broncho-pneumonia with influenza	9,686
Lobar pneumonia with influenza	4,451
Influenza, single cause	1,888
Pneumonia (undefined) with influenza	903
Pregnancy/labor with influenza	278
Heart disease with influenza	274
Pulmonary tuberculosis with influenza	122
Bronchitis with influenza	103
Meningitis with influenza	102
Whooping cough with influenza	78

Source: Office of the Secretary of State of Massachusetts 1918.
Note: "Bronchitis" includes both acute and chronic. "Pregnancy" combines "accidents
of pregnancy" and "other accidents of labor."

report published the current version of the codes for the International
Classification of Causes of Death.

As 1918 drew to a close and the state Department of Health grappled
with the many continuing cases of influenza, it was time to take stock
of the year and begin assembling the department's annual report. It
is easy to imagine an overworked department, with little remaining
money, strained to exhaustion and unsure whether the epidemic was
actually passing.[26] Outwardly, this issue of the annual report would
appear much like the previous year's, with reports and supplements from
each of the department's divisions, but special attention was devoted
to the influenza epidemic and to activities related to the war. Unlike
the Office of Vital Statistics, the Department of Health devoted several
paragraphs to the discussion of influenza.

At this early stage, it projected that total deaths in Massachusetts
would come to at least 15,000, from a conservative estimate of 400,000
cases. The authors described the inadequate supply of physicians and
nurses as a result of the war and their appeals to neighboring states
and the federal government. The governor had appointed an epidemic
emergency committee, which coordinated services and established
several emergency hospitals throughout the state to accommodate the
overflow of patients. The Department of Health commissioned the
same Dr. Timothy Leary mentioned earlier, a professor of pathology at
Tufts, to produce an influenza vaccine, which he did. There was great

hope for it, but after several trials the vaccine effort was abandoned. One trial was conducted in an unnamed state "institution," in which a slightly larger number of those vaccinated were taken sick and died than those in the unvaccinated control group.

The Massachusetts Department of Health (1919: 200) concluded the following:

From the lack of knowledge of the etiology, the lack of knowledge of prophylactic vaccines, the lack of knowledge of the exact modes of transmission, no definite measure of control could be formulated that would be applicable to all communities, but it did seem to be the general opinion that the following measures were best adapted to aid in the control of influenza—

1. Compulsory reporting of cases of patients ill with influenza.
2. Isolation of patient and quarantine if necessary.
3. Disinfection of discharges from the nose and throat.
4. Wearing of masks by attendants in sick room.
5. Care of the hands of patients.
6. Care of food utensils.
7. General closing orders, especially those places where crowding was most liable to occur.
8. Education and publicity.

As in the report of the Office of Vital Statistics, numerous tables were produced and included from the various divisions within the health department. Especially informative was one showing the incidence of communicable disease by month and another on the cases and death rates for the reportable diseases of 1918. From these two tables it is possible to track influenza cases and see them in the context of other infectious diseases.[27]

In the department's report for 1919, influenza was included among the diseases "dangerous to the public health." A total of 40,222 cases of influenza was reported for the year: 25,579 in January, 6,380 in February, and then a rapid decline in numbers over the remainder of the year. Altogether, 3,052 Massachusetts residents died of influenza in 1919 (Massachusetts Department of Health 1920). For 1920 the Department of Health noted another influenza epidemic, prevailing in January through March, with the vast majority of cases in February. A total of 35,633 cases was reported, with 1,660 deaths. The department dismissed the apparently high fatality rate, concluding that many mild cases of influenza went unreported and thus inflated the death rate. The format for reporting cases was similar to that in the previous two years. The department commented that had it not been for the 1918 epidemic, the 1920 epidemic would have been considered an "unprecedented disaster." "It is difficult to state just why such a complete reversal of sentiment occurred. The war and the influenza epidemic [of 1918] have perhaps accustomed our people to death in the mass to such an extent that the public poise is not shaken by occurrences that a few years ago would have produced almost a public hysteria" (Massachusetts Department of Public Health 1921: 13).

Rethinking Plague Time

In my reading of the archives and documents about the 1918 influenza in Massachusetts, I have focused on the local and not on the global. My aim has been to understand perceptions of the epidemic in the state, the county, and the community. By getting a sense of how the epidemic was experienced locally, I have attempted to build my understanding from the "bottom up." By backgrounding the *pandemic* and foregrounding the local *epidemic*, I focus on which other diseases and countervailing forces were in play. Is it possible, by doing so, to (re)contextualize the flu of 1918?[28]

Franklin County, Massachusetts, in the late nineteenth and early twentieth centuries had a mixed economy and a rural character at a time when most parts of the country were also considered rural, agricultural, and to have mixed economies. In this way the county may be more representative of a large cross section of Progressive Era America than might be perceived at first glance. Yet Massachusetts, as a state with historically high rates of literacy and a long tradition of vital registration and health surveillance, also has data that are virtually unequaled and a population comfortable with statistical summary. Consequently, the estimation and reconstruction of epidemiological events there hold some advantages over those for other states. With these points in mind I offer the following observations:

1. In the experience of most American communities at the time, the influenza epidemic of 1918 lasted not a year or a season but approximately a month. In the case of most Franklin County towns, it was the month of October. The temporality is important.
2. Whereas a few communities were hit hard and suffered many deaths, a large number of small communities may have had several cases

but very few or even no deaths. Such differences could occur in communities directly adjacent to one another.

3. Health professionals at the local level had to react in extreme ways during the height of the epidemic, but they were also preoccupied with the usual load of other infectious diseases, including the causes of infant mortality, childhood fevers, pulmonary tuberculosis, and poliomyelitis. By the time these people were fully mobilized, flu cases were already on the decline.

4. Propaganda and news of World War I dominated people's thoughts on the national level and took precedence over the epidemic. Unlike the observations Briggs and Herring (this volume) each report about the media's overplaying a disease threat and blaming and stereotyping those "at risk," in the Franklin County case the local media conveyed optimism and minimized fear.

5. Because of the previous two years' experience with polio, townspeople in Franklin County were somewhat accustomed to voluntary and forced closings of public meeting places, and children were acquainted with school closings because of scarlet fever outbreaks.

It is also easy in our twenty-first-century haze of logistic regressions, hazards models, and network analyses to forget how sophisticated and pioneering the mundane studies by nascent epidemiologists actually were. In them we see the underlying structure of the complex multivariate models, sophisticated time series, and likelihood estimates that were to come. The tables, charts, and graphs that preceded and then followed on the heels of the 1918 pandemic were more complex and informative than we sometimes give them due. As I have illustrated elsewhere (Swedlund 2010: chapter 8; Swedlund and Ball 1998), the analysis of infant mortality in the early decades of the twentieth century incorporated and weighted virtually all the variables that epidemiologists deploy in third world settings today, except for the microbiology. A look at Raymond Pearl's (1919) articles in *Public Health Reports* and A. J. McLaughlin's (1920) synopsis of research in the *Boston Medical and Surgical Journal* reminds us of the rich analyses that followed soon after 1918. If anything, there may have been a period of declining sophistication in conceptualizing disease causality during the immediate post-antibiotic era, as Herring has suggested. There is in these state reports and early studies much to enhance further exploration of Singer's syndemics, Noymer's selective mortality, Briggs's communicability (each in this volume), and other innovative approaches to the way we frame plagues.

Contrary to the impression I initially drew from Crosby (2003), Barry (2004), and their sources, influenza-pneumonia deaths in Franklin County were not neutral with respect to class and race (ethnicity). The hardest-hit neighborhoods in Franklin County were working class and located in factory villages in Greenfield, Montague, and Orange. The names of the dead were overwhelmingly eastern European, Irish, and French Canadian, with far fewer white Anglo-Saxon Protestants among them. The commercial elite residents of towns and the prosperous farmers outside the town centers *appear* to have been proportionally greater among the survivors. When one couples this with the fact that population density was a big factor in the 1918 flu epidemic (as always) and that Native Americans and First Nations peoples died at very high rates, as Barry (2004) attests, then this epidemic begins to look much more like most other epidemics from the past in terms of race and class (also see Noymer, this volume).[29]

I believe a large number of people in 1918 were poised to believe in Progressive Era positivism, and their own experiences suggested to them that their family's and the community's health was improving. They were able to recover that sense quickly after the epidemic passed and the war ended. In Massachusetts the crude death rate had been on a steady decline, from a high of about 21 per 1,000 in 1858 to about 15 per thousand in 1917. In 1918 it jumped back to 20 per thousand, but it fell again in 1919.

At the same time, death was no stranger to families in 1918. Despite the decline in infectious disease since the 1880s, infant mortality was still high in Massachusetts and the United States. There were almost 11,000 infant deaths in Massachusetts in 1918, compared with what the state thought at the time was about 13,800 deaths from influenza.[30] Almost 2,000 additional deaths were caused by measles, scarlet fever, diphtheria, and whooping cough together. Tuberculosis claimed 6,000 lives, and more than 800 women died from complications of childbirth. From this cluster of diseases alone it is easy to imagine losing a family member in any given year around the decade that included 1918. I suggest that people's feeling as if things were improving even while living in a time of high mortality served to dampen anxieties about and memories of influenza. Today's low mortality rates in the West, coupled with our recognition of virulent emerging and antibiotic-resistant diseases, now raises our anxiety over flu viruses such as H5N1 and H1N1 and projects it back to an earlier era (see Herring, this volume). Our postmodern sensibilities no longer provide the comfort given by a Progressive Era discourse.

Everyday mortality in 1918 was caused by infant diarrheas, child-hood fevers, tuberculosis, workplace accidents, war, cancer, and heart disease. At each stage in the life course there were significant risks to life.[31] They competed with influenza for people's attention in 1918. They interacted with flu to affect morbidity and mortality. Reminding ourselves of everyday mortality in small places, reconstructing domin-ant discourses, and recognizing the hard work of early investigators are all means by which we may be able to reenvision the 1918 flu and other historical plagues.

Afterword

On November 9, 2009, as I return this chapter to the editor, the world is experiencing the H1N1 "swine flu" pandemic of 2009. As in 1918, some flu cases were reported worldwide in April, and the largest numbers of cases so far have been reported for October and surely for November. The Centers for Disease Control reports approximately 22 million cases of the flu in the United States to date, with approximately 4,000 deaths (www.cdc.gov/H1N1FLU/). The population most at risk is reported to be children under four years of age and pregnant women. All evidence so far suggests that this will be a far milder experience with H1N1 than that which befell the world in the fall of 1918.

Notes

I would like to thank Reba-Jean Shaw-Pichette from the Education Department and Shirley Majewski of the Library of the Pocumtuck Valley Memorial Association, Deerfield, Massachusetts, for their help in providing research materials for this chapter. I thank D. Ann Herring for her helpful comments on a draft of this chapter.

1. The character Henry Chiver in Holman's historical novel had trained and been implicated with the notorious grave-robbing doctors Burke and Hare of Edinburgh, Scotland.

2. In 1918 the Russell Cutlery Factory was located in Turners Falls, Massachusetts. Employing several hundred workers, it was at one time in the late nineteenth century the largest cutlery factory in the world. Tuberculosis

was exacerbated among the workers because of the high level of particulate matter in the air, and respiratory disease was common.

3. This story is embellished and based loosely on a composite of scenes from the novel *Wickett's Remedy* (Goldberg 2005), a fictional account of the 1918 flu epidemic in Boston, Massachusetts.

4. This is not to say that there are not several outstanding exceptions to both observations. The Massachusetts Office of Vital Statistics and the Massachusetts Board of Health, for example, were by 1918 collecting quite detailed data and were capable of making complex inferences.

5. Portraying past experience is itself a thorny problem about which much has been written by historians, so I use the term advisedly. In this I have been influenced by the writings of Joan Scott, Herman Rebel, Barbara Bender, and others.

6. This point has also been made by Barry (2004), Kolata (1999), and many others.

7. Admittedly, these are popular accounts, but most critics agree that both Crosby's and Barry's research of the literature is of high caliber.

8. My mother was one of them; she was seven at the time. Her aunt died and two of her uncles were very ill. She remembered scores of people being sick and that she herself felt ill and had nosebleeds, but she was unsure whether she actually had the flu.

9. For overviews, see Barry 2004; Crosby 1976; Kolata 1999.

10. The fatality rate was estimated at 7.6 percent for all of Massachusetts in 1920. Massachusetts State Department of Health 1920: 231.

11. Estimates range as high as 675,000 deaths for Massachusetts. See, e.g. the Web site 1918.Pandemicflu.gov.

12. Of course the fatality rate would be lower if a larger number of cases were accepted.

13. Recent genetic analysis of the 1918 virus suggests an avian-to-human form that was both novel and particularly virulent. See, for example, Belshe 2005. Early studies (e.g., McLaughlin 1920) even suggested that females might have been at greater risk, but this may have stemmed from the problem of getting accurate age-specific sex ratio data by community during wartime.

14. There was as yet no mention of the flu in the local newspapers at this time.

15. For a discussion of the virulence of scarlet fever, inducing strep infections in the mid-nineteenth century, see Swedlund and Donta 2003.

16. See Oshinsky 2005. Polio first became a reportable disease in Massachusetts in 1909.

17. What I mean by "new age" is the combination of progressivism and scientific positivism that was the prevalent, if not dominant, discourse in 1918 America.

18. The following is adapted for this chapter from Swedlund n.d.

19. Rates for childhood fevers and tuberculosis are rates per 100,000 population, averaged over five years and centered on the census year (Office of the Secretary of State of Massachusetts 1915: table 64, 211). The report shows the distribution of deaths by age groupings and offers an extensive analysis of infant mortality, but no extensive analyses of deaths among other age groups. All rates are subject to errors due to underenumeration, misclassification of diseases, and changing age structure of the population at risk, but general trends are valid.

20. There were other newspapers, including the *Gazette and Courier* in Greenfield and the *Turners Falls Recorder*, but the *Greenfield Recorder* had a far larger circulation. Radio, although invented, was not a factor.

21. The first influenza deaths in Greenfield took place on 22 September, and the first official reporting on 26 September. Massachusetts State Department of Health 1918: 198.

22. Sunderland, Deerfield, and Conway had outbreaks in December 1918. These towns had managed to avoid large numbers of cases in the fall. *Greenfield Recorder*, 1 January 1919.

23. Information from Reba-Jean Shaw-Pichette, based on interviews at the Anchorage Nursing Home, and from quoted interviews in a *Greenfield Recorder* article on the 1918 flu, 27 October 2001.

24. All Franklin District Medical Society reports are taken from the minutes of the Franklin District Medical Society, PVMA archives.

25. Note the discrepancies between the towns' and the state's estimates for Greenfield and Montague. There were assuredly more than 201 deaths for Franklin County, but this estimate may not be too far off.

26. In fact, out of the state's appropriation of $253,950, the department managed to leave a balance of $11,655, not counting special appropriations. Massachusetts State Department of Health 1919: 36. In today's dollars, $253,950 would be equivalent to about $3 million.

27. A third table provided the number of cases and deaths for seventeen "diseases dangerous to the public health" for all 364 towns of Massachusetts, grouped by population size. It also included Camp Devens and the State Infirmary. The table did not include influenza but did include lobar pneumonia.

28. In Phillips's (2004) historiographic review of literature on the 1918 flu, he notes that many urban accounts have been written and several local accounts of other cities and towns as well, but the impression is that these tend to censor the communities' broader encounter with disease and social process.

29. McLaughlin (1920) mentions Slavs. Jones (2005) notes that in Canada, recent immigrants were not stigmatized in 1918 as they had been during

previous smallpox and cholera epidemics. More typical for New England would probably be the results reported by Fanning (2008) for Norwood, Massachusetts. Tuckel and co-workers (2006) suggest that the distribution of flu deaths in Hartford, Connecticut, can be explained largely by location of ethnic neighborhoods.

30. This estimate missed many of the deaths due to pneumonia, but not all of them. Office of the Secretary of State of Massachusetts 1918: 98–107.

31. For morbidity we would certainly have to add venereal disease and polio.

The Coming Plague of Avian Influenza

D. Ann Herring and Stacy Lockerbie

In 1997, a new strain of avian influenza virus, identified as H5N1 by the antigens sprouting from its surface coat, emerged in Hong Kong Special Administrative Region. It infected eighteen people and killed six. The World Health Organization ordered the slaughter of all chickens in the territory because it was believed that human infections resulted from direct contact with infected poultry. Images of masked officials killing poultry were transmitted around the world. The year 1997 thus represents the moment when avian influenza, now referred to as H5N1 HPAI (highly pathogenic avian influenza), can be said to have emerged as a human disease.

Diseases that emerge are rarely new; rather, they have "come into view" in the communities threatened by them. Outbreaks of avian influenza in poultry farms and wet markets had been reported in Hong Kong earlier that year, as well as in Guangdong Province, China, in 1996 (WHO 2007). Early recognition of the Hong Kong epizootic was facilitated by the fact that the territory has been a center for research on influenza ecology since the 1970s (Shortridge, Peiris, and Guan 2003). Highly pathogenic avian influenza is not a new disease; it has been known to affect poultry since 1878 (Martin et al. 2006). The newest strain of HPAI came into view, however, during an era of viral panic (Tomes 2000), a period in which a narrative about "the coming plague" had already been constructed and anchored to past epidemics (see Briggs, this volume; Herring 2008; Wald 2008). Described as "the single greatest threat facing the world" (Waltner-Toews 2007: 6), avian influenza is feared to be the coming plague.

179

In this essay we consider the story line for the coming plague, as expressed through fears about avian influenza, and the widespread communication of this story line through official international bodies such as the World Health Organization and through other media. International worries about avian influenza and the development of international health and agricultural standards have been translated into national policy and practice and have come to circumscribe the lives of people living at the disease's epicenters. To illustrate who is actually being plagued by avian influenza, we consider the case of farmers in Vietnam whose livelihoods are being undermined, reshaped, and transfigured because of global worries about the pandemic of influenza that has yet to come.

Situating Avian Influenza

> It all begins in Asia.
>
> —A. Mandavilla, "Report on Bird Flu"

Killing the chickens in Hong Kong may have stopped the epizootic of avian influenza in 1997, but it failed to stamp out the virus. H5N1 HPAI remains endemic in poultry in many parts of Asia and continues to evolve under the conditions of the third epidemiologic transition, conditions that bring human and avian hosts together in unprecedented concentrations, in new, age-related demographic configurations, and in a context of rapidly globalizing and urbanizing economies in which networks have expanded and transportation times are short because of air travel (Barrett, this volume; Morse 1993; Waltner-Toews 1995). Scaled-up versions of agricultural systems, responding to ramped-up urban market demand for low-cost protein in the twenty-first century, increase the chances of the emergence of new strains of avian influenza (Waltner-Toews 2007). Aquaculture, an ecologically efficient and ancient system of agriculture commonly practiced in Southeast Asia, brings ducks, pigs, and humans together in close contact, creating opportunities for the transmission of influenza strains across species (Hollenbeck 2005; Ito et al. 1998; Scholtissek 1992, 1994).

Scientific and media attention have linked the threat of a global human flu pandemic to Southeast Asian farming practices, especially aquaculture. Because most of the laboratory-confirmed human deaths from HPAI have occurred in Southeast Asia (WHO 2009), international strategies for dealing with the disease are focused on this region (FAO

2007). As the regional origin of most new influenza viruses and the source of SARS in 2003, Asia has been excoriated in the international media for its agricultural and health practices. China, in particular, has been labeled "the incubator for a global epidemic of avian influenza" (Kaufman 2008: S9).

Communities affected with avian influenza are depicted as filthy, backward places (lacking modernity) where subsistence farmers live in poverty, close to animals, and shop in crowded live-animal markets. These stigmatizing images convey the conjoined ideas that Asian farms and markets are dangerous to global health and that Asian farmers and market vendors are irresponsible citizens of the world (Herring 2008; Lockerbie and Herring 2008). In the aftermath of the 2003 SARS epidemic, Southeast Asia has become imbued with what Ungar described as the mutation-contagion package of fear (Ungar 1998). Its people suffer disproportionately from the disease itself and from condemnation for creating the context that allowed both SARS and H5N1 HPAI to emerge. Yet the poultry (chicken) industry has intensified worldwide, which means that a pandemic could erupt anywhere HPAI occurs (Shortridge, Peiris, and Guan 2003), not just from viruses circulating in the foreign, faraway reaches of Asia.

Generating Viral Panic: The Pathogen

All the prerequisites for the start of a pandemic have been met save one.

—K. Stöhr, "Avian Influenza and Pandemics"

Apart from the classic representation of the coming pandemic as an external threat, originating elsewhere (Slack 1992: 4), anxiety about HPAI is magnified by the mysteries that surround the mutable virus itself. Details of its evolution and spread dominate much of what is written about an impending plague. Considerable media attention accompanied the announcement in 2003, for example, that a more highly pathogenic strain of H5N1 HPAI, known as the Z strain, had been identified. Deadly to a wider range of species, including mammals and birds that normally harbor less pathogenic strains, the Z strain was also resistant to first-line antiviral drugs (Monto 2005). Announcements in rapid succession of outbreaks of H5N1 highly pathogenic avian influenza in Southeast Asian countries and of another deadly strain in the Netherlands, a wealthy Western nation, reinforced the sense of expanding, imminent danger.

Experience with the SARS outbreak seemed to confirm the strong suspicion that an avian influenza pandemic among humans had the "potential to slip past extensive surveillance and control mechanisms" (Weir 2005: 870). Mounting concern over a pandemic is reflected in a shift in 2003 in the number of newspaper and wire service articles in the United States that covered the threat of pandemic influenza: the volume more than quadrupled, to 746 items, in comparison with a relatively stable coverage of about 160 items in each of the intervening years since the Hong Kong outbreak in 1997 (Trust for Health 2006).

Diseases that travel and cross boundaries evoke fear because "the edge of safety cannot be defined" (Humphreys 2002: 847). To keep medical officials and the general public informed, the official WHO Web site for avian influenza presents regularly updated maps showing the cumulative cases of avian influenza worldwide (WHO n.d.). Although mapping—especially participatory mapping—can be an effective way of studying spatial aspects of disease and engaging community interest in local health issues (Nichter 2008: 165–167), historical studies show that tracking the path of a disease serves to increase panic (Humphreys 2002: 850). By 2006, the Z strain was reported to have spread west through the Middle East, Africa, and Europe (WHO 2006). In November that year, the World Health Organization issued an alert that the H5N1 bird flu virus could precipitate a pandemic for which most nations were unprepared (*Nature* 2006). In January 2007, H5N1 was reported in the United Kingdom on a farm in Norfolk (*Nature* 2007). Scientific and media reports presented the story line of a new, untreatable virus, spreading inexorably from Asia to the rest of the world (Herring 2008; Lockerbie and Herring 2008).

Despite this frightening image, the documented human cost of avian influenza as of May 2009 was a mere 423 confirmed cases and 258 deaths (WHO 2009). This relatively small toll accrued over the course of seven years of reports (2002–2008) from fifteen countries— slow progress for a simmering plague, a plague about to be (Trostle, this volume), a "virtual epidemic" (Rosenberg 2008: S6). Compare this with the situation for malaria, which in 2006 alone gave rise to an estimated 247 million cases and 881,000 deaths (WHO 2008). Most countries affected by epizootics of avian influenza have experienced fewer than five human deaths, and most of the reported deaths have been concentrated in five nations: China, Egypt, Indonesia, Thailand, and Vietnam. The history of epidemics shows that the panic engendered by a disease bears no relation to the level of morbidity and mortality it produces (Humphreys 2002: 846). Epidemics, however, are "sited in time and place" and configured by social values, collective experience, medical knowledge, and demographic and ecological circumstances (Rosenberg 2008: S4).

One of the dominant themes in contemporary writing about avian influenza is worry about its potential to evolve into a pathogen dangerous to human life on a global scale. "Sloppy, capricious and promiscuous" (Weir 2005: 869), avian influenza crosses the species barrier with ease as co-infected hosts become unwitting "mixing vessels" for a new strain (Palese 1993; Scholtissek 1992, 1994). It is unpredictable. Apprehension about an avian influenza pandemic seems undiminished by evidence that the majority of human HPAI occurs through direct infection from live or dead birds (WHO 2007). There are documented cases of person-to-person spread (see Rosenthal 2006; WHO 2007), but the virus's preference for cells in the deepest tissues of the human lung seems to constrain its ability to be broadcast by coughs and sneezes (Shinya et al. 2006).

So far, HPAI is engaged in "viral chatter," generating sporadic outbreaks of a zoonotic disease among people who are in close contact with its primary animal reservoirs. Many of these people are young and play a role in poultry farming, such as culling and defeathering birds, or in food preparation (WHO 2006: 256; see Barrett, this volume). Yet it is feared that natural evolutionary processes, outside the control of laboratory science, threaten the world: "All the prerequisites for the start of a pandemic have been met save one—namely, genetic changes in this virus that would allow it to achieve efficient human-to-human transmission" (Stöhr 2005: 4).

Generating Viral Panic: Anchoring Avian Influenza to the 1918 Pandemic

Fears about the potential damage of avian influenza—well beyond its small count of human infections and deaths—are augmented because it has been anchored to devastating epidemics of the past (Herring 2008; Lockerbie and Herring 2008; Rosenberg 2008). Scholarly and media accounts of the coming plague of avian influenza almost invariably make reference to the 1918 influenza pandemic, which is estimated to have killed from 50 million to 100 million people worldwide (Johnson and Mueller 2002). This shackles avian influenza to "the catastrophe against which all modern pandemics are measured" (Pandemics and Pandemic Threats since 1900: 1), even though other, more recent, less virulent influenza pandemics are available as models (Barrett, this volume; Herring 2008).

Rarely mentioned, moreover, is the considerable heterogeneity in mortality from the 1918 pandemic, which disproportionately affected tubercular persons, immigrant and economically disadvantaged neighborhoods, marginalized communities that lacked access to health care, and countries with developing economies (Johnson and Mueller 2002; Jones 2005; Lux 1997; Mamelund 2006; Noymer, this volume; Noymer and Garenne 2000, 2003). That said, there are relatively few national histories of influenza that place the 1918 pandemic within that history (Phillips 2004: 130–131); neither are there careful considerations of the way in which the influenza virus interacted with locally variable, co-circulating pathogens. Preoccupation with the detailed genetics of the influenza virus, its phylogeny and mutability, has overshadowed the fact that even in the pre-antibiotic year of 1918, most influenza sufferers survived, recovering within about a week. Those who succumbed did so because they also had secondary infections that gave rise to fatal pneumonia (Burnet and Clark 1942: 88; Frost 1919; Jordan 1927; Kilbourne 2006). The next pandemic of influenza, whether avian or some other strain, will therefore likely take its greatest toll in parts of the world where social circumstances promote clustering, transmission, and interactions between co-circulating pathogens, thereby giving rise to syndemics (Singer, this volume; Singer and Clair 2003).

The selectively described story of the destruction of the 1918 pandemic, which leaves out many important details of its variability and ignores the complicated environments of risk that affected its manifestations, justifies the search for the killer virus that waits to be unleashed. The chain linking avian influenza (H5N1) to the 1918 pandemic (H1N1) was shortened in October 2005 with the publication of the genome for the H1N1 strain associated with the pandemic. At one time, H1N1 was believed to have resulted from genetic recombination of human and swine influenza strains. Polymerase chain reaction analysis of lung tissue sampled from three people who died during the autumn 1918 wave of influenza called this interpretation into question. Instead, the new analysis suggested that the 1918 variant descended from an ancestor that originally infected birds, because its genome appeared to be primarily avian (Taubenberger et al. 2005). This interpretation met vigorous challenges (see Gibbs and Gibbs 2006; Hollenbeck 2005), but it helped bind avian influenza even more closely to the iconic 1918 pandemic as the idea that the pandemic most likely resulted from bird-to-human transmission gained traction in the scientific literature (see Hollenbeck

2005; Kristensson 2005; *Nature* 2007). When several macaques were experimentally injected with the reconstructed H1N1 virus in 2007, researchers reported observing a "cytokine storm," an overreaction by the immune system that overwhelmed the monkeys' lungs (Kawaoka 2007). This suggested to some observers that the lethality of the 1918 pandemic had little to do with secondary bacterial infections or the quality of medical care at the time; the virus itself was responsible for the virulence of the 1918 pandemic (Chatterjee 2007: 1; for an alternative point of view, see Brundage and Shanks 2008; Noymer, this volume).

Generating Viral Panic: Harnessing Avian Influenza to Bioterrorism

Publication of the genome of the 1918 virus in October 2005 also served to harness concerns about bioterrorism to avian influenza. The announcement in the top-ranked science journal, *Nature* (2005: 794), that "the 1918 flu virus is resurrected" gave rise to the sickening realization that a new, effective bioweapon was now available. Panic demand drove up prices for influenza drugs such as Tamiflu, which in October 2005 sold for as much as US$174 per packet on public auction sites such as eBay (*Nature* 2007). Highlighting influenza's place on the list of potential weapons of mass destruction, along with the scarcity of influenza chemoprophylaxis, added more layers of worry about avian influenza, global safety, and biosecurity.

It is perhaps unsurprising that these worries were fueled by and, in turn, fueled media and public attention. In the aftermath of publication of these events in 2005, news items covering pandemic influenza in the United States soared to 8,998—a remarkable, sixtyfold increase over the 165 newspaper and wire service articles on pandemic influenza published in 1997, at the time of the Hong Kong outbreak (Trust for Health 2006). The search volume index for "bird flu" on Google Trends shows a similar burst of global Internet traffic in the last quarter of 2005 and the first half of 2006. Peaks in traffic occurred on 18 October 2005, when the European Union announced that bird flu was a global threat; on 6 January 2006, when bird flu was reported to have spread to Turkey; and on 20 February 2006, when it was identified in Nigeria. This was a remarkable reaction to a plague that had not yet happened but for which a well-developed story line was circulating widely (Briggs, this volume; Wald 2008). The story itself had become contagious (Nichter 2008: 5).

Generating Viral Panic: Pandemic Preparedness

The identification of an epidemic hinges on who decides what evidence is acceptable, who does the counting, and who interprets and communicates the situation to the public. Epidemics are, by their very nature, products of bureaucratic processes and biopolitics (Briggs, this volume; Nichter 2008; Trostle, this volume). Ironically, immediate, comprehensive, and responsible reactions by national, regional, and international public health bodies aroused concerns about the potential for a human pandemic of HPAI. H5N1 viruses have been monitored closely since the 1997 Hong Kong outbreak to determine whether they are coming closer to causing a pandemic (Layne et al. 2001). The control and prevention of avian influenza is a top priority for the World Health Organization, which introduced a pandemic preparedness plan in 1999. In 2002, WHO introduced a global agenda on influenza to guide, support, and coordinate influenza research, control, and surveillance (Webster, Plotkin, and Dodet 2005). These initiatives led to more comprehensive reports of avian influenza from fifty countries (WHO 2007). Many nations have invested heavily in pandemic planning (WHO 1999), signifying the success of the international health bureaucracy in communicating its priorities to national political bodies.

More frequent reports of cases are an inevitable outcome of enhanced surveillance and wider coverage, leading to the unavoidable impression that the threat of avian influenza is on the upswing. It is worth remembering, however, that most of the outbreaks of HPAI were epizootics that occurred among poultry and wild birds. Human cases have been reported in only fifteen countries, ten of which have each accumulated fewer than twenty cases during the past seven years (WHO 2009). But even single cases of infected birds, such as the parrot imported to the United Kingdom that died from H5N1 avian influenza in October 2005 (BBC 2005), have come to be treated as ominous, internationally newsworthy events and as potential threats to global human health.

Avian influenza has become part of a growing list of emerging, re-emerging, and antimicrobial-resistant diseases that nourishes a twenty-first-century obsession with killer germs, bioterrorism, biosecurity, and coming plagues (Mattix et al. 2006; Tomes 2000). Influenza's shape-shifting and promiscuous qualities and its ability to cross boundaries rapidly and devastate communities at great distances, coupled with its links to the 1918 pandemic, make it a potent metaphor for the risks of globalization. The story of the coming pandemic of avian influenza follows Priscilla Wald's "formulaic plot that begins with the identification of an emerging infection, includes discussion of the global networks throughout which it travels, and chronicles the epidemiological work that ends with its containment" (Wald 2008: 2). Viral panic about avian influenza has its origins in technoscientific medicine, international laboratories, projections based on the experience of the 1918 pandemic, the experience of SARS, fears of bioterrorism, the policies of international organizations, and news accounts. It now circulates around the world. This narrative about an imminent pandemic plagues the lives of ordinary people who are subject to international protocols designed to save the world from H5N1 HPAI.

Generating Viral Panic: The Marketplace

Avian influenza is not simply a health issue; it has significant implications for world trade, domestic economies, and the marketplace. Asia contributes a large proportion of the more than 88 million tons of chicken produced annually (Waltner-Toews 2007: 103). Between 1994 and 2004, its poultry industry increased from 4 billion to 16 billion birds (Nikiforuk 2005), part of an ever-larger demand for low-cost animal protein, particularly among growing urban populations (Waltner-Toews 2007: 109). The 2003 avian influenza outbreak associated with the Z strain of H5N1 HPAI devastated trade, and poultry markets melted down in response to consumer fears about poultry product safety. International demand plummeted in the wake of import bans on trading partners affected by HPAI. Purchasers shifted away from Asian suppliers, especially Thailand and China, and turned to South American sources (FAO 2007). In 2003, for example, Thailand was a leading international poultry exporter, mostly to Japan and the European Union; chicken production, feed, and processing was a central sector in the national economy. In 2004, thousands of tons of its poultry exports were rejected and sent back from Europe, Japan, and South Korea, giving rise to a national agropolitical crisis (Chanyapate and Delforge 2004). Investors were warned that avian influenza could precipitate a global financial crisis (Cooper and Coxe 2005: 4).

The main method used to stop the spread of infection was, and is, killing infected flocks. More than 250 million chickens have either died from avian influenza or been exterminated (FAO 2007). Beyond the effect on the birds themselves, the effects of avian influenza have been felt most keenly by rural farmers whose livelihoods have been shattered by the disease and by international policies, enacted locally, aimed at limiting its spread. The 250 million chickens that have been culled came primarily from family farms in rural communities, because chicken is often the cheapest animal protein in developing countries. Avian influenza eradication policies therefore place a large economic burden on rural farmers, who are the most vulnerable to economic failures, food insecurity, and nutritional inadequacies (Chanyapate and Delforge 2004; FAO 2007; Waltz 2006).

We now turn to the case of Vietnam to consider some of the other ways in which anxiety about avian influenza, impelled by the outbreak narrative and put into practice through international policy, is felt in the day-to-day lives of people who raise poultry in an HPAI epicenter (for a more detailed discussion, see Lockerbie and Herring 2008).

Avian Influenza in Vietnam

An island of viral suppression in a sea of transmission ...

—Maryn McKenna, "Vietnam's Success against Avian Flu
May Offer Blueprint for Others"

Vietnam was one of the first countries affected by avian influenza H5N1; its first human infection was identified in December 2003. With 106 confirmed human cases and 52 deaths in the subsequent six years (39 of which occurred in 2004–2005), it ranks second only to Indonesia among countries currently most severely affected by HPAI (WHO 2009). Outbreaks of infectious disease are international embarrassments that draw attention to government failures to enact effective social and public health policies (Farmer 1999).

The international strategy for preventing a human pandemic of avian influenza targets the control of HPAI in poultry (FAO 2007). The outbreaks of avian influenza in Vietnam prompted the Vietnamese government to introduce preventive measures to preserve trade and foreign investment, rid itself of the stigma of avian influenza (see Barrett and Brown 2008), and rehabilitate its international image. Officials actively participated in international meetings designed to develop protocols for ensuring the safety of the poultry industry and in 2005 hosted the regional meeting of the UN Food and Agriculture Organization (FAO) and the International Epizootic Office (OIE) on avian influenza control in Asia in Ho Chi Minh City (FAO 2007: ix). Vietnamese government officials implemented a stringent policy of culling and vaccinating flocks and an intensive disease surveillance program that monitors poultry at every phase of production (*People's*

Daily Online 2007). In 2004, approximately 66 million birds were culled, and Vietnam was the first nation to implement mandatory poultry vaccination after the 2005 outbreak. This "island of viral suppression in a sea of transmission" was achieved because thousands of small farmers were willing to comply with government orders (McKenna 2006a: 1).

The practice of keeping poultry is widespread in Vietnam, and raising birds bolsters the household economies of about half of all rural and urban households. In the northern regions, 90 percent or more of households keep poultry. Most are small-scale operations, falling within the UN Food and Agriculture Organization's smallest category, one to fifty kilograms of poultry production per year, with a per capita household income of less than US$200 per year. Only about 1 percent of the flocks exceed one hundred birds (Otte, Roland-Holst, and Pfeiffer 2006; Pfeiffer 2006). As a result, the food sources and incomes of Vietnam's rural poor were badly battered when 66 million birds were exterminated in 2004 and mandatory poultry vaccination was instituted after the 2005 outbreak (Rivière-Cinnamond, Cuc, and Wollny 2005).

Represented in the international discourse as reservoirs of global infection, household flocks are reservoirs of family savings in the event of unexpected difficulties or shortfalls. For small farmers, poultry is a buffer against food insecurity, an investment and economic hedge. Eaten occasionally, often as prescribed by the lunar calendar, backyard birds also make up for long-term nutritional deficiencies and contribute to family health. Family birds have important social meanings beyond nutrition and household economics. Birds are slaughtered to commemorate special occasions such as weddings or saved to be slaughtered and eaten during festivities that honor ancestors. Even in fishing villages, where chicken has little effect on the daily diet, it is greatly missed as a food for special occasions (for a more detailed discussion, see Lockerbie and Herring 2008).

Another plank in Vietnam's strategy to limit avian influenza, guided by WHO and FAO recommendations, involves phasing out live bird markets and replacing them with Western-style supermarkets that sell dead birds, killed in government-sanctioned slaughterhouses (FAO 2007; McKenna 2006b). Supermarkets are expensive, urban places, patronized largely by the elites. By their very nature and location they exclude the large portion of the Vietnamese population that lives in rural communities—the people most directly affected by restrictions on poultry. People who regularly frequent live bird markets establish trading relationships with specific vendors to ensure both a fair price and that they are buying food that is safe to eat. These markets are not only centers for social life in rural communities but also places where a carefully nurtured system of trust and commitment among market sellers and market goers is enacted (Lockerbie and Herring 2008).

A major plank of the Vietnamese government's policy to control avian influenza, informed by FAO strategy, involves eliminating backyard operations and reorganizing poultry production along a Western model into large, biosecure farms (McKenna 2006a: 2). Government-sanctioned and commercial farms are promoted as safe and clean, even though these are the settings in developed countries where avian influenza erupts. Much of the research points out, indeed, that the large-scale, international poultry industry—not small-scale poultry farmers—creates favorable conditions for the emergence of new strains of avian influenza. The economies of scale for chicken production and disease are the same: "Small farms have outbreaks, big farms breed epidemics; globalization of big farms creates pandemics" (Waltner-Toews 2007: 104). The influenza virus spreads slowly among small village chicken flocks and fades out under low-density conditions, but it amplifies rapidly in densely packed factory farms. Factory farms will not solve the HPAI problem when "some of the largest outbreaks of avian influenza have been in some of the best-managed poultry operations in the world, in some of the wealthiest countries" (Waltner-Toews 2007: 111). Even Thailand, where backyard poultry operations have largely been replaced by a contract farming system that produces chicken mainly for export (about 90 percent), was not immune to avian influenza (Chanyapate and Delforge 2004).

Finally, the poultry-rearing practices being suppressed to achieve control over HPAI and prevent an influenza plague are precisely those promoted for decades as the solution to economic development in Vietnam. An export-based economy that focused production on particular food items (such as chicken, rice, and farmed shrimp) in specific regions was introduced to improve the incomes of the rural poor as well as the nation's domestic economy as a whole (Lockerbie 2006). The avian influenza problem stretches beyond the sphere of health to draw attention to the unintended consequences of development initiatives once promoted as sustainable economic improvements (Lockerbie and Herring 2008).

Plagued by a Plague-Yet-to-Be

Avian influenza (H5N1 HPAI), whose origin is understood to be Southeast Asian, is a central element of global panic about "the coming plague."

With its shape-shifting coat, ability to acquire genes from other viruses, and likelihood of traversing biological and geographical boundaries, it is a potent symbol of the fears of globalization. It has "mirrored our fears, stoked our xenophobia about non-Western societies being alien and dangerous" (Rosenberg 2008: S6). Anchored to the story line of the 1918 influenza pandemic, H5N1 avian influenza contributes to a deep foreboding that a global cataclysm lurks in the farming communities and markets of Southeast Asia, waiting to be unleashed. Attempts to control avian influenza in Southeast Asia, guided by policies and reports from sentinel international organizations, are embedded in a climate of viral panic in which the relatively small count of human deaths from H5N1 HPAI has gained enormous significance in the accounts of its coming destruction. The power to define a plague lies in the hands of these organizations. Countries such as Indonesia that snub international health regulations and signed agreements with the World Health Organization in the name of "viral sovereignty" are censured as morally reprehensible mavericks and dangerous to global safety (Holbrooke and Garrett 2008: 1).

Yet the people who are most plagued by the pandemic yet-to-come are rural farmers living at the epicenters of avian influenza. In Vietnam and elsewhere (Chanyapate and Delforge 2004; GRAIN 2006), it is the rural poor, whose livelihoods are sustained or supplemented by small household flocks of poultry, who bear the cost of international policies aimed at protecting global biosecurity and the future of humanity.

Past into Present

History and the Making of Knowledge about HIV/Aids and Aboriginal People

Mary-Ellen Kelm

There are many histories of AIDS. One such history is characterized by an enormous crevasse of consciousness (Gilman 1988; Grmek 1990; Shilts 1987). This is the story we all know—the story of a generation's first confrontation with death, of a time when the promise of sexual freedom appeared ruthlessly withdrawn by a mysterious disease affecting our brothers in the gay community just at the moment when the "moral majority" was claiming a voice at the highest levels of American politics. It is also a story of change in medicine. The emergence of new infectious diseases such as AIDS marked an end to the so-called golden age of medicine brought about by the application of antisepsis, antibiotics, and vaccines. It is a story, too, of patient activism so strong and so effective that the nature of clinical trials was forever transformed (Rothman 2003). It is a story, we are told, of political inaction, even scientific disdain, forced to account to a populace activated by the enormous force of AIDS-aware cultural production (Berridge and Strong 1992; Crimp and Roston 1990; Patton 2002). It is the story of the movies *And the Band Played On* and *Philadelphia*, of Liz Taylor and Bronski Beat, of red ribbons. This is the story we all know, this story of rupture.

Another story is characterized not by rupture but by resonance. This is the story that the historian hears as health professionals, representatives of international development agencies, municipal politicians, and members of political organizations of dissent speak of AIDS in Africa, in Asia, in urban zones of poverty and despair, and in "Indian country" across North America. The two stories are neither distinct nor discordant, for they overlap, sometimes harmonizing, in many ways. One story of resonance is that of HIV/AIDS in Aboriginal communities in North America. The disease has been characterized over the last fifteen years as an "emerging epidemic," and substantial government funding, health research, and surveillance of Aboriginal communities have been devoted to monitoring the spread of HIV in First Nations (Lachmann 2002; McKenna 1993).

The picture that emerges is alarming not so much because it is new as because it is so old. History appears to repeat itself, not just in the reemergence of infectious disease as a factor in Aboriginal mortality but also as an influence on the knowledge produced about Aboriginal people. Health research about Aboriginal people and HIV/AIDS is built on a scaffolding of past research (medical, historical, and anthropological) that characterized Aboriginal communities as spaces of pathogenic behavior and Aboriginal bodies as highly mobile vectors of transmission, always on the verge of destruction. This chapter intersects with Briggs's discussion of biocommunication (this volume) in that it is clear that concern about HIV/AIDS among First Nations pre-dated elevated rates of infection and was rooted, in part, in a historical awareness of epidemic disease in Aboriginal history.

I begin the chapter with the role played by history in instigating research that anticipated AIDS in Aboriginal communities. I proceed with an exploration of the relationship between historical ideas about Aboriginal vulnerability, health disparities, and definitions of risk. At the center of the story is a profound crisis of representation (Hammond 1997). How do we talk about AIDS—a disease for which the principle preventive measure is education—in populations that have been, through colonial discourse, repeatedly sexualized and pathologized, without playing into, replicating, and reifying those old stereotypes? I propose that the first step may be to use the historian as interlocutor to help uncover the historical scaffolding that surrounds contemporary health research involving Aboriginal people and HIV. I experiment with the historical methodology of "reading against the grain" as a way to answer the call of some Aboriginal epidemiologists for a strength-based approach to HIV/AIDS research.[1] I offer no sustained critique of health research involving Aboriginal people, but I do offer a historian's reading of that work, one that might help locate and then disrupt the patterns of the past that are imbedded in the present.

Anticipating AIDS

It took nearly two decades for HIV/AIDS to appear at statistically significant levels in Aboriginal communities in Canada and the United States. The first reported AIDS case in an Aboriginal person came to the attention of the US Centers for Disease Control and Prevention (CDC) in 1982.[2] But throughout the 1980s, the number of AIDS cases involving American Indians and Alaska Natives (as the CDC calls Aboriginal people in the United States; hereafter AI/ANs) remained small, at only 272 (235 males, 38 females) reported to the CDC by 30 June 1991. This figure stands in comparison with 182,561 reported AIDS cases in the United States by the same date. Cumulative incidence rates in the United States also remained relatively low, so that by the beginning of the second decade of AIDS, the incidence rate for AI/ANs was 13.7 cases per 100,000, relative to an American incidence rate of 74 cases per 100,000 (Conway 1992; Sullivan 1991). The situation was similar in Canada. In 1994, there were only 93 reported AIDS cases among First Nations people, accounting for only 1.6 percent of all of Canada's approximately 2,000 AIDS cases and a miniscule number in the context of a worldwide AIDS epidemic of an estimated 4 million cases and 16 million HIV-infected people (Du Bois 1996; Tseng 1996). Moreover, Aboriginal people were not disproportionately represented. In 1997, AIDS cases in the AI/AN population numbered 1,783, making up about 0.3 percent of all cases, less than the 1 percent of persons that AI/ANs contributed to the national population in the United States. Incidence rates at mid-decade, moreover, were very similar to those affecting "whites" and were seven times lower and three times lower, respectively, than rates for the African American and Hispanic populations (*Morbidity and Mortality Weekly Report* 1998).

Health researchers and Aboriginal leaders were wary of such numbers. History seemed to suggest that if HIV/AIDS had not yet hit First Nations, it soon would. Indeed, health researchers cited historical examples of epidemic devastation, the culpability of settler societies in the spread of disease, and the failure of government to act effectively on behalf of First Nations. George Conway began his study of HIV infection among Aboriginal people by reminding readers that "AI/AN are a minority population that has suffered disproportionately from infectious disease epidemics" (Conway 1992: 803). Irene Vernon, summarizing the place of HIV/AIDS among Native Americans by the year 2000, reminded readers of government incompetence when dealing with smallpox in the nineteenth century and wrote that "today, many refer to AIDS as the new smallpox" (Vernon 2001: 1). Christina Mitchell and a team of researchers from the Rosebud (Sioux) reservation made a similar connection: "Indigenous peoples have historically suffered disproportionately from epidemics of infectious diseases such as smallpox, measles, and tuberculosis, which have weakened and in some cases completely destroyed entire nations. As a result of this history of devastating epidemics, HIV and AIDS are of special concern to a number of AI communities" (Mitchell et al. 2002: 402). Others talked about the perception that "AIDS is another form of germ warfare on Indians" and used terms such as *ethnocide* and *genocide* to describe the history of Aboriginal people in North America (Simoni, Sehgal, and Walters 2004: 33). Health researchers used such references to the past to raise alarms about a not-yet-emerging epidemic of AIDS among Aboriginal people.

How might the "new smallpox" be avoided? The answer has been research. Researchers writing in anticipation of an Aboriginal AIDS epidemic called for more surveillance and a review of the procedures then in place to signal its emergence (Crown et al. 1993; Hall et al. 1990; Mill 2000; Ramirez et al. 2002) Indeed, the concern among health researchers that critical moments of AIDS prevention were being lost while they waited for HIV to appear among Aboriginal people prompted studies of the classification and surveillance systems that some suspected might be underestimating HIV/AIDS among American Indian populations. A Los Angeles County study concluded that Native Americans were underrepresented by as much at 50 percent in surveillance statistics, and an Oklahoma study speculated that incidence rates for other sexually transmitted diseases (STDs) would increase by as much as 57 percent if racial misclassification was corrected (Bertolli et al. 2004; Lieb 1992). All this work tended toward the conclusion that the apparent low incidence of HIV/AIDS in Aboriginal populations of North America was the result of poor surveillance. The corollary was that greater surveillance and better classification were needed. That such classification was built on a scaffolding of historical policies that defined who was and who was not an Indian, and that such policies were themselves crafted in particularly political, economic, and gendered ways, was not acknowledged in this literature but is a point to which I return momentarily (Duster 2003).

Anticipating an AIDS epidemic among Aboriginal people also focused attention on sentinel infections, particularly STDs (Bullock et al. 1993, 1996; Calzavara et al. 1998; Lee et al. 1987; Orr et al. 1994; Romanowski et al. 1991). Research has generated considerable knowledge about STDs and sexual practices among First Nations people. Studies reported high rates of chlamydia, gonorrhea, and syphilis among Aboriginal women in both Canada and the United States (McNaughton et al. 2005; Mitchell et al. 2002; Tseng 1996). Health care workers worried that these STDs would facilitate the spread of HIV once it was introduced to the population (Sullivan 1991). Researchers raised levels of concern even higher through studies of condom use, sexual activity during travel, and sexual activity between Aboriginal and non-Aboriginal partners. A study conducted in the mid-1990s in which a team of non-Native researchers employed Aboriginal investigators to interview nearly seven hundred reserve residents about their sexual practices found that 61 percent never used condoms. In a small study of Aboriginal people living in New York City, 73 percent of those involved said they had not used condoms in the previous six months (Calzavara et al. 1998; Walters, Simoni, and Harris 2000). Aboriginal people interviewed in Montreal in the mid-1990s indicated that men traveling to the city from remote communities tended to "sleep around," and an Alaskan study from the same period showed that non-Native drug-using men refused condom use when engaging in sex with Aboriginal women (Baldwin 2000; Du Bois 1996).

By the turn of the twenty-first century, health professionals had amassed a considerable archive of data related to the sexual lives of Aboriginal people, before an AIDS epidemic among Aboriginals had emerged. Politicians and health care workers, drawing on more than a decade of health research, were still warning against "erroneous over-optimism" based on "current statistics" (Ramirez et al. 2002: 29) and expressing fear that Native Americans could be "the next brush fire in the HIV epidemic" (*AIDS Alert* 2001: 27; see also Garmaise 2003b: 27; Waldram, Herring, and Young 2006).

It seems, then, that an awareness of history and a refusal to see Aboriginal people as isolated populations stimulated significant surveillance even before HIV/AIDS was epidemic in that population. Certainly, identifying First Nations as a population at risk has been crucial to obtaining research funding. In the United States, tribal leaders and Native organizations have pressed government to see beyond their relatively low infection rates, in comparison with other minority populations, and to invest in research on American Indians and Alaska Natives separate from other "people of color" initiatives (Vernon 2001). Support from the Centers for Disease Control for research on Aboriginal AIDS, for example, emerged in 1988 and has been renewed, most recently, in two initiatives begun in 2003. These were the Minority HIV/AIDS Research Initiative (MARI) and Research Fellowships on HIV Prevention in Communities of Color. Both are intent on steering junior scientists to study AIDS in minority populations in the United States (Dean et al. 2005; Holman et al. 1991). In Canada, a focus on Aboriginal AIDS emerged soon after the turn of the twenty-first century, when the National Aboriginal Council on HIV/AIDS (NACHA) was created to increase collaboration among, and in consultation with, Aboriginal communities and to advise the federal government on the development of a national Aboriginal HIV/AIDS strategy (Waldram, Herring, and Young 2006). In 2007, the Canadian Federal Initiative on HIV/AIDS announced a doubling of government funding for research and prevention programs, some of which will target First Nations (Garmaise 2003b).

Although politicians such as Congresswoman Barbara Lee (D-Calif.) could still win applause at the American Foundation of AIDS Research in Oakland, California, in 2005 for promises to "spotlight neglected populations and underserved communities," including Native Americans, in fact the number of publications on Aboriginal health has grown exponentially in the AIDS era, spurred in part by new funding initiatives such as those just mentioned (*AIDS Policy and Law* 2003: 9). A retrospective review of articles published in medical and health-related journals showed a leveling off in the late 1970s of the number of articles published on Aboriginal health, following a sharp decline after 1971. A tremendous increase in published material, however, is apparent after 1991, since when at least 450 articles have been published on Aboriginal health each year. This trend mirrors the number of articles published on AIDS in Aboriginal communities on both sides of the border.[3]

Because of this surge in research, surveillance mechanisms were already in place when it became clear, at the turn of the twenty-first century, that the penetration of HIV/AIDS into North America's Aboriginal population had been delayed, not averted. But if history can prompt knowledge production in health research, what influences does it bring? These are not always so salubrious, for the historical and anthropological scaffolding upon which contemporary health research regarding Aboriginal people rests is not always sound. Without a historical awareness of the materials used to build that scaffolding, twenty-first-century health research may find itself replicating the colonial discourses of the past.

Pathologizing Aboriginal People

Aboriginal health had long been the subject of missionary, traveler, and government observations, but systematic medical research involving

Aboriginal people did not get under way until after the turn of the twentieth century. There were some specific reasons for this delay. Public health–oriented epidemiological research tended to focus on communicable diseases affecting urban and industrial areas, and the belief that rural lands were bucolic and relatively free of disease no doubt distracted researchers from remote Aboriginal communities. Settler colonialists did not, for the most part, envision Aboriginal people as disease threats, so a North American equivalent of "tropical medicine" did not develop. Finally, the placing of Aboriginal people in distinct administrative categories, in both Canada and the United States, cut them off from the kinds of public health interventions that others of the time (immigrants and schoolchildren, for example) experienced. Still, knowledge about Aboriginal health was produced. Missionaries and traders wrote of the devastating epidemics that swept through Indian country, and beliefs at the time accepted that primitivism made Aboriginal people vulnerable to the "diseases of civilization" (Benson 1999; Jones 2004; Kelm 1998; McCallum 2005).

It was not until the early decades of the twentieth century that public health researchers began to study Aboriginal people. Some public health advocates were dismayed that the field was "practically completely ignorant" of the "importance of the Indian population problem" (Hoffman 1930: 612). Others were excited by the prospect of studying a population over which government had complete authority (Fox 1927). Public health researchers conceived of Indian reserves as laboratories. One researcher wrote in 1932: "The Indian, without his knowledge or consent, offers us a human experience in immunology as well as epidemiology which we can ill afford to ignore. The material is conveniently located, the data are or should easily be made available for record and study, and the results applied to regulative measures of control" (Burns 1932: 498).

Of particular interest was the study of tuberculosis, since Aboriginal people continued to have high rates of the disease even after it was in decline in the general population. Public health writers of the 1930s increasingly raised the concern that Aboriginal people were inherently tubercular and posed a health threat to the non-Native population. Native sufferers of tuberculosis were reconfigured from being victims of an imported disease to being agents infectious to white populations just as the public health movement, exposed to eugenic ideas, was turning to increasingly invasive methods of contagion control (Korns 1937; Richards 1932). A writer for *Canadian Public Health Journal* warned in 1941: "Each province has a share of the Indian problem. Every tuberculosis death represents a focus of infection with from eight to ten latent or actual cases. Such an estimate is conservative and the danger of transmission from the Indian to the white population is very real" (*Canadian Public Health Journal* 1941: 38).

Indian reservations were pathologized as centers of infection, and public health researchers referred to them as "important reservoirs of infection which must be controlled to prevent the spread of the disease to the non-Indian population" (Burns 1932: 506). Aboriginal mobility became the way in which diseases could be spread from these reservoirs to the general population. Researchers in the last century therefore decried labor practices that encouraged the employment of Aboriginal workers, Indian policies that forced people to relocate away from reservations, and the allegedly natural inclination of Aboriginal people toward transience (Burns 1932: 507; Kelm 1998; Mawani 2001; Wall 1934: 279). Although tuberculosis and trachoma formed the main focus of these fears, venereal disease attracted attention as well. When American and Canadian troops swelled the population of Prince Rupert, British Columbia, in the 1940s, for example, the government assigned special social workers to monitor and, if deemed necessary, arrest and compel to treatment any Native woman suspected of venereal disease.[4] Vital statistics collected by the province did not confirm this fear, but medical practitioners, working for the government of the day, conflated mobility, sexual contact, and disease (British Columbia Ministry of Health 1945). First Nations were transformed, in medical minds, from victims to vectors of disease. As such, they joined the ranks of the polluting "other."

Looking back, it seems clear that in these early decades of medical research on Aboriginal people, medical observations about First Nations were built on a scaffolding of preexisting ideas about sexuality, primitivism, and pathology. Is this happening today? In the published research on HIV/AIDS among Aboriginal people, three themes are particularly resonant to the historian's ear. These themes involve the understanding of alcohol use, mobility, and Aboriginal status as risk factors for HIV/AIDS.

Substance abuse dominates health research on AIDS in Aboriginal people. Sixty percent of all new HIV infections among Aboriginal people in Canada at the turn of the twenty-first century were the result of transmission via intravenous drug use (Craib et al. 2003). But the discussion of substance abuse as a risk factor for HIV/AIDS among Aboriginal people goes beyond intravenous drug use, a mode of transmission that can be eliminated by safe injection practices. Instead, health research has focused on substances as disinhibitors contributing to unsafe sex. Studies of condom use among Aboriginal people, for example, showed that they were less likely to use condoms when they had been drinking, so alcohol was considered a co-factor for risk (Du Bois, Brassard, and Smeja 1996).

Why, then, the literature asks, do Aboriginal people drink? How are they particularly affected by alcohol? In this regard, one finds nearly a century's worth of alcohol studies about Aboriginal people, all grounded in the assumption that Aboriginal people suffer disproportionately from addiction and that particular Aboriginal drinking styles exist, a body of work that some social science researchers now dispute (Waldram 2004: 135–165). Still, some health research takes higher rates of drug use, alcoholism, and solvent inhalation to be a characteristic of Aboriginal populations (*Morbidity and Mortality Weekly Report* 1998). One study reported that Aboriginal people had a rate of death from alcoholism seven times the national average in the United States (Aguilera and Plasencia 2005). The risk-factor literature characterizes Aboriginal people as binge drinkers who consume large quantities of alcohol during drinking episodes, usually in nearby towns, and who bear a heavy weight of consequences, being more often involved in motor vehicle accidents and in violent or suicidal acts while under the influence (Aguilera and Plasencia 2005; Hall et al. 1990; Mitchell et al. 2002; Simoni, Sehgal, and Walters 2004; Spittal et al. 2002; Sullivan 1991; Tseng 1996).

As James Waldram (2004) has convincingly argued, little in the literature actually explains how all these factors are distinctly Aboriginal (indeed, anyone who has lived in a northern Canadian, rural, or remote town would recognize them as the behaviors of rural youths, fishers, logging camp workers, and the like) or how they are linked to conditions of endemic poverty, historical oppression, and cultural loss. The literature that links substance abuse with HIV/AIDS *assumes* social disorganization among First Nations and posits it as a precondition. Although this may be so, as Waldram points out, "seldom is it determined first that [social disorganization] exists, and then [that] alcohol abuse is the cause, the result or related in some way" (Waldram 2004: 166). Furthermore, this literature tends to ignore evidence that contradicts these assumptions about Aboriginal drinking, including evidence for higher rates of abstinence than rates in nearby non-Native towns.[5] The literature on Aboriginal alcoholism as a risk factor for HIV builds on a scaffolding of historical assumptions about Aboriginal drinking that have not always sufficiently questioned definitions of alcoholism and have homogenized Aboriginal people.

Mobility is another risk factor identified in the literature as important for Aboriginal people. Aboriginal people, some write, naturally live semi-nomadic lifestyles, traveling to urban centers for school or work and repeatedly returning to the reservations for family and cultural reasons (Sullivan 1991). Others portray travel to cities as a mechanism by which to cope with abusive living situations on reserves, hence propelling psychologically damaged individuals into pathogenic street culture, replete with intravenous drug use and sex trade. Continued connections with home reserves, explained as an essential Aboriginal characteristic, completes the epidemiologically dangerous cycle, bringing urban-acquired HIV/AIDS to virally naïve reserve communities (Du Bois, Brassard, and Smeja 1996; Tseng 1996). HIV-infected Aboriginal people, moreover, might come home for traditional healing treatments and, in the process, infect remote communities, which would be devastated (Conway 1992; McKeown, Reid, and Orr 2004; Mitchell et al. 2002; Mitchell, Kaufman, and Beals 2004). Surprisingly few studies show that this has occurred, but researchers predict dire consequences (Hall 1990).

Why the focus on mobility? On one hand, studying the movement of diseases and their vectors is just what epidemiologists do. Tracking "patient 0" and the spatial distribution of HIV/AIDS was a key part of epidemiological work in the early days of the disease. Subsequent studies have identified other people—bisexual men and sex tourists, for example—who, through their movement within and between communities, become depicted as people who are "dangerous to health" (Patton 2002). A 1984 case involving the transmission of HIV to a small non-Native community in Newfoundland was instructive and alarming. In this case, a single male, incarcerated in Conception Bay, Newfoundland, infected two women with HIV, despite a court order prohibiting him from sexual activity. Within ten years, there were forty-one cases of HIV in a town with a population of about fifty thousand (Tseng 1996). Clearly, tracking the movement of human populations and how they may spread disease is well within the remit of health research.

But the historian cannot help recalling that settlers and government officials have always seen mobility among Aboriginal people as dangerous. Reservations (in the United States) and reserves (in Canada) were designed to be places where Aboriginal people could reside and be contained, out of the way of settlement. Those who left the reservation in the early days of this policy were considered "hostile" and could be shot. Even years later, violence could follow anyone who left the reservation, because settler communities feared "outbreaks" of violence (Deloria

2004). In Canada, a pass system was enacted whereby leaving the reserve required the permission of the Indian agent. As many historians have pointed out, the lines around reserves were far from impermeable, and Native people often left their reserves to work, sell goods, and participate in celebrations (Miller 1990). But whenever government officials began to worry about how much time people were spending off-reserve, it was health concerns that they raised. Early public health ordinances in Victoria, British Columbia, were aimed at discouraging Aboriginal people from visiting from up coast (Barman 2005). When Indian agents tried to keep Aboriginal women from working at canneries on the Pacific Coast, they cited fears that tuberculosis might be passed from workers to the canned fish. Government officials and missionaries justified banning the potlatch, the sun dance, and other Native ceremonial gatherings on the grounds that such congregations naturally spread disease (Kelm 1998; Pettipas 1994).

At the same time, government policy on both sides of the border encouraged and even forced relocation and mobility. Reserve lands in both Canada and the United States were often too small to support their populations, forcing Aboriginal people into nearby towns to work and often to live. Economic deprivation worsened for Aboriginal people in Canada in the 1930s, when the provinces took control of Crown lands, areas that had previously been open to Aboriginal hunting, trapping, and fishing. Treatment of disease further encouraged Aboriginal people to move to larger centers. In Canada, although a number of experts advocated tuberculosis sanitariums that would treat Aboriginal patients close to their own communities, the government instead advocated large hospitals close to or in urban centers. Tuberculosis sanitariums and "Indian hospitals" opened in Edmonton, in Hamilton, and near Vancouver, for example, drawing patient populations from the Arctic and from rural and remote areas across the country. Not only did this draw Aboriginal people who were sick with tuberculosis into urban centers, but it also encouraged families to visit and sometimes to relocate in order to be close to their afflicted relatives. Finally, postwar policies forced urbanization on many First Nations as hydroelectric development flooded reserve and traditional lands (Barber 2005; Dawson 2001). In the United States, the policy of termination of tribal recognition, along with assisted urban relocation, resulted in an Aboriginal population that is now about 70 percent urban (Fixico 1986).

What is troubling, then, about the depiction of mobility as a risk factor in the spread of HIV/AIDS in Aboriginal populations is not that mobility is discussed but the extent to which it is naturalized as an essential Aboriginal characteristic and is shorn of its relationship to government policy and socioeconomic conditions. If Aboriginal people are particularly mobile today, it is as much because of limited opportunities on reserves and the effects of previous forced relocations than because of historical, seasonal economic cycles (Dickason 1997: 331, 335–342; Fixico 1986; Harris 2002; Kelm 1998: 19–82, 129–152; Trennert 1998; Waldram, Herring and Young 2006: 68–70, 178, 188–209).

Repeatedly, many studies simply depict Aboriginal culture as complicit in the spread of HIV/AIDS. In this sense, they have much in common with early public health analyses that situated the unhealthiness of First Nations in their "primitive cultures" (Montgomery 1933, 1934; Moore 1941; Richards 1932; Wall 1934). As one writer put it in the 1930s, "ignorance, superstition, ancient habits and customs, indifference, poverty, unfavorable environment, lack of knowledge of the English language, and frequent lack of industrial ambition— all have to be combated in order to effect any marked or permanent improvement" (*American Journal of Public Health* 1915: 271). Studies that link HIV/AIDS to Aboriginal culture tend to have three things in common: a poorly articulated definition of culture, a tendency to conflate Aboriginal behavior and attitudes with Aboriginal culture, and a sense of history as a broad sweep rather than as specific explanatory frameworks.

The quest for culturally competent prevention work has stimulated health researchers to include "culture" in their analyses (Baldwin 1996; Dawkins 1996). But few seem to have engaged with the detailed discussions of culture that have preoccupied anthropologists and historians for the last two decades. As a result, health researchers acknowledge that they have little specific information about the precise interplay between culture, history, and health-related behaviors among Aboriginal people. Some are clear that the results of their work should not be taken as representative of all Aboriginal people (Connors et al. 1992; Du Bois, Brassard, and Smeja 1996). Others, trying to find broad applicability for microstudies, seek to make just such generalizations.

Some health researchers seem to relate current behavior to a baseline called "tribal society," as in Carol Sullivan's work on AIDS vulnerability among the Navajo. Sullivan (1991: 241) wrote: "Certain characteristics common to tribal societies distinguish them from modern societies and influence tribal disease rates and epidemiology ... these features make their vulnerability distinct ... Navajo exhibit ... greater resistance to spontaneous changes, and a greater vulnerability to external influences."

For this reason, she said, tribal leaders would be resistant to AIDS education and might endanger their people. This is a kind of evocation of the ethnographic present, in which Aboriginal people are thought to exhibit cultural norms untouched by centuries of government policy and cultural change.

Another study (Mill 1997) tried to situate the troubled sexual relations of late-twentieth-century urban Cree women in the context of David Mandelbaum's 1940 ethnographic study, *The Plains Cree*, which depicted gender relations as hierarchical and hostile. The author suggested that sexual abuse and low self-esteem might have been the result of Cree culture, but her informants, eight Cree women in a treatment center, situated their behavior in the context not of Cree culture but of their personal experiences of abuse.

In other instances, researchers have depicted certain attitudes as inherently "Native" that surely could have come from other sources. For example, a study of Native schoolchildren interviewed in 2000 found that these students did not want to talk about sex with their parents and that they held many false beliefs about HIV transmission, according to which they perceived many more behaviors as risky than actually were (e.g., toilet seats and drinking fountains were places where these students thought HIV was contracted). Therefore, the authors concluded, "fatalism and family communication"—both described as expressions of Native culture—"may be more important than socioeconomic status in predicting variations in HIV knowledge" (Ramirez et al. 2002: 37). That all the students in the study attended a Catholic day school was not considered a significant factor in the knowledge and behaviors the researchers discovered. In other instances, Aboriginal culture has been described as having been perverted by interference from non-Natives, particularly from churches and boarding schools, producing a new Aboriginal culture that is homophobic and hence a risk factor in the spread of AIDS because it stigmatizes men who have sex with other men (Conway 1992; Gilley and Co-Cke 2005; Sullivan 1991). In these reports, Aboriginal culture, almost always sketchily defined by the researchers, is pathologized.

Increasingly, health researchers are entering the category "Aboriginal status" into their analyses without discussing the extent to which "Aboriginal status" itself is historically constructed. Canadian and American government officials used measures such as the Indian Act and blood quantum theory to determine who was and who was not an Indian under the law. This was not an abstract, legalistic process but rather determined where one lived, what educational opportunities one had available, and whether one could use certain natural resources, own land, and vote in elections. Hence, ethnic "status" influenced socioeconomic status in very specific ways. It became reified in the lives of Aboriginal people (Frohlich, Ross, and Richmond 2006). But it is still an unnatural categorization. For much of the previous two centuries, particular and localized affiliations were often more important to Aboriginal people's individual identities than overarching pan-Indianism (Fixico 2006; Ray 2002). Furthermore, in both Canada and the United States, a great many Aboriginal people have been denied "Indian" status and have had to struggle to be considered Indians under the law (Fiske 2006). For this last reason especially, health researchers of the last decade included self-identified Aboriginal status rather than, or in addition to, legal Indian status as a category of analysis. But what does self-described Aboriginal status mean? This is not always made clear in the health research that uses it.

Nonetheless, in recent years some studies have concluded that Aboriginal status is predictive of certain health-diminishing behaviors. Alex Chan, in a 2004 article, used multivariate regression analysis to determine that "aboriginal ethnicity" was an "independent risk factor for discharge AMA [against medical advice]" (Chan 2004: 57) Similarly, Fu-Lin Wang (2005) described Aboriginal status as a significant factor in determining which women would decline prenatal testing for HIV. Taken on their own, these studies seem to essentialize Aboriginal status and to conclude that such behaviors are rooted somehow in that status. But the *reasons* pregnant Aboriginal women may be twice as likely to decline prenatal testing, for example, are not explored. An Edmonton-based study might have provided researchers with some clues. Of the HIV-positive women in a drug rehabilitation program, 98 percent feared that knowledge of their HIV status would result in social services personnel seizing their children (Houston 2004). The long history of state control over Aboriginal children, first through residential schooling and then through social services, clearly contributes to the unwillingness of Aboriginal women to consent to prenatal testing for HIV. By focusing only on Aboriginality as a factor in testing refusal, researchers confirm stereotypes that Aboriginal patients will be resistive and noncompliant. One can imagine the kinds of expectations that emergency room physicians, having read such articles, might bring to their interactions with drug-addicted Aboriginal women with HIV.

Unwillingness to look at specific social, economic, and historical reasons for Aboriginal behavior, concluding instead that Aboriginal status produces negative health outcomes, contributes to a long history of such assumptions about Aboriginal people. These assumptions justified residential schooling on the grounds that Aboriginal women did not adequately address the sanitary and nutritional needs of their children. Such assumptions led to the denunciation of Aboriginal healing as either useless incantations or as contributing to mortality by traumatizing already ill patients. Such beliefs alienated elders and grandparents from the treatment of the young because they were thought to disrupt the authority of the doctor (Kelm 2004). For many medical writers a century ago, Aboriginality, found in either bodies or culture, was the root of disease. It is difficult not to hear resonances of these assumptions in the literature on Aboriginal people and HIV/AIDS and to wonder at their source and their effects on Aboriginal people seeking treatment.

Toward a Postcolonial Epidemiology

Bonnie Duran and Karina L. Waters (2004) articulated a two-pronged approach to an indigenous postcolonial epidemiology. It included the use of specific "effective histories" of medicine to situate Aboriginal interactions with Western medicine and the examination of "culturally protective" factors. I have hinted at the efficacy of such historical grounding, and there now exists a significant body of work that demonstrates the embeddedness of Aboriginal health in historical contexts (Hackett 2005). In addition to using history in this way, those advocating postcolonial epidemiologies look to a focus on the strengths that Aboriginal people bring to their struggles with disease. We know from work in social pathologies that the more social capital a community has at its disposal, the greater the likelihood that they will avert epidemics of suicide, for example (O'Neil and Mignone 2005). But the dominant trends in the literature on HIV/AIDS and Aboriginal people in Canada and the United States previously discussed suggest that there are few strengths to report on. Here is where reading "against the grain" can come in handy. Used for decades in historical research, reading against the grain has been a way to find information about groups who do not generate their own data. In this case, we find a significant quantity of data on strengths through a reading of "counterfactuals" that appear in the health literature on HIV/AIDS in Aboriginal communities.

The first point worth making is that despite myriad risk factors, HIV/AIDS has been slow to penetrate Aboriginal communities. Nearly a decade after the identification of the human immunodeficiency virus, studies among Aboriginal populations indicated that they were not being disproportionately affected. A 1992 study conducted in prisons, for example, showed "no association between HIV status and Aboriginal status or age group"; indeed, the rate for Aboriginal inmates was slightly lower than that for the general correctional population (Martin and Matthias 2002: 107). In 1993, a paper presented at the ninth International Conference on AIDS in Berlin reported that there were no cases of HIV among the eleven thousand Cree of northern Quebec, but that the Cree, because of their control over public health education in their communities, had already launched AIDS education in all nine Cree villages and hoped to prevent the spread of the disease to their communities (Valverde and Smeja 1993). A 1995 study using blood samples obtained from First Nations drug and alcohol treatment centers did not find that Aboriginal people had higher rates of HIV seropositivity than other intravenous drug users, a situation that remained unchanged when followed up in 2000 (Martin and Matthias 2002). A 1998 study in Calgary of participants in a needle exchange program, many of whom were Aboriginal, also found that HIV prevalence remained low, even though high-risk behaviors were common (Guenter et al. 2000).

The need to avoid conflating Aboriginal status with specific risk factors is something that some health researchers stress when they say that "race/ethnicity is not a risk factor for HIV" (McNaughton et al. 2005: 66). Drug dependency, unsafe injection practices, and gendered power and control issues within the world of injection drug use and the sex trade all emerge as factors in HIV transmission, and despite the "statistically significant" place of "Aboriginal status" in some studies, the linkages between that status and these risks is implied more than proved.[6] Rather than looking only for reasons why Aboriginal people are affected by HIV, researchers may wish to start asking what has prevented the spread of HIV from urban street populations, which include Aboriginal people, to Aboriginal populations more generally. They may want to examine some of the success stories of early intervention, such as the study presented in 1998 that showed how a multifaceted prevention program launched in 1990 in Arizona had clearly reduced new cases of HIV and all other STDs so that no new cases of HIV had been reported for the rural Arizona Aboriginal community using the prevention program after 1995 (Yost 1998).

Some demographic characteristics described as risk factors may also confer health benefits. Whereas one study identified the male sexual commuter who drank to excess and engaged in unprotected sex in the city, far away from his reserve home, as a potential path of transmission, other studies have pointed out that men commonly find that they have less sex, rather than more, when they are drunk or high (Myers et al. 1994, 1997). In some studies, the youthfulness of Aboriginal populations was considered a risk factor, but one Alaska study showed that youths and women had significantly higher CD4 cell counts than men and older patients, indicating a more fully active immune system (Diamond et al. 2001).

Similarly, youth and participation in traditional culture have been shown to decrease the prevalence of risk behaviors, even when traditional cultural activities promote mobility. For example, young people in Northern Plains Indian communities who were described as coming from "traditional homes" showed a high degree of personal efficacy in decision making around sex, particularly in their use of condoms. On these reservations, risk behaviors such as exchanging sex for gifts, money, or drugs, injection drug use, and unprotected anal sex were found to be quite low (Mitchell et al. 2002; Mitchell, Kaufman, and Beals 2004). Once infected, some Aboriginal women spoke explicitly of their sense of responsibility toward their home communities to prevent the spread of the disease. They turned to traditional healing as well as Western allopathic medicine and sought treatment for underlying psychological, drug, and alcohol problems (Mill 2000). Simoni and co-workers argued that stronger American Indian identity may be a protective factor against HIV, because engaging in community practices decreased other risk behaviors (Simoni, Sehgal, and Walters 2004). Stevan Hobfoll and colleagues (2002) found that the "communal culture" of many Native Americans, with its emphasis on social support, was a mediating factor discouraging child abuse and high-risk sexual behavior later in life. These studies show that Aboriginal communities, particularly those with strong senses of culture (both Aboriginal and in terms of "values and norms of trust, reciprocity and collective action"), rather than exhibiting "fatalism," a "terrible apathy," or poor communication, have been proactive in their response to the threat of HIV.[7]

In the years since 1997, although it was clear that incidence rates of HIV/AIDS for American Indians and Alaska Natives were increasing, it was equally clear that AI/ANs were not denying the threat of HIV/AIDS. Rather, the opposite was true. A study published in 2003 showed that Aboriginal people perceived themselves to be at greater risk and were more likely to be tested than any other group of Americans (Denny, Holtzman, and Cobb 2003). Indeed, if the research proves anything, it is that Aboriginal people have responded with anything *but* apathy. In a time when all research involving human subjects must be conducted with informed consent and when any deception, including placebo trials, must be justified or disclosed, Aboriginal people are consenting to be studied at drug treatment centers, at injection sites, on reserves, and in outpatient settings. Prevention education appears to be getting to the right people and influencing behavior. A study of condom use by Aboriginal people in Canada that was generally pessimistic nonetheless reported that condom use was highest (greater than 80 percent) among youths considered at high risk for HIV infection, in comparison with low-risk youths, who had a condom use rate of less than 40 percent (Calzavara et al. 1998). A study of fourteen hundred injection drug users in Vancouver found that those at greatest risk of HIV infection were young, female, survival sex trade workers who received help to inject heroin, cocaine, or speedball daily. Yet these young women, half of whom were Aboriginal, reported consistent condom use (Miller 2002).

Aboriginal people tend to view themselves as being at higher risk than their behavior actually suggests and are more likely to be tested and to take preventative action (Denny, Holtzman, and Cobb 2003; Mitchell, Kaufman, and Beals 2004). In a study of hepatitis C and HIV infection among emergency room patients, designed to help health care workers protect themselves from infection, Aboriginal people were found to be most likely among all those who presented at an Edmonton emergency ward to know that they were HIV positive and to disclose that information to staff (Houston 2004). They were as likely as any other HIV-positive persons to reach out for help. A sophisticated study that matched Aboriginal HIV-positive people with non-Natives having the same demographic profile showed that there were "no statistically significant differences between the two groups for HIV exposure category, CD4 count, substance abuse problems, being homeless, [or] likelihood to receive medical care, mental health or substance abuse treatment/counseling, dental care, food, emergency financial and transportation assistance as well as client advocacy" (Ashman, Perez-Jimenez, and Marconi 2004). Indeed, with respect to housing, this urban American study suggested that needs of Native people were met better than those non-Natives. Advocates of postcolonial epidemiology stress that it is this kind of information that must be discussed along with that which focuses on risk factors, so that fear and helplessness are not the predominant messages. Some AIDS educators argue that education based on risk factors, fear, and, especially, essentializing discourses that link AIDS with Aboriginal bodies or culture discourages prevention, especially among young people (Aguilera and Plasencia 2005; Clarke 2005; Mill 2000).

Placing history in conversation with health research reveals the ways in which the past helps to make the present. Historical thinking was often invoked by health researchers who worried, when the numbers were not high, that officials would ignore Aboriginal people as if they were not at risk for HIV. The desire to understand risk factors before HIV/ AIDS was statistically significant among Aboriginal people generated a significant archive of data that probed Aboriginal people's lives for risk factors. Historical thinking may affect the way health researchers study Aboriginal people and what they conclude.

Alcohol, as a disinhibiting factor, was predicted to be significant in the transmission of HIV through unprotected intercourse, but intravenous drug use accounts for the majority of new infections. In order to understand the role that mobility might play in spreading HIV in Aboriginal populations that are both urban and reserve based, an understanding of how that mobility has been historically produced through specific government policies is needed. Finally, the historically contingent nature of Aboriginal status itself cannot be ignored, lest we return to essentialized notions of race. Without these historical considerations, much health research on Aboriginal people and HIV/ AIDS produces accounts that pathologize Aboriginal people. Understanding as we do that this itself can undermine prevention work, we must engage ourselves in searching through the counterfactuals to find out how Aboriginal people are fighting history and fighting this disease called AIDS. By doing so, we find women in Edmonton who take care not to infect others in their home communities with HIV. We find Aboriginal youths who, recognizing their high-risk status, use condoms. We find Sioux young people who, through engagement with their cultural forms, find their self-efficacy in matters involving sex and substances grow. And by finding these strengths upon which to build, we begin to refuse the legacies of history.

Notes

1. This chapter is based on a literature review that uncovered some 428 citations of work on HIV/AIDS in Aboriginal communities in Canada and the United States. Detailed content analysis was performed on 45 of these articles (roughly 10 percent, randomly sampled) and on 146 published abstracts of conferences that ran between 1992 and 2006.

2. For the most part, health research in Canada employs self-identification to determine Aboriginal status, although earlier work used Department of

Indian Affairs definitions of "status" and "non-status" according to the Indian Act. The Centers for Disease Control uses the definitions of the Indian Health Services in the United States for American Indian and Alaska Native.

3. Sean Carleton, "Aboriginal Health Findings" (unpublished literature search), part 1. Carleton used Medline and its predecessor Index Medicus, as well as AIDSearch and Althealth Watch/Health Source. Total publications rose steadily from 1927 to 1943, declined sharply until 1947, spiked in the early 1950s, and rose steadily until 1971, when another sharp decline took place. The number then increased steadily and dramatically until it more or less leveled off from 1975 to 1991.

4. J. Gillett to Headquarters, 1945, Library and Archives of Canada, Department of National Health and Welfare, Indian Health Services, Record Group 29, vol. 2782, file 823-1-A984.

5. In a study by Carol Sullivan (1991), drinking rates among Navajo were found to be 30–42 percent, whereas the drinking rate for the nearby non-Native towns was 71 percent.

6. A good example in which ethnicity is added to the analysis is Estrada et al. 1990, but the similarities among individuals who use intravenous drugs, whatever their ethnicity, cautions against drawing conclusions on the basis of ethnicity. For a contrasting article that implies the importance of Aboriginality, see Heath et al. 1999.

7. The definition of culture as "values and norms of trust, reciprocity and collective action" comes from O'Neil and Mignone 2005: S51. "Fatalism" and "terrible apathy" are predicted as Native responses to HIV in Sullivan 1991 and Ramirez et al. 2002, respectively.

Accounting for Epidemics
Mathematical Modeling and Anthropology

Steven M. Goodreau

Mathematical modeling has been used to explore the nature of epidemics for a century, but the contributions of social scientists to this field are of much more recent origins. These contributions have been growing in recent years, resulting in an increased focus on the ways cultural and behavioral variation channels infectious disease and accounts for population-level disease disparities. Although the approach may seem mechanical to outsiders, modelers inevitably make numerous theoretical decisions—about what to model (or not), what assumptions to make in the process, how to interpret their results, and how to communicate these to the larger world. In this chapter I examine some of the features that characterize modeling as a "way of knowing" about epidemics, particularly as conducted by anthropologists.

I begin with a brief explanation of what epidemic modeling is and give a quick history of its development, including anthropologists' role in that history. I then discuss the philosophy of mathematical modeling in the sociobehavioral and biological sciences generally. Using this as a springboard, I consider the additional ways in which epidemic modeling as done by social scientists contributes to the production of knowledge about disease and its disparities among individuals and populations. I rely on two case studies from the HIV/AIDS modeling literature, one from Uganda and one from Peru, to illustrate many of my points.

Among the things I do *not* do in this chapter is to teach the methods of epidemic modeling—for this the interested reader should peruse the classic tomes on the topic (Anderson and May 1991; Bailey 1975) or more recent texts (Daley and Gani 1999; Diekmann and Heesterbeek

2000). I also do not review what modeling has taught us about epidemics generally, except through a few key examples. Let me provide the additional caveat that I am by no means a trained philosopher of science or a critical medical anthropologist. As a biological anthropologist and practicing modeler, my goal is simply to step back and contextualize the work my fellow modelers and I conduct. This volume presents a variety of ways of knowing about plagues and epidemics; my hope is that this chapter will help readers understand how modeling, often so seemingly esoteric to outsiders, can be a useful and complementary tool with which to explore the causes and consequences of the many phenomena highlighted by these diverse theoretical approaches.

Epidemic Modeling: What and Why?

The basic motivation for epidemic modeling can best be explained through a simple example. Imagine two black South African women, both age thirty-five, both married and with no sexual partners besides their respective husbands. They live in the same village, come from the same ethnic group and speak the same language, have the same economic status and overall health. Each woman's husband has an ongoing sexual relationship with one other woman during his many months a year spent away at the mines. In one case, the female partner at the mining camp has additional sexual partners with whom she does not use condoms; in the other case, she does not.

The first two women are at very different risks for acquiring HIV, yet they appear exactly the same when one considers only their personal situations; individualistic explanations are of no help. At the other end of the spectrum, cultural, economic, and political factors play a strong role in putting them both at risk in the first place, by creating a system in which men are away from home for long periods and in which it is generally culturally acceptable for men to have two partnerships simultaneously. But these factors do not directly explain the difference in risk between the two women. That difference is determined by their positions in a complex sexual network, which is itself shaped at one end by the behavioral decisions of individuals and pairs and at the other by the cultural, political, and economic contexts that constrain those decisions. In this situation, everyone's risk is jointly affected by the behavior of everyone else in a complex feedback system.

The elements of such a network that most determine an individual's risk are not always intuitive, especially when small changes in behavior by people two or three degrees removed makes a big difference. Even less intuitive than the factors creating individual risk are those generating disparities among populations, especially when the population risk factors differ from individual ones (we see such an example later in the chapter). Modeling aids in exploring all these questions, as a tool for linking individuals and populations through the intermediate level of personal interactions, using the common language of mathematics. One theme that runs through this volume is the relationship between "counting" and "accounting"; epidemic modeling is, quite straightforwardly, a tool with which to account for the intertwining of processes at all levels, using relatively advanced methods of counting.

Complementing modeling's ability to clarify what creates differential risk is its role in identifying potential effects of behavioral, biological, or structural interventions that might reduce risk. In that sense, modeling can represent a kind of epidemiological laboratory where no other exists, in which "experiments" can be run *in silico*. There are, of course, many cases in which modeling is unnecessary; no fancy mathematics are needed to understand that increasing condom use within existing sexual contacts will decrease the incidence of sexually transmitted diseases (STDs). However, it is not uncommon that, although the *direction* of some effect may be obvious beforehand, the likely magnitude is not. A 10 percent increase in condom use might generate a 5 percent decrease in STDs in one network and a 20 percent decrease in another. In other cases, even the direction of the outcome may be unclear, as when a single change has two countervailing effects. For instance, increasing access to a treatment that extends life but neither provides a cure nor reduces infectiousness will save many lives in the short term. Having infected people remain alive longer, however, could lead to a larger number of new infections down the line and, perversely, to a long-term increase in deaths. Although taking action in such a case would focus on ethical considerations about access to treatment, modeling can at least provide a clearer picture of the expected outcomes in each case.

The practical value of a model is only as good as the assumptions it makes. This oft-repeated critique of modeling is absolutely true, but it is also true of all forms of knowledge production. The general response of modelers when they receive this critique is that modeling makes no more assumptions than other approaches; it simply communicates them more explicitly, which is preferable to having them hidden. Exploring some of the trends in the assumptions made in epidemic models in practice, whether explicitly or implicitly, is another goal of this chapter.

A Brief History of Epidemic Modeling

Lisa Sattenspiel (1990) provided a thorough, though now dated, introduction to the history of epidemic modeling for an anthropological audience. In brief, the field emerged in the early twentieth century with the work of epidemiologists such as William Kermack and Anderson McKendrick (1927), who formalized deterministic models, and Lowell Reed and Wade Hampton Frost, who explored stochastic epidemic models in a series of unpublished lectures. Early work focused on developing a basic understanding of epidemic dynamics for relatively simple models. Among the key advances was a formalization of the "herd immunity" concept—the realization that not all members of a population needed to receive vaccination (or other intervention) in order for a disease to die out and for all to benefit. Another was the development of the critical population size, the size of an interacting human population necessary to sustain various infectious agents, a concept central to the idea of the first epidemiological transition accompanying the adoption of sedentary agriculture (see Barrett, this volume). These and other early insights emphasized the interdependent nature of epidemics—the fact that demographic structure plays a major role in channeling disease and that the health consequences of actions taken by some become felt by all.

From its origins until the 1970s, epidemic modeling remained populated mostly by applied mathematicians and parasitologists. The result was that the greatest attention was paid to the biological features that distinguished pathogens from one another and the way these affected the resulting disease dynamics. Questions of human biological variation were less in focus, and issues of human behavioral and cultural diversity even less so.

By the 1980s, two changes led to massive growth in the field of epidemic modeling overall, and especially in the role of social scientists. The main one was the explosion of STDs in the West, most notably the HIV epidemic. These diseases, perhaps more than any others, are channeled by contacts under strong, culture-specific control. The second development was the rise of large-scale computing, which freed modelers from many of the practical constraints on their models and made it easier to consider new forms of complexity.

In these early years, Sattenspiel was almost single-handedly responsible for representing the field of anthropology in epidemic modeling. She, her students, and her collaborators in other fields produced early work on the effects of behavioral heterogeneity on HIV transmission (Sattenspiel et al. 1990), geographical subdivision and mobility (Sattenspiel 1987b; Sattenspiel and Dietz 1995), local community structure in the form of day-care groups (Sattenspiel 1987a), and short-term behavior change (Sattenspiel and Castillo-Chavez 1990). Given that epidemic modeling is a realm in which biology and culture clearly intersect, it is perhaps surprising that more biological anthropologists in particular were not drawn to the field, although the need for advanced mathematical training was likely a major hindrance.

In recent years, more anthropologists have begun to publish in the realm of epidemic modeling. As might be expected, one aspect that links much of this work is a focus on cultural practices. For example, anthropologist Eric Roth and his mathematician colleagues (McCluskey, Roth, and Van Den Driessche 2005) looked at the role that male age sets play in shaping sexual network structure among the Ariaal of Kenya and the way this accounts for the propagation of gonorrhea over the generations. I have worked with a team of epidemiologists (Goodreau, Goicochea, and Sanchez 2005) to explore the issue of sexual role (exclusively insertive, exclusively receptive, or versatile) among homosexually active Peruvian men and the way it affects HIV transmission (more on which later). In a series of papers, anthropologist James Jones and statistician Mark Handcock (Handcock and Jones 2004; Jones and Handcock 2003a, 2003b) reevaluated the theoretical appropriateness and statistical fit of an approach that led a team of physicists to conclude that sexual networks from very different settings could be described using a single model (Liljeros et al. 2001). At the same time, Sattenspiel has continued work in the field, primarily with her colleague Ann Herring and others on issues of settlement structure and quarantine in the Canadian Arctic during the 1918 flu pandemic (Sattenspiel and Herring 1998, 2003; Sattenspiel, Mobarry, and Herring 2000).

One of the main hallmarks of the new generation of epidemic models has been a gradual movement toward more "agent-based" models, as opposed to earlier "mass-action" models. Social scientists have played a major role in this development. Agent-based models entail the representation of every individual in the population of interest as a distinct entity, so they more easily account for the elaborate social processes at work within populations of highly diverse and dynamic individuals. Many of the agent-based models in use in the epidemic modeling literature also fall into the category of network modeling, in which both individual members of a population and their pair-wise contacts are explicitly represented. This approach is especially valuable for diseases transmitted through rare, memorable, highly nonrandom contacts, conditions typified by STDs. The downside of agent-based models is that they require computationally intensive simulation, making them more difficult to implement and less attractive to those who prefer analytical solutions. Anthropologists, however, are probably among those most easily convinced of the value of jettisoning simple solutions when these require one to treat individuals as largely identical, static, and rational instead of diverse, dynamic, reactive, and constrained. The approaches are particularly useful when one wants to consider multiple interacting forms of diversity simultaneously, such as demographic and behavioral diversity (Clark 2006) or behavioral and genetic diversity (Goodreau 2006).

Nevertheless, the initial development of epidemic modeling within mathematics means that the very abstract language of this field—the language of counting (quantification generally) and accounting (determining causation statistically)—tends to dominate the approach. The term *epidemic* predominates, rather than the more emotionally laden *plague* or *outbreak*. As articulated elsewhere in this volume (e.g., Anderson; Littleton, Park, and Bryder), the latter terms carry heavy connotations—of chaos, blame, pollution—all of which are generally outside the modeler's direct purview. In modeling, people are referred to as *actors* or even as *nodes*. *Risk* and *responsibility* are frequently discussed, but purely in their statistical senses, as concepts of probability and causation, with connotations of blame typically avoided. All these terms (which I myself employ virtually automatically throughout this chapter) aid in making questions of epidemic dynamics highly abstract. This has value during modeling itself, when abstraction is a useful tool, but as we will see later, extreme care must be taken that it does not inhibit the communication of the model to the broader world or the contextualizing of its implications.

The Philosophy of Modeling

One piece of the theoretical grounding of epidemic modeling that has been well explored is the philosophy of mathematical modeling generally. Good introductions to this topic can be found in the philosophy of science literature (Giere 1999) and in more practice-oriented textbooks (Haefner 2005). In brief, epidemic modelers typically conceptualize their work (implicitly or explicitly) as part of the *hypothetico-deductive* model of scientific inquiry and thus as but one piece of a larger system for producing knowledge about the causes and effects of epidemics. The field is literally hypothetico-deductive in that it first proposes a set of hypotheses about the phenomena underlying a disease and then uses mathematics to deduce the epidemic patterns that must logically flow if the hypotheses are true. Returning to the case of AIDS in Africa will help here.

AIDS, Concurrency, and Hypothetico-Deduction

In the early 1990s, it was still unclear why HIV was spreading among heterosexuals in Africa at a level much higher than anywhere else in the world, and whether this phenomenon would ultimately occur elsewhere. Indeed, the former question is still hotly debated. What was becoming clear by then was that most people in the worst-hit areas of Africa reported no more sexual partners over the course of their lifetime than did the average American heterosexual (see, e.g., Buve et al. 2001; Laumann 1994). Sociologist Martina Morris and mathematical epidemiologist Mirjam Kretzschmar explored the possibility that the key factor might be long-term sexual partner concurrency (Kretzschmar and Morris 1996; Morris and Kretzschmar 1995, 1997). Concurrency means having multiple relationships that overlap in time, as opposed to having sequential relationships. It is virtually given that having multiple partners will increase HIV spread relative to having only one partner; the issue of concurrency is one not of numbers of partners but of timing—that is, having the same number of partners sequentially or concurrently, since this appears to represent a main difference between African sexual networks and those elsewhere. There were intuitive reasons to believe that this timing might account for some major disparities within the AIDS epidemic: from the virus's point of view, simultaneous partnerships imply less time waiting for someone to change partners, from the one who infected them to a new one who is susceptible. Initial mathematical work (Watts and May 1992) confirmed this intuition. Intuition, however, is less clear about how strong this effect will be in general or in any particular population, which is why modeling was of particular use here.

In effect, Morris and Kretzschmar considered a hypothetical scenario, using data that Morris had been involved in collecting and analyzing from Uganda. If two "Uganda-like" populations were identical in nearly every way, including overall levels and types of unprotected sexual activity, and differed only in the sequential versus concurrent nature of partnerships, then how differently would the HIV epidemic play out in them? The question is hypothetical, because of course no populations are identical except for this single factor; in the real world, any two populations differ in countless ways. The process is hypothetico-deductive because it begins from these hypothetical scenarios ("hypotheses") and then deduces, through either analytical mathematics or simulation, the patterns of disease transmission that would necessarily flow from them. Morris and Kretzschmar demonstrated that concurrency could amplify the HIV epidemic under "Uganda-like" conditions. Combining this knowledge with the empirical knowledge that concurrency is high in Uganda and HIV is high in Uganda, they lent strong support to the hypothesis that long-term concurrency helps account for the particularly large heterosexual HIV epidemic in Uganda and perhaps elsewhere in sub-Saharan Africa. They did so without claiming to estimate perfectly how much concurrency mattered in any specific population; they knew this would be an overstatement given the simplifying assumptions they had needed to make.

Simplicity and Generality

One of the most thorough explanations aimed at an anthropological audience for the value of using models in this way is that offered by Peter Richerson and Robert Boyd (1987). The world is too complex ever to be understood in its entirety, so attempts to develop knowledge about it require the selection of some section of it to be considered in relative isolation. For entities amenable to representation in a mathematical model, the authors argue that a collection of relatively simple models is the best approach for maximizing understanding. A single simple model can explain only one small part of a complex system, which is insufficient if one's goal is to gain some overall picture of the system, however imperfectly. But a single overcomplicated approach that tries to explain everything at once is akin to building a map of an area as large as the area itself. Complex models are especially dangerous in social science, Richerson and Boyd argued, because they are "most likely to be scientifically justified when phenomena are complex but not diverse"—that is, when a system's many parts are effectively identical or fall into a small number of categories. Although many physical systems might be described this way, no real social systems could be accurately described as consisting of essentially identical people.

Instead, Richerson and Boyd advocated approaching a system with a wide range of models, each of which was individually simple but which collectively shed more light on the problem than either any single small model or one large meta-model. This is analogous to the idea that no one approach to knowledge (postcolonial, human ecological, etc.) accounts for all facets of any phenomenon, but combining them all into a single meta-view would actually confuse more than elucidate.

Richerson and Boyd's approach is effectively what developed in the field of epidemic modeling, whether planned or not. Morris and Kretzschmar's model is but one of many exploring the effects of different elements of cultural, behavioral, and biological complexity on the HIV epidemic around the world. Each necessarily includes things that others exclude, and vice versa. And HIV is certainly not unique—at least thirty-five papers modeling some aspect of the interpersonal transmission of tuberculosis, each somewhat differently, have been published (Achterberg 2009). Perhaps this approach was inevitable, given the difficulty of building complex models, the wide range of questions of interest to modelers, and the diversity of disciplinary training of those in the field. In that case, the fact that Richerson and Boyd argued that this was actually the best way to proceed was merely a boon.

Richerson and Boyd (1987: 36) further advocated that these collections of simple models be generalized—that is, that each model try to explain not only a single case but a whole class of cases:

> Generalized [models] are useful because we do not seem to be able to construct models of social and biological phenomena that are general, realistic, and precisely predictive… That is, evolutionary biologists and social scientists have not been able to satisfy the epistemological norm derived from the physical sciences that holds that theory be in the form of universal laws that can be tested by the detailed predictions they make about the phenomena considered by the law. This failure is probably a consequence of the complexity and diversity of living things.

Were I to create my own version of this quotation, I would remove the word "probably" from the last sentence. I would also modify the underlying universality of the idea that generalized models are always the ideal. Epidemic modeling is an applied field, and epidemic models are built with one of two goals in mind: sometimes to account for general trends in epidemics and their determinants across a range of populations, and sometimes to provide information for guiding specific interventions in specific cultural settings. The former clearly lends itself better to generalized models. Morris and Kretzschmar accomplished these dual goals by exploring the specifics of concurrency in Uganda in some papers and concurrency's effects more generally, using the same basic model, in other papers.

Epidemic Modeling and Social Theory

In the hypothetico-deductive view of modeling, one way to define "theory" is as any set of heuristics that provides guidance in deciding what to include or exclude in a model, and what simplifying assumptions to make in doing so. In this view, modeling as a whole is officially atheoretical (or perhaps pan-theoretical), because it places no absolute limits on what can be considered in a disease model. Any specific model, however, is an instantiation of a particular theoretical alignment. Of course in practice certain phenomena are easier than others to operationalize in the language of mathematics, so that modeling in practice is not truly as pan-theoretical as modelers might wish. For example, it is generally easier in epidemic models to examine actual behaviors than to model the psychological motivations behind behaviors. The latter is not impossible, but the former is sufficiently easier that it typically comes to the forefront. As a whole, then, modeling tends to emphasize the "what" of human contacts over the "why," with potential consequences for our understanding of the latter's role in shaping the former.

Structuralism and Interdependence

For epidemic modeling, one piece that is always included, quite centrally, is the notion of interaction among members of the population. Because of this interest in relationships and their structure, epidemic modeling bears some resemblance to the British structuralist school of anthropology. The motivations for understanding these relationships were different, however, for A. R. Radcliffe-Brown and the Manchester School than for epidemic modelers. Typically, the British structuralists wanted to understand how relational patterns emerged to fill functional roles in maintaining the social organism. For epidemic modeling, the goal of elucidating social structure—to understand how infectious disease spreads on it—is more immediate. Yet the underlying focus on individuals, relations, and populations leads to a number of shared methodological and technical issues. This similarity is strongest in epidemic models using social network methods, because this approach is directly descended through a clear lineage from the Manchester School.

British structuralism fell out of favor for many reasons, perhaps most crucially because its proponents were perceived as overconcerned with regularities, ignoring both exceptions and conflicts. They were also limited by the technology available at the time, which prevented deep exploration of models of heterogeneous agents, even though this was what structural anthropologists were seeking to understand. Today's models are better equipped to deal with the messiness of actual social systems. And with a less lofty goal than trying to define the ultimate causes of social structure, epidemic models are perhaps more immune to some of structuralism's critiques.

Integrating Other Theoretical Approaches

This central focus on contact and interaction does not preclude modelers from considering other factors in the perpetuation of disease; it is simply a way of accounting for all the diverse factors in a unified framework. One way to see this is to consider how actual transmission events are structured in most epidemic models, for any disease transmitted directly from person to person. These events have four key elements: (1) the existence of a person susceptible to infection; (2) the existence of an infectious person; (3) contact between these two people, under whatever definition of contact is relevant for that disease; and (4) actual transmission, given that such a contact has occurred.

The number of the first element, susceptible people, at any time is shaped by birth rates and death rates from causes other than the disease itself. It may also be shaped by genetic factors affecting susceptibility to a particular pathogen and by the existence of and access to vaccines against that agent. For a disease that can be contracted only once, the number of susceptible persons depends on the ways in which people previously avoided infection. For the second item, an infectious person, we see a similar logic: What chain of events led to someone's becoming infected but neither recovering nor dying?

The third item, contact, involves numerous anthropological considerations, in terms of understanding people's overall propensity to interact but also with whom, and how these propensities affect the likelihood of an infected and a susceptible person's coming into contact. The considerations include public health interventions such as quarantine and the many aspects of social structure that obtain prior to such interventions. When disease rates vary by age, how often do people of different ages interact? How does race channel with whom we shake hands or have sex? How about geography, gender, and class? Finally, the fourth item, transmission given contact, is affected by factors such as the immunological states of the two actors, their genetics, their underlying health and nutrition status, and their attempts to prevent transmission—for example, by covering their mouths when coughing or using condoms during sex. All these considerations, affecting all four items—from issues of global inequality down to immunology and genetics—can be placed side by side in a mathematical model of epidemic spread, in the common language of mathematics.

Of course some things are easier to represent in the language of counting than others. One piece of human social experience that mathematical models are relatively good at incorporating is heterogeneity among actors. It is generally a straightforward matter to account for different types of actors in models and allow them to behave differently, and some form of real-world heterogeneity is present in virtually all applied models these days. Common variations include age (Morris and Dean 1994), geographic or social group membership (Sattenspiel 1987a, 1987b), and behavioral variability (Goodreau 2006). This basic idea underlies both mass-action models (in which compartments are defined by types of persons) and agent-based models, although the latter are more easily capable of handling higher levels of heterogeneity. Mass-action models are also constrained to consider heterogeneity as discrete, which may force the modeler to categorize people more coarsely than is truly relevant.

Agency

Despite the name "agent-based models," one feature that is actually less commonly seen in epidemic models is agency. The very concept of agency is difficult to pin down for virtual beings defined only within a computer program. What I mean by the term is the ability for individuals to change their characteristics or behaviors in the face of changes occurring around them. One example would be engaging in lower rates of contact as the prevalence of some disease increases around one. Models addressing heterogeneity among actors, however, often fix many of those characteristics at the outset or allow them to change randomly rather than as a function of the environment. Again, this is typically done for simplicity and not realism. One counterexample from the anthropology literature (Sattenspiel and Castillo-Chavez 1990) modeled a gay male population in which men had individual propensities for engaging in risky behavior, which could change temporarily depending on whom they interacted with and under what conditions.

Individual agency is of course shaped by culture and political economy, as seen in chapters throughout this volume (e.g., Castro, Khawja, and Johnston; Kelm; Lepani; Lindenbaum). We saw in an earlier section that one of anthropologists' main contributions to epidemic modeling has been to bring in more culture-specific information when relevant. Another recent trend has been an increased interest in accounting for political and economic systems' effects on infectious disease. For example, recent work has sought to measure population risk for HIV from the very scenario I started with—the labor migration system of southern Africa (Coffee, Lurie, and Garnett 2007). Another example considered the provision of services within the UK national health care system and the way this amplified the spread of gonorrhea under some conditions and dampened it under others (White et al. 2005). One long-standing concern has been the amplifying effects of multiple epidemics in resource-poor settings. Called "syndemics" in the medical anthropology literature (see, e.g., Singer, this volume; Noymer, this volume), the same ideas can be found explicitly in the epidemic modeling literature, even when not described in the language of medical anthropology. In one recent example, epidemiologists modeled the syndemic effects of malaria and HIV in Africa (Abu-Raddad, Patnaik, and Kublin 2006). Work bridging modeling and medical anthropology on the topic of syndemics has recently appeared (Herring and Sattenspiel 2007) and, it is hoped, will lead to increased dialogue between those with similar questions but different terms and tools.

Communicating Models

For most models that deal with topics of culture or political economy, those contexts are highly abstracted in the model itself but play a strong role both in framing the question in the first place and, most important, in shaping how the results are interpreted and translated into potential action. Not all modelers are equally adept at ensuring that this final step occurs, and another great contribution of the social sciences to epidemic modeling has been to strengthen that connection. The use of mathematical language can sometimes hinder this process. For instance, one paper discussed the value of "destruction of the best-connected nodes" in an epidemic as a strategy for interrupting transmission (Liljeros et al. 2001). When one realizes that nodes represent people, then the idea of any public health intervention that "destroys" nodes becomes meaningless. Public health approaches might try to differentially reduce the contacts of the best-connected nodes or reduce the probability of transmission on those connections, something the authors did subsequently discuss. Yet the former wording is precisely the sort of disconnect that can cause modeling to be ignored by the rest of the epidemiology community or, worse, to be used to justify interventions whose ethical, practical, cultural, or economic implications are not addressed in implementation, solely because they were not addressed in a model of that implementation. As a counterexample, the work on concurrency of sexual partners by Morris and Kretzschmar was solidly grounded in local understandings of why concurrency existed in Uganda and what efforts to change it might be successful, a process aptly explored in a recent popular book on the politics of AIDS in Africa (Epstein 2007).

Role Versatility and HIV in Peru

The issues I have discussed so far can be seen in a single case study of HIV among men in Lima, Peru (Goodreau, Goicochea, and Sanchez 2005). In this study my colleagues and I sought to answer a seemingly simple question: What effect does sexual role segregation have on the spread of HIV among men who have sex with men, or MSM? (Note that I avoid the term *gay*, because in this setting many MSM do not identify as such.) The motivation for this question stemmed from a few related observations, the main one being that HIV is more easily transmitted from insertive to receptive partner during penile-anal sex than vice versa. MSM who engage in anal sex may adopt one of three sexual roles over time: always the insertive partner, always the receptive partner, or some mixture of the two. The first two are referred to as types of "role segregation," and the last, as "role versatility." It seems reasonable to believe that high role segregation may act as a barrier to HIV transmission in a population, because the virus cannot move through the population without passing through transmission "bottlenecks" from a receptive man to an insertive man. In a culture with high role versatility, men can become infected easily, through receptive sex, and then transmit easily, through insertive sex.

Considerable ethnographic work has been conducted on MSM in Latin America (Carrier 1976, 1995; Carrillo 2002; Gutmann 2003; Murray 1995a; Parker 1999), including work on MSM in Peru specifically (Arboleda 1995; Cáceres and Jiménez 1999; Cáceres and Rosasco 1999; Murray 1995b). Questions of sexual role are major themes of the literature, with a common observation that role segregation has been high in Latin America (at least relative to the United States and western Europe) but that role versatility may be on the rise. The selection of sexual role is a deeply symbolic act with connotations of reconstructing male-female gender distinctions; it also intersects with issues of wealth, age, class, and power, not to mention personal desire. Most strikingly, it is intertwined with questions of cultural globalization, because for some men versatility represents the adoption of a Northern perspective on gay identity, represented lexically in the words for *versatile* in Peru (*moderno*) and Mexico (*internacional*). Cáceres and his colleagues have shown how all these processes play out in Lima specifically, within a diverse and fluid set of sexual cultures.

Given the high but possibly changing level of role segregation in Peru (and elsewhere in Latin America), we sought to gain more insight into the degree to which role segregation was affecting the HIV epidemic. Following the philosophy of beginning with simple models, we kept much of the rich contextual complexity regarding *why* men select the roles they do in the background. Instead, we used relatively descriptive data on the counts of men who had been exclusively insertive, exclusively receptive, or versatile during unprotected anal sex during the recent past among Lima MSM. We then compared this scenario with two hypothetico-deductive cases: What if all those men had had the same rates of sexual encounters, but everyone had been versatile? And what if they had had the same level of encounters, but everyone had been role segregated?

With simplicity in mind, we introduced the unrealistic assumption that individual men never changed their role class—once versatile, always versatile, and once segregated, always segregated. We also made no attempt to model the way men changed their level of sexual contact or condom use as they aged or acquired HIV, or as HIV levels changed in the population. Our agents were entirely lacking in agency.

The only forms of heterogeneity in the population, then, were three roles and two disease statuses, uninfected and infected. In all other respects the members of our populations were indistinguishable. In essence the model reduced people's life trajectories into a small number of events: entering the sexually active MSM pool; having a contact and not seroconverting; having a contact and seroconverting; and leaving the sexually active pool through aging or death. One additional piece we considered was whether or not versatile men preferentially chose other versatile men as partners. If versatility represents a Northern worldview, then it is reasonable to imagine that such men would be more likely to be connected in the sexual network, and the degree to which this was true was expected to play a strong role in shaping versatility's effects.

Despite these simplifications, the model resulted in a set of equations requiring half a page to write down and that was solvable only using high-powered computational algorithms. Reassuringly, our "Lima-like" population generated an HIV epidemic among MSM very similar in prevalence to the actual one. We saw that a comparable all-versatile population would have an HIV epidemic about twice as large as that of a "Lima-like" population during the epidemic's first few decades, and in a completely segregated population the epidemic would be only marginally smaller than in the Lima model. The widespread practice of role segregation seemed to be having an enormous effect in protecting this population from HIV.

One interesting twist was that in both cases, HIV prevalence according to our model was higher among receptive-only men, lowest among insertive-only men, and intermediate among versatile men, who had an HIV prevalence about equal to that of the overall population. This alone is unsurprising, but it means that versatility can be a population-level risk factor and simultaneously *not* be an individual-level one. Generating knowledge about such counterintuitive processes can be nearly impossible without modeling.

Mindful of Richerson and Boyd's call for generalized models, we also sought to demonstrate that versatility's effects could be strong across a range of scenarios, not just those observed in Peru. We approached this by conducting sensitivity analyses, varying some of the features of the model that we had held constant earlier. In total we ran 605 simulations for populations that diverged in different ways from the behavior reported in Peru. Versatility levels remained important throughout in determining the level of HIV prevalence in a population. But what determined whether versatility became an individual risk factor or not— that is, *who* got infected rather than *how many* got infected—was the degree to which versatile men chose each other as partners, forming a cohesive subset within the sexual network.

The rich ethnographic work that has been conducted on male sexuality and role reappeared in allowing us to interpret our results and translate them into potential public health considerations. A purely ungrounded approach might have said: "Role versatility dramatically increases HIV, placing the entire community at higher risk; therefore, the public health community should encourage role segregation over role versatility." The research into the meaning of role and all its intersecting currents told us that this would be inappropriate; it could be interpreted as a suggestion that MSM perpetuate gendered power differentials or that they be dissuaded from actively redefining what it means to be gay in modern Latin America. Two very different ways of knowing about epidemics were thus able to come together.

Unfortunately, there was no clear intervention we could point to as a result of this work, in the sense of an alternative message that could incorporate the epidemic importance of versatility but that would not have the problems just mentioned. All we could conclude was that versatile men were indirectly responsible (again in the strictly epidemiological sense) for a disproportionate amount of the epidemic in settings where role segregation was common. Thus, any efforts that reduced numbers of partners or increased condom use would have an extra (but probably never directly detectable) population-level effect if they included a disproportionate number of versatile men.

Harnessing this knowledge meant getting a sense of who versatile men were. To do so, we examined the ethnographic literature and conducted some quantitative analyses of our own data (Peinado et al. 2007). We found that there were two largely distinct clusters of versatile men: those with high levels of education, income, and travel; and sex workers. Both groups match the ethnography and common sense, the former because it fits the idea that versatility represents flow of cultural norms from the North, and the latter because it fits with reasons of economic necessity. Interestingly, because so many characteristics of the two groups are opposed to one another, simple analyses examining a wide range of individual predictors of the probability of being versatile showed no effect. Again, the ethnography directed us toward additional ways to analyze the data in order to tease apart these observations and gain a richer understanding of the structure of individual and population risk for HIV in this community.

Conclusion

The seemingly mechanical practice of mathematical modeling for epidemics engages productively with other ways of knowing, particularly when the modeling is performed by anthropologists and other social scientists. I end with two simple hopes for the future. First, that epidemic modelers, social epidemiologists, and medical anthropologists can learn to communicate more effectively about the commonalities in their approaches to understanding disease, and that this essay may play a role in that. Second, that more social scientists, and especially more anthropologists, will enter the world of epidemic modeling. The latter would almost certainly aid the former. Together these developments will ensure that epidemic modeling remains firmly grounded in social theory and in specific cultural experiences and thus best able to be of practical use in the human battle against epidemics.

Acknowledgments

I thank the Wenner-Gren Foundation, especially Leslie Aiello and Laurie Obbink, for the opportunity to participate in the plagues symposium. I also thank the symposium participants, organizers D. Ann Herring and Alan C. Swedlund, and William Stanford.

Social Inequalities and Dengue Transmission in Latin America

Arachu Castro, Yasmin Khawja, and James Johnston

Thus, whereas plague by its impartial ministrations should have promoted equality among our townsfolk, it now had the opposite effect and, thanks to the habitual conflict of cupidities, exacerbated the sense of injustice rankling in men's hearts. They were assured, of course, of the inerrable equality of death, but nobody wanted that kind of equality. Poor people who were feeling the pinch thought still more nostalgically of towns and villages in the near-by countryside, where bread was cheap and life without restrictions. Indeed, they had a natural if illogical feeling that they should have been permitted to move out to these happier places. The feeling was embodied in a slogan shouted in the streets and chalked up on walls: "Bread or fresh air!" This half-ironical battle-cry was the signal for some demonstrations that, though easily repressed, made everyone aware that an ugly mood was developing among us.

—Albert Camus, *The Plague*

The threat of dengue, initially looming most heavily over Southeast Asia, has come to weigh profoundly on Latin America as well, through both socioeconomic processes and the natural history of disease. A review of the literature shows frequent references to the effects of historical processes, unplanned rapid urbanization, population growth, failure of public health programs, increased air travel, lack of adequate biodegradable waste disposal, poor water quality, and underfunding of prevention and control programs on the increase of dengue transmission, although the mechanisms by which these factors interact in their social context are not well documented. A biosocial approach to dengue research—which includes analyses of the interaction between viral, immunological, epidemiological, and social factors accounting for varying disease incidence, severity, and distribution—contributes to better elucidation of the mechanisms that propel dengue in Latin America.

The principal vector for dengue virus is the mosquito species *Aedes aegypti*, thought to have originated in Africa (Gubler 1997). The female mosquito transmits the virus from person to person through daytime bites. The mosquito likely adapted to the domestic environment prior to the slave trade initiated during the sixteenth century, by feeding on humans and breeding in water containers (Gubler 1997). Once part of the domestic habitat, *Aedes aegypti* followed human migrations to urban settlements throughout the world (Ehrenkranz et al. 1971; Gubler 1997). The origin of dengue virus itself is more controversial. Most agree that dengue evolved as a mosquito's virus prior to human transmission. Although some researchers dispute its place of origin (Holmes and Twiddy 2003), several trace it to Asia (Gubler 1997, 2004a). Dengue exhibits considerable genetic diversity, existing in four distinct serotypes (Den-1, Den-2, Den-3, and Den-4) and numerous phylogenetically defined genotypes (Holmes and Burch 2000; Rico-Hesse 1990). The virus also appears to be growing progressively more diverse (Zanotto et al. 1996).

Epidemiological Overview of Dengue

Dengue is the most important mosquito-borne viral disease affecting human populations (CDC 2007). Two and a half billion people in one hundred countries live in dengue-endemic areas (WHO 2004) and are at risk for developing dengue disease (fig. 13.1). Each year in the early twenty-first century, between 50 million and 100 million people are newly infected with dengue virus, of whom an estimated 250,000 to 500,000 develop dengue hemorrhagic fever (DHF) and about 24,000 die (Gibbons and Vaughn 2002; Guzmán and Kourí 2002; WHO 2004). Most dengue infections go unnoticed, with mild symptoms or none at all and, when symptomatic, dengue is usually self-limiting, with no known permanent sequelae (Burke et al. 1988; Gubler 1998; Rigau-Pérez et al. 1994). In the Americas alone, the World Health Organization (WHO) reported more than 1 million cases of dengue in 2002 (Nathan and Dayal-Drager 2007).

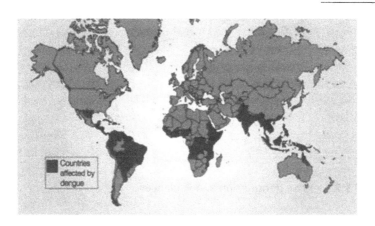

Figure 13.1 Countries affected by dengue, 2004. Source: Kroeger, Nathan, and Homback 2004.

Dengue hemorrhagic fever and dengue shock syndrome (DSS), the most severe forms of dengue, occur in only a small percentage of people infected with dengue but have a high case-fatality rate: 10 to 20 percent in untreated DHF (relative to 0.2 percent in treated DHF) and more than 40 percent in cases of DSS (Gibbons and Vaughn 2002; Guzmán and Kourí 2002). Reported cases of severe forms of dengue have increased rapidly since the 1980s. This is due in part to better recognition and reporting, but it is also due to increased epidemic transmission and hyperendemicity in urban environments (Gubler 2004b; Monath 1994). The emergence of severe forms of dengue is most striking in Latin America, where the number of reported DHF cases per year has increased more than twentyfold, from about 60 cases before 1980 to 75,000 cases in 2000 (PAHO 2001).

Viral and Immunological Factors

Several factors have been associated with increased risk for developing severe forms of dengue, including the viral strain, the patient's age and genotype, his or her immune response, and the infection sequence (Guzmán and Kourí 2003; Halstead 1997). Figure 13.2 shows some of these interactions. Although all four serotypes of dengue virus can induce the severe forms of dengue, a Den-2 and Den-3 strain combination is more commonly associated with severe disease (Guzmán and Kourí 2002). The sequence of serotypes also plays a role in dengue pathogenesis (Guzmán and Kourí 2003), with severe forms more likely

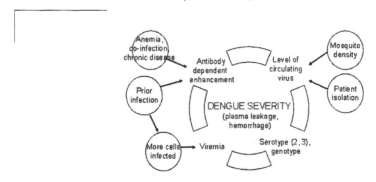

Figure 13.2 Dengue transmission and virulence.

when the secondary viral strain is of Southeast Asian origin (Chungue et al. 1993; Deubel et al. 1993; Guzmán et al. 1995; Rico-Hesse et al. 1997; Sariol et al. 1999).

Viral diversity can influence dengue epidemiology in multiple ways. First, greater viral diversity can increase the chance of heterotypic antibody production—an infection with a dengue serotype different from the serotype of a previous infection—which could lead to more cases progressing to DHF. Second, some dengue strains appear to be more virulent than others, and third, certain sequences of viral infection may be more harmful than others (Guzmán and Kourí 2002). The possibility that specific dengue strains will be selected for properties such as increased virulence and epidemic potential is a palpable concern.

The relative risk of experiencing a severe form of dengue during a heterotypic secondary infection may be one hundred times greater than the risk experienced with a primary dengue infection (Monath 1994), because of a process known as antibody-dependent enhancement (ADE), in which antibodies that develop after the primary infection, during a heterotypic secondary infection may enhance dengue replication (Halstead 1988). Antibodies produced in response to primary dengue infection provide long-term immunity to the infecting dengue serotype. Reinfection with a second dengue serotype, however, can generate non-neutralizing heterotypic antibodies. These antibodies facilitate entry of the virus into receptors such as monocytes and macrophages, that mediate signaling events essential for host defense, but they fail to neutralize the new dengue serotype. The virus is then able to replicate further in the monocyte lineage. This pathological immune response is thought to be exacerbated by the release of cytokines—proteins involved in chemical signaling between cells in immunological, inflammatory, and infectious diseases—which can lead to vascular permeability (Rothman 2004; Rothman and Ennis 1999). Severe forms of dengue, however, have also been shown to occur in the absence of prior infection or enhancing antibodies (Holmes and Burch 2000).

The highest risk of ADE is found in people capable of mounting a secondary immune response—that is, among people over one year of age with a previous infection and among infants with a primary infection who have dengue-immune mothers (Burke et al. 1988; Halstead, Nimmannitya, and Cohen 1970; Halstead et al. 1967). Children appear to be at greater risk for developing the severe forms of dengue than are adults (Guzmán and Kourí 2002), with a modal age between eight and ten years (Kourí et al. 1989). Young infants and the elderly have been shown to have the highest hospitalization and case-fatality rates among those affected with the severe forms (Guzmán et al. 2002). It has been suggested that populations of African descent may be less susceptible than others to, and even resistant to, advancing to the severe forms of dengue (Bravo, Guzmán, and Kourí 1987; Deubel et al. 1993; Guzmán et al. 1990; Halstead et al. 2001; Morier et al. 1987; Valdés et al. 1999; Vaughn 2000). Further research is needed to elucidate whether the association is due to genetic or social factors.

Some studies point to a syndemic relationship (Singer, this volume) between dengue and nutritional status, reinforcing the idea that better immune response, mediated through better nutrition, increases the risk of ADE. In a study conducted in Bangkok, Thailand, researchers found that malnutrition was less prevalent among children with DHF than among children with other infectious diseases and even children classified by the researchers as healthy (Thisyakorn and Nimmannitya 1993). Other researchers found that in Bangkok, children with malnutrition had a lower risk than obese children of contracting dengue infection, although malnourished children infected with dengue had a higher risk of developing shock than other children (Kalayanarooj and Nimmannitya 2005). Other researchers have reported that among children with DHF in Bangkok, obesity and Den-2 increased the risk of developing the most severe forms of DHF (grades 3 and 4) (Pichainarong et al. 2006). In Vietnam, researchers found that among 245 infants with dengue infection, the proportion of those with low height and weight was smaller than among 533 uninfected controls (Nguyen et al. 2005). Studies conducted in India and in Bangladesh, on the other hand, have shown no association between severity of malnutrition and severity of dengue (Ahmed et al. 2001; Kabra et al. 1999).

Social Conditions and Increased Dengue Transmission

The dengue epidemic has been linked to increased population movement and rapid urbanization (Gratz 1999; Gubler 1998; Knudsen and Slooff 1992; Narro-Robles and Gómez Dantes 1995; Pinheiro and Corber 1997), although the mechanisms by which such associations exist are not well documented. The discontinuity of vector control programs, which follows the disinvestment in and the collapse of public health infrastructure (Gubler 1998; Guzmán 2001), coupled with increased inequalities in access to health care, are contributing factors to the increased transmission of dengue in Latin America, where urbanization and greater human density offer a perfect breeding ground in which the mosquito and the virus can thrive and spread.

Increased Population Movement

Increased international trade in persons and goods, migrations, displacement, and tourism result in the circulation of dengue serotypes and increased viral diversity. These factors are associated with an increase in heterotypic secondary infections.

The advent of the transatlantic slave trade, transnational commerce, and the global shipping industry hastened the spread of both *Aedes aegypti* and dengue (Ehrenkranz et al. 1971; Gubler 1997). *Aedes* populations thrived in the squalor of slave-trading vessels, while slaves and their captors served as prime viral hosts. Commercial shipping also fueled the urbanization of port cities, drawing migrants from rural villages. High population density and poor hygienic conditions in urban areas, along with the constant influx of susceptible hosts, nurtured both vector and virus. Eight pandemics of dengue-like disease were recorded between 1779 and 1916, each spreading from seaports (Gubler 1997; Howe 1977). The Caribbean slave trade was considered the cause of the 1827 pandemic (Ehrenkranz et al. 1971), and in 1870–1873, a dengue pandemic spread from Dar Es Salaam and Zanzibar, two known slave trading ports, to what are now Saudi Arabia, Mauritius, Reunion, India, China, Taiwan, and the United States. The Asian slave trade continued well into the twentieth century, potentially extending dengue's spread throughout Asia (Ehrenkranz et al. 1971).

By the early twentieth century, dengue was endemic in India, Southeast Asia, and the Philippines, with epidemics generally affecting immigrant populations (Howe 1977). In the Americas, dengue was intermittently active, with occasional large outbreaks. In a 1922 outbreak in Galveston,

Texas, for example, more than forty thousand cases were reported (Rawlings et al. 1998; Rice 1923), and as many as 2 million people were affected (Ehrenkranz et al. 1971).

There is evidence that the resurgence of dengue in Asia and the modern dengue pandemic are linked to disruptions that took place in the 1940s during World War II (Ehrenkranz et al. 1971; Gubler 1997; Howe 1977; Monath 1994). Water supplies and sewage systems were destroyed during the war, accompanied by an increase in war scrap and water storage. These events led to a surge in *Aedes* populations. Water-filled tires and water storage containers were popular vehicles for the vector. Troop movements presented a continuous supply of susceptible hosts and rapidly spread different dengue serotypes to new territories. By the end of World War II, the majority of Southeast Asian countries had evolved from being areas of low-level endemicity to being areas of hyperendemic dengue (Gubler 1997, 2002b; Monath 1994). During the postwar period, millions of poor rural peasants in Southeast Asia moved to urban areas, and most were immunologically susceptible to dengue. Unplanned urbanization, coupled with poor housing and inadequate water and waste management, sustained dengue hyper-endemicity, with annual outbreaks in many Southeast Asian cities. The trend of urbanization and crowding was further fueled by Asian economic expansion during this period (Gubler 1997; Monath 1994).

In this context of epidemic transmission, urban hyperendemicity, and the mixing of serotypes, a more severe form of dengue emerged in Southeast Asia. The first recorded case of dengue hemorrhagic fever occurred in 1953 in Manila, Philippines. Since then, epidemic DHF has expanded throughout Southeast Asia and beyond, to China and throughout the Pacific islands, India, Pakistan, Sri Lanka, the Maldives, and Latin America (Gubler 1997; Monath 1994). In many Asian countries, DHF epidemics recur every three to five years (Gubler 1997), in contrast to previous centuries, when epidemics erupted in cycles of ten to forty years (Gubler 2002, 2004a). DHF is now a leading cause of pediatric hospitalization and mortality in several Asian countries (Gubler 2002; Pinheiro and Corber 1997).

Discontinuity of Vector Control Programs

The political structures and financial commitments of many govern-ments are such that large, vertically organized programs for the control of infectious diseases have become difficult to implement and sustain (see Cueto, this volume). In some areas, the erratic nature of underfunded control programs has been associated with the spread of insecticide resistance in mosquitoes. In lieu of vector control strategies, many countries have developed emergency response programs, which have proved largely ineffective (Gubler 1989).

In the Americas, periodic dengue epidemics were recorded from the nineteenth century and soon afterward, although they were relatively rare (Agramonte 1906; Bernal 1828; Ehrenkranz et al. 1971). The purpose of early *Aedes aegypti* control efforts was to combat urban epidemics of yellow fever, a virus hosted by the same mosquito. By 1933, Brazilian public health officials had succeeded in eliminating *Aedes* from several Brazilian cities. This was followed by the elimination of the vector from Bolivia in 1941. These campaigns employed classic source-reduction techniques: water containers were inspected for larvae and breeding places were covered with oil (Camargo 1967; Soper 1965a). By 1946, dichlorodiphenyltrichloroethane (DDT), the first modern pesticide and among the best-known organic pesticides, was proven effective in the reduction of *Aedes* populations (Camargo 1967; Gubler 2004a). Consequently, from the late 1940s to the 1960s, *Aedes aegypti* control campaigns focused on using DDT to reduce larvae (Reiter and Gubler 1997).

This method appeared to be effective and, together with the success of the eradication programs in Brazil and Bolivia, led to the Pan American Health Organization's (PAHO) initiation of a program to eradicate yellow fever in the Americas in 1947 (Monath 1994; Reiter and Gubler 1997). This regimented, DDT-based eradication strategy was successful for more than a decade. Between 1947 and 1963, epidemic dengue was not reported in the region (Ehrenkranz et al. 1971), and nineteen countries were reported free of *Aedes aegypti* by 1964 (Camargo 1967; Gubler 1989; Reiter and Gubler 1997). But although eradication of *Aedes aegypti* was achieved in most of South and Central America, many Caribbean countries, along with the United States, Guyana, Venezuela, and French Guiana, were unsuccessful in achieving full eradication and remained reservoirs of *Aedes aegypti* (Camargo 1967; Gubler 1989; Istúriz, Gubler, and Brea del Castillo 2000). In 1953, the first laboratory-confirmed case of dengue in the Americas was documented in Trinidad, followed by more cases over subsequent months (Anderson, Downs, and Hill 1956; Ehrenkranz et al. 1971).

Eradication campaigns faced several obstacles. First, many countries failed to organize programs. The United States initiated an eradication program only in 1965 and terminated it four years later because of an alleged lack of funds (Slosek 1986). Resistance to insecticides also developed, particularly in the Caribbean, and several countries experienced reinfestation, often with insecticide-resistant mosquitoes (Slosek 1986). Meanwhile, the availability of a yellow fever vaccine diminished interest in eradication programs, particularly in the United States, where dengue and yellow fever posed no immediate threat (Slosek 1986). The success of vaccine research shifted funding from preventive field programs to heavily laboratory-based activities (Gusmão 1982). Finally, the long-term health consequences of insecticides had surfaced. These factors led to the dismantling of eradication programs in the early 1970s and subsequent spread of *Aedes aegypti* throughout the Americas over the subsequent decades (Monath 1994; Reiter and Gubler 1997; Soper 1965a; Sweeney 1999) (fig. 13.3).

In 1963–1964, Den-3 serotype was isolated in Jamaica and Puerto Rico before spreading to the Lesser Antilles and Venezuela (Ehrenkranz et al. 1971). Haiti and Cuba were not affected during this epidemic. Some writers have suggested that in the 1960s these countries were relatively isolated from the flow of international commerce; when Haiti became reengaged in Caribbean commerce, epidemic dengue reappeared (Ehrenkranz et al. 1971). In 1968–1969, a second epidemic, mainly of Den-2 virus, swept through the Caribbean basin (Pinheiro and Corber 1997). In 1970, the PAHO eradication campaign was suspended, despite the fact that it had not yet achieved its goals (Gubler 1989, 2002a; Pinheiro and Corber 1997).

The Den-2 and Den-3 serotypes resurfaced in Colombia during epidemics in 1971–1972 (Den-2) and 1975–1977 (Den-3) (Groot 1980; Pinheiro and Corber 1997). In 1977, a third dengue serotype, Den-1, was introduced to the Americas, resulting in a three-year pandemic in the Caribbean and Central and South America (Mas 1979). The 1977

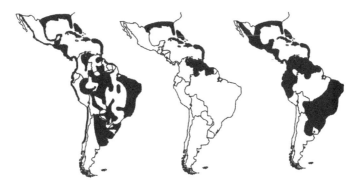

Figure 13.3 Reinfestation of *Aedes aegypti* in the Americas, 1930, 1970, and 2007. Source: PAHO 2007.

outbreak was noteworthy for its size: conservative estimates reported 702,000 infections, and some claimed more than 5 million infections when Venezuela, Cuba, and Colombia were included (Kourí et al. 1989; Mas 1979; Pinheiro and Corber 1997).

The 1980s witnessed continued expansion of epidemic dengue as well as the emergence of epidemic DHF in the Americas. In 1981, Den-4 was introduced, causing outbreaks in South America, the Caribbean, Central America, and Mexico (Gubler 1987; Istúriz, Gubler, and Brea del Castillo 2000). Den-1 spread to five previously dengue-free countries in South America—Peru, Brazil, Bolivia, Ecuador, and Paraguay—causing explosive epidemics in several of them (Pinheiro 1989; Pinheiro and Corber 1997). Figure 13.4 shows the distribution of dengue serotypes in Latin America and the Caribbean.

DHF may have been present in the Americas in the early twentieth century, for hemorrhagic manifestations had been documented in outbreaks in Havana (1897) and Texas (1920) (Guzmán and Kourí 2003). But the first reported DHF epidemic in the Americas was registered in Cuba in 1981 (Guzmán et al. 1992). Until then, DHF was largely a disease confined to Southeast Asia, with only sporadic case reports in the

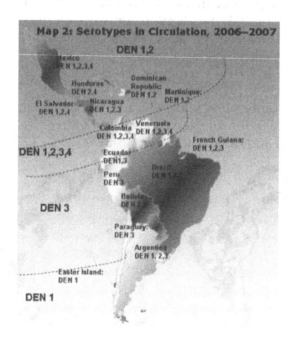

Figure 13.4 Distribution of dengue serotypes in Latin America and the Caribbean, 2006–2007. Source: PAHO 2007.

Americas (Kourí et al. 1989; Pinheiro 1989). During the Cuban epidemic, 344,203 cases were diagnosed, and 116,151 people were hospitalized. Of these, 10,312 patients met the criteria for DHF and DSS, and 158 deaths were recorded. The Cuban epidemic seems to have been caused by the arrival of a Southeast Asian Den-2 strain four years after a milder outbreak of Den-1 in 1977 (Guzmán et al. 1995; Kourí, Guzmán, and Bravo 1986; Kourí et al. 1989).

Since 1981, confirmed or suspected cases of DHF have been reported in every year except 1983 (Isturiz, Gubler, and Brea del Castillo 2000; Pinheiro and Corber 1997). In 1989, a Venezuelan epidemic resulted in 3,108 cases of DHF and 73 deaths (Anonymous 1990; Istúriz, Gubler, and Brea del Castillo 2000). Den-1, Den-2, and Den-4 serotypes were isolated, but all fatal cases were infected with Den-2 (Gubler 1997; Lewis et al. 1993). Other epidemics have taken place in Colombia (1990), French Guiana (1991), and Brazil (1992–1994) (Gubler 1997). The disease is likely endemic in several countries where viral hyperendemicity exists (Gubler 1997).

During the 1990s, dengue arrived in Latin America's only remaining dengue-free countries, Panama and Costa Rica. In 1994, Den-3 was re-introduced after seventeen years of absence, causing several outbreaks, such as in Nicaragua (Guzmán et al. 1996). Dengue outbreaks became more frequent, with a Den-2 outbreak with DHF cases in Puerto Rico in 1994–1995 (Rigau-Pérez, Vorndam, and Clark 2001) and a second large Den-2 outbreak with DHF cases in Cuba in 1997 (Guzmán et al. 2000). In 1998, Den-3 and Den-1 reappeared in Puerto Rico after a twenty-year absence (Rigau-Pérez et al. 2002).

The incidence of dengue in the Americas has increased at an alarming rate. Whereas in 1980 the total number of recorded dengue cases was 66,000, in the year 2002 alone, 1,025,074 dengue cases were reported, including 14,272 cases of DHF and 254 deaths. The United States records 100 to 200 dengue cases annually in people who have traveled in endemic countries (CDC 2003). Between 1977 and 2004, a total of 3,806 suspected cases of dengue were reported in the United States, 864 of them having been laboratory confirmed. Many more are expected to go unreported each year (CDC 2007). The Southern states have indigenous *Aedes* populations, which predisposes the region to autochthonous dengue transmission and outbreaks—of which six occurred in south Texas between 1980 and 2004 (CDC 2007).

Since the early 1980s, *Aedes aegypti* control programs have aimed to achieve control instead of eradication of the vector. Most countries with dengue have *Aedes aegypti* control programs (Lloyd 2003a; Reiter and

Gubler 1997), but except for Singapore and Cuba, governments are not maintaining the programs (Gubler 1989; Gubler and Clark 1996; Reiter and Gubler 1997). Through government-regulated house sprayings, Cuba has successfully used insecticides to limit vector resistance (Bisset 2002).

In the 1980s, the goal of the Pan American Health Organization became the "cost effective utilization of limited resources to reduce vector populations to levels at which they are no longer of significant public health importance" (PAHO 1985; Reiter and Gubler 1997). Insecticide use has continued in the form of sprays, the most popular method being the application of ultra-low-volume malathion (Gubler and Clark 1996). But it has become clear that space spraying is ineffective: several studies have shown the absence of much effect on female *Aedes aegypti* populations. Moreover, the false sense of security created by reliance on vertically implemented interventions in the form of insecticide sprayings lowers the perceived risk of infection (Gubler 2002) and encourages passivity among community members (Knudsen and Slooff 1992; Narro-Robles and Gómez Dantes 1995). Source reduction has once again become the focus of mosquito control (Gubler 1989; Gubler and Clark 1996).

In 1994, PAHO promoted an "integrated, comprehensive dengue prevention and control program," with a greater emphasis on community-based strategies as an alternative to vertically oriented programs (Gubler and Clark 1996). In 1996 it promoted the Continental Plan of collaboration among American states (Cruz 2002). Community-based approaches to public health threats, however, downplay the idea of vector control as a governmental responsibility. They involve redefining safe and acceptable behavior—an intensive and slow process (Gubler and Clark 1996; Reiter and Gubler 1997) that relies on communities and individuals to take ownership of vector control after receiving appropriate orientation and education. The underlying assumption is that once people understand specific behaviors that generate larval habitats, they will consider these behaviors unacceptable (Lloyd 2003b; Reiter and Gubler 1997). Achieving these goals, however, appears difficult. To date, despite some successes, community-based programs have been largely ineffective in preventing dengue epidemics (Gubler 1989; Lloyd 2003b; Reiter and Gubler 1997).

Active epidemiological surveillance and case reporting are essential for successful control programs. Dengue surveillance requires the integration of clinical and entomological data for an appropriate response to reduce the disease burden, and it includes laboratory confirmation of dengue, mortality reporting, sentinel clinics, monitoring of fevers of undiagnosed origin, and continuous analysis of trends (Lloyd 2003b; PAHO 2001). Laboratory-based case reporting is essential to differentiate dengue from several clinically similar diseases (Gubler 1997) and to determine the viral serotype and molecular epidemiology of each outbreak (Gubler 1997, 2004b). Most surveillance programs, however, currently take clinical and vector control data in isolation (Lloyd 2003b). Moreover, clinical surveillance is usually passive, requiring physicians to report suspected cases of dengue, often without laboratory confirmation. Passive surveillance is not sensitive enough to detect dengue outbreaks, resulting in delayed responses to emerging epidemics (Lloyd 2003b).

Population and Urban Density Growth

As of 2007, half the world's population lived in urban areas (UNFPA 2007). Large, concentrated urban populations, particularly when poverty and inequality fuel migration to large cities, may give rise to dengue epidemics (Gubler 2004b). Rapid urban growth is associated with increased transmission of dengue because the proliferation of uninsulated homes, irregular access to running water, lack of proper sewage treatment and garbage collection, piling up of nonbiodegradable waste, and high human density create ideal conditions for increased *Aedes aegypti* densities and disease transmission (Gubler 1998; Guzmán and Kourí 2002). Nonbiodegradable plastic products, used automobile tires, and other artificial water receptacles—the preferred breeding grounds of *Aedes aegypti*—all of which proliferate in Latin America, increase vector density (Gubler 1989, 1998; Monath 1994). As a result, cities become the epicenters of dengue epidemics. Urban areas appear not only to act as sources of dengue transmission but also to generate strains with greater epidemic potential (Cummings et al. 2004; Gubler 2004b). A study conducted in Thailand demonstrated the emergence of virulent epidemic strains that traveled in waves from Bangkok outward to other locations in the country (Cummings et al. 2004).

Over the past decades, enormous demographic shifts have taken place in the regions where dengue has emerged (Gubler 2004a; Gubler and Trent 1993; Reiter and Gubler 1997). In 1930, Latin America had a population of 100 million, of whom 20 million were considered urban. By the close of the twentieth century, 350 million of 470 million Latin Americans lived in cities (Green 1997), and between 2000 and 2030, the urban population of Latin America and the Caribbean is expected to increase from 394 million to 609 million—already representing

77 percent of the population in 2005 (UNFPA 2007). Moreover, urban areas in Latin America are much larger than those in high-income countries. Rural-to-urban migration has concentrated populations in megacities—cities of 10 million or more inhabitants—such as Mexico City, São Paulo, and Buenos Aires and in smaller cities, which usually have fewer resources to address shortages in housing, transportation, piped water, waste disposal, and other services (UNFPA 2007). Population growth, added to rural-to-urban shifts, has led to the development of overcrowding, squatter settlements, and inadequate public health responses in many urban areas (PAHO 2001). This urban redistribution has occurred in all dengue-endemic countries. Moreover, the changes in the urban environments have occurred at a time when many governments have been unwilling or unable to undertake large-scale mosquito control measures (Monath 1994).

Latin American cities display marked disparity between the rich and the poor. In 1980, 118 million people in Latin America were considered poor; ten years later, the number had jumped to 196 million, with 80 percent of the newly impoverished living in cities (UNDP 1995). The growth of the urban poor was not due to population growth alone. During the 1980s, the growth rate of those living in poverty was 42 percent, nearly twice the general population growth rate of 22 percent (UNDP 1995).

The extent of urban poverty is exemplified by the proliferation of informal settlements, or shantytowns, in Latin American cities. The first slums were recorded in Rio de Janeiro in 1920. Today, more than six hundred slums, or *favelas*, exist in Brazil. Meanwhile, in 2001, 135 million people—35 percent of the urban population of Latin America— lived in slum housing (United Nations Human Settlements Programme 2003). Such settlements are usually established by building temporary shacks from plastic and scrap metals, then resisting often violent attempts at eviction. Once established, settlers begin slowly transforming their homes into more permanent dwellings (Gilbert 1994). Informal settlements are fraught with health and safety problems (Gilbert 1994; Hall and Pfeiffer 2000). They are often built on dangerous, desolate, or unsanitary land. Clean water and adequate sanitation are usually nonexistent, not to mention other basic services such as electricity, garbage collection, health centers, schools, and transportation. Slums are also characterized by high population density. The combination of poor location, high population density, lack of sanitation, and illegal status renders residents extremely vulnerable to disease and death. Yet despite the vulnerability of informal settlements, cities often offer immigrants greater access to resources such as schooling, health care, and employment than is available to them in rural areas (Angotti 1995; Gilbert 1994). The prospect of new resources and basic social services appears to outweigh the vulnerability of urban life (Angotti 1995; Hall and Pfeiffer 2000), particularly when, by moving to the city, rural people escape environmental degradation, loss of land, employment, or income, or political persecution and violence.

Many of today's Latin American cities were established during the sixteenth or seventeenth century as centers for colonial administration (Gilbert 1994). Early cities served as gateways for export-based colonial economies and forged the link between urbanization and economic growth. This link has since been strengthened: in the mid- to late twentieth century, as agricultural practices became mechanized, subsistence farming declined and urban industry grew (Angotti 1995). Meanwhile, Latin American governments, in conjunction with international institutions, restructured their economies to encourage urban-based economic growth. The social patterns created by these economic policies have accelerated rural flight to urban areas.

Two types of economic programs greatly affected the urbanization of Latin America: import substitution industrialization programs and structural adjustment programs (SAPs). Import substitution industrialization programs were developed in several Latin American countries between the 1940s and 1970s to encourage production from within the country in an effort to promote self-sufficiency. One component of such strategies was to reduce food prices below market levels in order to offset the costs of urban living. These policies increased rural poverty while encouraging urban growth (Roberts 1995). The pattern established by import substitution industrialization—that of rural poverty and urban investment—intensified as a result of external SAPs imposed on Latin American countries by international organizations.

SAPs were developed in response to the debt crisis of the late 1970s and early 1980s (Gershman and Irwin 1999; Watkins 1995). In 1979, rising oil prices and a worldwide recession led to increases in US interest rates, sometimes to 18 percent or higher (Gershman and Irwin 1999; Watkins 1995). This, combined with falling commodity prices, pushed much of Latin America toward bankruptcy. The crisis culminated in 1982 when Mexico stopped debt payments to international banks (Gershman and Irwin 1999; Watkins 1995). The International Monetary Fund (IMF) and the World Bank intervened in response to the debt crisis. Their response, in the form of SAPs, was aimed to restore the balance of payments from developing countries (Gershman and Irwin 1999).

The influence of SAPs on the Latin American economy should not be underestimated. During the 1980s, there were 107 World Bank–IMF programs in 18 Latin American countries (Watkins 1995). Although SAPs vary from country to country, they have several common characteristics. One is liberalization and deregulation: SAPs reduce the role of the state in regulating the market economy. This includes reducing rural subsidies, food subsidies, and labor protection while removing tariffs on imports in order to liberalize trade. A second common characteristic is privatization: SAPs reduce the role (and spending) of the state by selling state-owned assets and shifting social services—health care, education, and social security—to the private sector (Gershman and Irwin 1999; UNDP 1995; Watkins 1995).

IMF and World Bank programs were designed, according to their architects, to return developing countries to growth while they continued to service their foreign loans. However, the burden of SAPs fell disproportionately on the shoulders of the poor (Gershman and Irwin 1999; UNDP 1995; Watkins 1995). Stabilization plans decreased funding for social services and subsidized commodities, thereby affecting those most in need of such assistance. Meanwhile, poverty and social inequality increased in Latin America during the 1980s (UNDP 1995; Watkins 1995). The number of impoverished people, which increased by 88 million during the 1980s, reversed a twenty-year trend during which the percentage of impoverished Latin Americans had been reduced (UNDP 1995).

Under SAPs and integration into the global economy, farm programs, subsidies, price supports, environmental protection, and supply management were all removed. Rural farmers were exposed to competition from high-volume agribusiness—and to low global market prices. This exposure to global market forces was particularly damaging during the 1980s, when the value of traditional exports fell by 17 percent in Central America (Torres Escobar 1994). The fall in market prices further undermined the self-reliance of rural subsistence farmers, a trend already developing under import substitution industrialization programs.

Wages in Latin America fell during the 1980s without increasing employment (Watkins 1995). In 1987, a "strong and consistent pattern of reduction in labor's share in income" during this period was reported (Pastor 1987). Likewise, the 1990s saw no substantial gains for the working poor (Gershman and Irwin 1999). As a result, the employment opportunities that do exist remain in high demand. Export-oriented industrialization, which is used to generate much-needed foreign capital (Watkins 1995), has led to the proliferation of assembly plants throughout Latin America and to a concentration of investment within cities. Some argue that labor market deregulation enables countries to attract assembly industry through lower wages while workers receive much-needed employment. Few rural migrants, however, can find regular employment in export-based industry, leaving a surplus of unemployed laborers (Gilbert 1994). Without a social safety net, migrants are forced to find work in the informal economic sector, such as street selling, casual construction labor, or other temporary, unstable employment (Gilbert 1994). Moreover, the deregulation of industries and spread of subcontracting is shrinking the sparse formal sector (Gilbert 1994). The surplus of poor urban workers keeps demand for jobs high and wages low (Angotti 1995).

Social Inequality and Access to Health Care

Fragmentation of primary health care contributes to lack of epidemiological surveillance, inadequate diagnostic capacity, underreporting, inadequate clinical management, limited health promotion activities, overemphasis on dissemination of individually focused prevention information (as opposed to community-based prevention interventions), and increased barriers in access to health care, all of which contribute to increased dengue transmission. Lack of access to health care in general, to trained clinicians who can diagnose and manage dengue, to diagnostic tests, and to health facilities where patients can be isolated and receive palliative care also shape the epidemiology of dengue (fig. 13.5). In most of Latin America, a shrinking commitment to public health care and a push for its privatization have led to growing inequalities in access to quality care. Moreover, the number of trained specialists who understand dengue prevention, diagnostics, and treatment may be insufficient.

Some researchers have addressed the relationship between dengue and socioeconomic status, reporting mixed results. Socioeconomic status has been shown to be strongly inversely related to dengue illness in Mexico (Dantes et al. 1988) and Puerto Rico (Meltzer et al. 1998), whereas one study in an urban Brazilian area found a uniform risk of dengue infection across socioeconomic groups (Teixeira et al. 2002). A study in Colombia (Kroeger et al. 1995) reported an increased risk of dengue among those with higher socioeconomic status, which was attributed to their ability to afford water tanks while the poorest populations could not. Therefore, it is difficult to link the increase of dengue transmission to poverty alone.

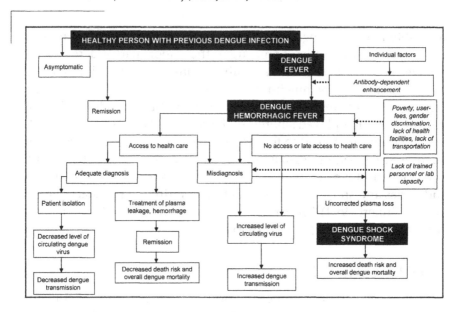

Figure 13.5 Effects of access to health care on dengue transmission.

As in the city of Oman described in *The Plague* (Camus 1947), dengue may operate with an "egalitarian and impartial ministration," spreading across social groups—to some because they have no running water and must collect it haphazardly and to others because they have plenty with which to water the plants and in other open spaces. Social inequality, however, operates through mechanisms other than poverty. Social inequality creates social exclusion, differential access to health care, and barriers such as lack of political interest in improving the social conditions of people living in poverty—which together create a disincentive to invest in public services. Social inequality is related to the transmission of dengue through indirect mechanisms: rapid urban growth, migration, and deterioration in access to health care—a genuine ecosyndemic process (Singer, this volume). As in the city of Oman, and as an example of a coming plague, dengue may spare no one, but its consequences highlight and reinforce existing social inequalities. As a result of dengue, poor and rich alike may be affected by the "lack of fresh air," but the privileged will not embody the unequally imposed "bread or fresh air" predicament brought by plague.

Note

The preparation of this manuscript was funded by grant number OD/AP-03-00235 from the Social, Economic and Behavior Steering Committee of the UNICEF/UNDP/World Bank/WHO Special Program for Research and Training in Tropical Diseases, made to Arachu Castro. We thank María Guadalupe Guzmán and Gustavo Kourí for their encouragement to explore dengue from a social perspective and for their many clarifications, provided throughout our analysis. We thank Paul Farmer for his contributions to an earlier version of the chapter and Johannes Sommerfeld for his overall support. Finally, the first author thanks the Wenner-Gren Foundation for Anthropological Research for having invited her to discuss an earlier version of this chapter at the symposium "Plagues: Models and Metaphors in the Human Struggle with Disease."

From Plague, an Epidemic Comes

Recounting Disease as Contamination and Configuration

Warwick Anderson

"The plague of kuru upon the Fore people has attracted the wonder, curiosity, sympathy, and imagination of the lay and medical world," D. Carleton Gajdusek observed early in 1963 (p. 151). The young American virologist was in London addressing the Royal Society of Tropical Medicine and Hygiene, loquaciously describing his investigations of the fatal brain disease afflicting the isolated Fore people of the eastern highlands of New Guinea, a territory entrusted to Australia. As he entertained his audience with stories of picaresque adventures among "primitives," the tragic dimensions of this plague ineluctably became clearer. Each year, 1 percent of the population died from kuru, most of them women and children, and the Fore feared extinction. Although the people blamed sorcery for the spasmodic movements and uncontrollable tremors to which so many succumbed, Gajdusek in his talk expatiated on possible genetic causes and the ecological background of the disease. Soon, however, he would begin transmission experiments at the US National Institutes of Health (NIH), in Bethesda, Maryland, seeking an infectious source for the bizarre neurological deterioration he had witnessed with such distressing frequency. The London address therefore took place at a pivotal point in his studies of the epidemic, as he shifted from ecological explanations of the disease toward efforts to discover an infectious agent. On first encountering the Fore in March 1957, Gajdusek had found their primitivism and isolation captivating: he quickly assumed the personae of ethnographer and geographer, discarding for a time his microbiological training. Six years later, he was contemplating a return to microbe hunting.

251

In 1948, delivering his presidential address to the American Association for the History of Medicine, Erwin H. Ackerknecht delineated three great divisions among nineteenth-century epidemiologists. There were those who sought evidence of physico-chemical or geographic causes of disease, trying to identify the environmental correlates of outbreaks, their association with miasma or filth. Others, some of them like Rudolf Virchow liberal in their politics, offered a sociological interpretation of disease patterns, arguing for the pervasive influence of economic injustice on the distribution of human pathology. Then there were the rising bacteriologists, who linked specific germs to specific diseases and proceeded to track these microbes through food, water, the earth, and the atmosphere, as well as through insects and animals, including human bodies. In theory one might be both a microbe hunter and a sociologist or environmentalist. But in practice bacteriologists focused ever more narrowly on germs—even as they tracked the microbes, ignoring what might be underlying social or ecological explanations for the organisms' distribution.

Some forty-five years later, one of Ackerknecht's students, Charles E. Rosenberg (1992a), elaborated further on modes of epidemiological reasoning. In viewing epidemic diseases, some chose to emphasize configuration, or structural and relational aspects, while others concentrated on contamination, the technics of transmission of microorganisms. Importantly, Rosenberg noted that the successes of germ theory had not completely suppressed the configurational impulse, even in the middle of the twentieth century. The configurations that continued to excite interest might be sociological or biological or geographical, and generally they revealed assumptions about fit and stress, about balance and mismatch, between humans and their milieu. Both configuration and contamination depended in part on knowledge of individual predisposition to specific diseases. Both styles of explanation could be rich sources of admonition and moral advice.

As a social historian of medicine, Rosenberg evidently favored configuration in accounting for disease. In *The Cholera Years* (1962) he treated the epidemic as a social "sampling technique," the responses to it revealing economic inequalities, patterns of behavior, and otherwise latent cultural assumptions and discriminations. The feared advent of cholera provided the historian with "materials for the construction of a cross-section of cultural values and practices at one moment in time" (Rosenberg 1966: 452). Later, Rosenberg expanded the indexical power of disease, claiming that it was "at once a biological event, a generation-specific repertoire of verbal constructs reflecting medicine's intellectual and institutional history, an occasion of and potential legitimation for public policy, an aspect of social role and individual, intrapsychic, identity, a sanction for cultural values, and a structuring element in doctor and patient interactions" (1992b: xiii). Shirley Lindenbaum, in her ethnographic study of kuru, once made a similar point: in eliciting Fore responses to their plague, she was inevitably tracing an "epidemiology of social relations" (Lindenbaum 1979: viii), uncovering social configurations of the disease.

At the beginning of his investigations of kuru, Gajdusek shared many of these configurational inclinations. He was an unusual virologist, to put it mildly. Attracted to exotic places and intractable, "primitive" peoples, the prodigious scientist spent most of the 1950s snooping on the margins of the medical map, drawing blood from tribesmen in South America, the Middle East, and the Pacific. Under the guidance of Joseph Smadel, first at Walter Reed Army Medical Center and then at the National Institutes of Health, Gajdusek imagined himself as a medical geographer, charting the environmental and biological relations of hemorrhagic fevers across the globe. Working with F. Macfarlane Burnet in Melbourne, Australia, confirmed this ecological mindset. Burnet always insisted on the need to develop an integrative, though never holistic, understanding of disease processes using Darwinian evolutionary theory (Burnet 1940). As a natural historian of disease, he sought to apply fundamental biological principles to microbiology. His interest in the dynamic and complex interactions of life forms in different environments distinguished him from reductionist biochemists and mere microbe hunters. Burnet convinced Gajdusek that colonial New Guinea represented an enormous laboratory for the study of disease ecology and human biology. The young American thus initially approached the Fore people with pronounced ecological and anthropological leanings. He would find, however, that his later focus on contamination, or microbial transmission, gave the bigger payoff—in this case the biggest of all, the Nobel Prize (Anderson 2008).

Throughout the twentieth century, some biomedical scientists and epidemiologists have drawn intermittently on two powerful integrative, or configurational, resources: evolutionary biology and the social sciences. Pragmatically, they have endeavored to give ecological and sociological complexity to their understanding of disease processes, employing broader disciplinary knowledge of life forms and their relations to the environment to enrich their analyses of the normal and the pathological. Although always minority interests, disease ecology and social medicine have never disappeared entirely (Anderson 2004b; Porter 1992). Not surprisingly, these two integrative approaches map roughly onto the geographical and sociological categories that Ackerknecht discerned in nineteenth-century epidemiological reasoning. But in the twentieth century, the older geographical determinism became much more animated and interactive—more ecological—and the older political economy was overlaid with functionalist sociology and cultural anthropology. A few leading epidemiologists thus took at least metaphoric recourse to evolutionary biology in their attempts to develop a more intricate and naturalistic accounting of disease patterns (Flexner 1922; Greenwood 1919; Mendelsohn 1998). Eventually, they managed to incorporate biological principles and insights into increasingly complex mathematical models (Anderson and May 1979; Fenner and Ratcliffe 1965; Sattenspiel 1990). Others sought to attract epidemiology back into the orbit of the social sciences in order to make visible again the social causes and correlates of illness (Galdston 1954; Krieger 2000; Reeder 1972).

In the remainder of this essay I follow Gajdusek and others as they strove to make sense of three relatively obscure diseases in out-of-the-way places. As they investigated kuru, Guam amyotrophic lateral sclerosis and Parkinsonism-dementia complex (ALS-PDC), and Viliuisk encephalomyelitis (VE), a motley crowd of microbiologists, epidemiologists, and anthropologists tried to fit these fatal ailments into various cognitive frameworks. While the sufferers of these phenomena experienced them intimately as plague, Gajdusek and fellow outsiders attempted literally to *re-count* the plague of others in terms of contamination and configuration, to reframe or specify it as controllable epidemic disease. These late-twentieth-century sentinel investigations—all of them hard cases—show us the rewards and pitfalls of seeking through various means to turn unbridled plagues into calculable epidemics.

Kuru

Reporting on kuru in 1963, Gajdusek noted that it "presents an unprecedented situation of an entire population (a sub-culture of Melanesians) afflicted by a lethal disease reaching hyper-endemic proportions, predisposition to which may be determined by a rather simple genetic mechanism" (p. 151). Although Gajdusek initially had assumed kuru was an infectious brain disease, its clinical features and the pathology findings suggested no inflammation, and all microbiological tests proved negative. Observing its ethnic delimitation, Gajdusek and others soon came to favor a genetic explanation. But no one was ever completely satisfied with the genetic hypothesis. In order to account for the special susceptibility of women, as well as children of both sexes, geneticists had to play with notions of gene expression and penetrance, with the result that their explanations became hedged with qualifications and inelegant. Nor could anyone understand how such a lethal gene, apparently without any accompanying survival benefits in its recessive form, could have been so effectively propagated in this isolated population, especially since so many of its victims died before reproducing. Evidently, the genetic hypothesis alone was insufficient to explain the prevalence and pattern of the disease.

In the circumstances, Gajdusek, whose expertise in genetics was minimal, resorted to further study of the ecological and social setting of the malady. His principal interest was in the biological characteristics (which for him included linguistics and behavior) of the Fore people. An anthropologist manqué, the virologist avidly took up studies of Fore social life, especially their practices of childrearing, assumptions about kinship, and sexual behavior. He observed the Fore closely, making copious notes on their ordinary customs and habits as well as their more unusual rituals, including the consumption of loved ones after death. What captivated him was the apparently primitive character of these people, a state of nature that licensed his sociobiological musings. In particular, it was the opportunity to engage with such primitives—to become entangled in their lives—that excited him. This personal quest animated his wide-ranging studies of the Fore and their unique plague. But obsessive attention to his own self-fashioning often made him a poor observer of others.

Gajdusek subjected the Fore to the most "intense medical surveillance" (1963: 153) during the late 1950s and early 1960s. With the help of patrol officers and other visiting scientists, he "enumerated" (p. 153) or registered the whole population each year. Most Fore had some blood taken. Medical investigators examined more than a thousand kuru sufferers during this period, carefully documenting their inevitable decline and death. Sometimes the investigators were allowed to conduct autopsies and send tissues out to Bethesda or to an Australian laboratory. At first they tried to find some infectious agent, toxin, or nutritional deficiency to account for the brain damage. Even after a genetic cause was proposed, they sought an environmental factor that might trigger kuru in the hereditarily susceptible population. Government dieticians analyzed Fore meals; aging Cambridge anthropologists collected cooking stones; botanists examined the local flora; entomologists looked for odd insects. In the absence of a simple infectious model, medical investigators turned to macrobiological processes for answers and became ecological entrepreneurs. But studies of human biology and environment provided no clue to the cause of kuru—though they did later inspire Jared Diamond, a young protégé of Gajdusek, to embark on his investigations of human adaptation (Diamond 1966).

In 1959, William Hadlow, a veterinary pathologist at the Rocky Mountain Laboratories in Montana, had pointed out to Gajdusek the similarity of kuru and scrapie brains. Veterinarians knew that scrapie, principally a disease of sheep, was infectious—its cause a mysterious "slow virus"—so Hadlow recommended transmission experiments in primates. Still vaguely attached to the genetic hypothesis and troubled by the logistical challenges of long-term primate experiments, Gajdusek would take another three years to begin inoculating chimpanzees with brain homogenate from kuru victims. Not until late 1965 could Clarence J. Gibbs Jr. and Michael Alpers report to Gajdusek, returning from a trip to Guam, that one of the inoculated chimps had succumbed to a neurological deterioration resembling kuru. Postmortem pathological studies confirmed their suspicions. To their amazement, the scientists had discovered the first human "slow virus"—although the agent remained puzzlingly immaterial, and its mechanism of transmission among Fore, conjectural. At the NIH, Gibbs proceeded to inoculate his laboratory animals with brain tissue from a vast array of other mysterious neurological disorders, eventually proving that Creutzfeldt-Jakob disease (CJD) was also transmissible. The laboratory thus became a sort of machine for minting out new slow-virus diseases.

In 1963, Gajdusek lamented that it was "impossible to reconstruct a fully reliable past history in the kuru region, where tradition and genealogical memory is shallow" (p. 158). Try as he might, the virologist failed to obtain more than a few accounts of earlier cases of the disease. But a couple of anthropologists sent to the region to ascertain kin relations were having more success in reconstructing kuru history. After living closely with the Fore and talking with them about the past, Robert Glasse and Shirley Glasse (later Lindenbaum) became convinced that kuru had made its first appearance only forty or so years earlier. They also heard that cannibalism had become fashionable as a mourning rite not long before the advent of the disease. Robert Glasse attempted to interest Gajdusek and other medical investigators in the temporal association of cannibalism and kuru. He argued, moreover, that patterns of postmortem consumption might account for the predominance of women and children victims. But it was not until the establishment of the transmissibility of the disease in 1965 that anyone could identify the mechanism that plausibly linked pathogenesis with culture and behavior.

Meanwhile, Shirley Glasse was carefully observing the response of the Fore to this devastating plague, compiling her "epidemiology of social relations" (Lindenbaum 1979: viii). In particular, she wanted to understand Fore beliefs about the cause of the catastrophe and how they attributed blame. She therefore focused on the proliferation of sorcery accusations and the social functions of divination, recrimination, and censure. Allegations of sorcery and oratory on the causes of the decline of the Fore people had become for some men the means to reconstitute and solidify their afflicted communities and to exert dominance over marginal figures. The inhabitants of the region were thus seeking their own way to explain and control this devastating and conceptually challenging phenomenon—this plague. Kuru was also transforming social roles during this period. With fewer women available, men began to care for young children and labor in the gardens. They spent more time with the few remaining women. For Shirley Glasse, the disease represented a complex sampling technique, revealing multiple cross sections of Fore social life and cultural assumptions. Above all, it was the sociological architecture of kuru that fascinated her.

As the Glasses continued their ethnographic research among the Fore, another young medical doctor entered the region, intending to conduct clinical and epidemiological studies of kuru. Michael Alpers, who later worked in Gajdusek's laboratory in Bethesda, studied anthropology before completing his medical degree. Like the Glasses, he soon became deeply entangled in Fore social life, forming intense bonds with his chosen community. Alpers was convinced that anthropological insights would complement his epidemiological investigations—which were, conveniently, ethnically bounded. He set about analyzing kuru mortality from 1957 to 1963 according to sex, age, village, and parish, using the records of the 1,450 cases accumulated in Bethesda. He was startled to find that the disease was now far less common among children under the age of ten than it had been earlier. The fall in childhood kuru deaths was most extreme in areas that had endured the longest contact with white people. Alpers predicted that the next cohort of young adolescents would soon show the same decline, and then progressively older age groups, leading eventually to the disappearance of the disease.

Field observations and laboratory experiments were converging. In Bethesda, Alpers alternated between statistical analyses of kuru, anthropological discussions, and care of the inoculated chimpanzees. By the beginning of 1966 it was evident that the pattern of kuru was changing, and the disease was transmissible. How did these deductions fit together? One morning Alpers suddenly realized that cannibalism must have spread the slow virus. Cannibalism explained why the disease was limited to the Fore, and its distinctive age and sex distribution. It solved the puzzle of how the *epidemic* began some forty or fifty years earlier and why it was now declining among Fore children, who since 1960 had been growing up in communities free of the practice. Moreover, it elucidated the rather tenuous linkage of disease disappearance with exposure to "civilization."

When Gajdusek was awarded the Nobel Prize in medicine or physiology in 1976, it was for his recognition of a new mechanism for the origin and dissemination of infectious disease, for his discovery of the first human slow virus. But the focus on the transmission experiments tended to obscure the contributions of ethnographers and anthropologically minded epidemiologists to unraveling the kuru story. Kuru made visible many otherwise hidden aspects of Fore society and culture, while social analysis and cultural sensitivity eventually illuminated the shape of the epidemic. Knowledge of transmissibility was never sufficient to explain kuru. The disease made sense only when human biology and social anthropology came to structure and inform its microbiology. But by then Gajdusek was moving on, sometimes suppressing earlier configurational inclinations or, more often, subcontracting anthropological and ecological studies to others, in his continuing quest for transmissible agents of other neurological disorders.

Guam ALS-PDC

Soon after World War II, US naval medical officers posted to Guam noticed that an unusual number of the island's inhabitants, the Chamorros, suffered from a distinctive neurological degeneration involving limb weakness, spasticity, twitching, and muscle wasting, leading inexorably to death. Chamorros called the condition "lytico," from the Spanish word *paralytico*, but the medical officers recognized it as a form of amyotrophic lateral sclerosis, with some atypical features such as sensory changes, forced laughter or crying, and eyelid tremor. The navy assigned Donald W. Mulder to investigate the disease. The nascent NIH sent out Leonard T. Kurland, chief of the epidemiology branch of the National Institute of Neurological Diseases and Blindness (NINDB), to assist in the fieldwork. A pioneer of neuro-epidemiology, and eager to extend the global reach of US medical research during the cold war, Kurland already had studied extensively the geographical distribution of multiple sclerosis. In 1953 the two investigators visited Guam and examined more than forty patients, reviewed autopsy reports, and conducted a house-to-house search for neurological disease, using a questionnaire Kurland devised (Kurland and Mulder 1954). They thus initiated an intensive NINDB research project, beginning thirty years of effort in clinico-pathological correlation, epidemiological surveillance, brain and serum banking, genetic registration, and detection of environmental risk factors (Chen 2004).

The most southern of the Marianas Islands in the south Pacific, Guam was poor and scrubby and routinely ravaged by passing typhoons. Once an isolated Spanish colony and now a massive US naval base, it was no tropical paradise. Mulder and Kurland found that in some villages on the island, ALS was a major cause of adult deaths. They also observed many cases of an unusual form of Parkinsonism, called "bodig," in which profound dementia rapidly supervened on the standard signs of slow or impeded movement, cogwheel rigidity, and resting tremor. It was not clear whether this Parkinsonism-dementia complex was a separate disease from ALS or part of a spectrum of related neurological disorders. Later, neuropathologists observed that ALS and PDC brains contained neurofibrillary tangles, implying a common pathological process (Hirano et al. 1961; Malamud, Hirano, and Kurland 1961). One thing was certain: Guam represented the perfect island laboratory for the investigation of mysterious, fatal brain disease.

From the beginning, Kurland attributed the neurological disorders on Guam to the presence of some unknown environmental or biological agent acting on the genetically susceptible population. Presumably, the victims were exposed over many years to something that incited their eventual deterioration. The clinical and pathological features did not suggest any typical infection. The diet, customs, and habits of sufferers did not appear to differ much from those of people remaining exempt from the disease. But epidemiologists turned up a few tantalizing leads. Investigators soon realized that ALS and PDC had emerged on Guam relatively recently, becoming more prevalent during the war years (Reed and Brody 1975). Yet by the 1970s, ALS and (to a lesser extent) PDC were in decline, with very few new cases in people under the age of fifty (Garruto, Yanagihara, and Gajdusek 1985). Chamorros who moved to California, adopting the mainland diet and lifestyle, were still succumbing to ALS many years later in exceptional numbers. Nor was the disease ethnically bounded, like kuru: some Filipinos who had worked for decades in Guam also fell victim to ALS (Garruto, Gajdusek, and Chen 1981). Kurland and others found themselves drawn irresistibly into the epidemiological maze. Although apparently recondite, the key to this etiological puzzle promised to unlock the mysteries of ALS, Parkinsonism, and dementia more generally.

In 1962, Marjorie Whiting, a nutritional anthropologist, studied food practices in a Guam village with many ALS victims, looking for any distinctive patterns or recent changes in consumption (Whiting 1963). She learned that during the war, Chamorros began eating large quantities of tortillas made from carefully prepared wild cycad seeds, but with Americanization they generally came to favor hamburgers and fries. The notion that cycad seeds might contain a neurotoxin enchanted Kurland. But monkeys fed the seeds showed no evidence of neurological damage, although they often developed liver impairment, epilepsy, and cancer. Even so, the cycad theory proved remarkably attractive and durable. It was revived late in the 1980s (Gajdusek 1989; Spencer et al. 1987) and then revised and reissued in the twenty-first century, this time allied with fruit bats.

Paul Cox, an ethnobotanist and expert on rain-forest ecology, proposed that the Chamorros' taste for fruit bats, or flying foxes, might explain the epidemic. He discovered some dead fruit bats whose tissues contained high concentrations of a potentially neurotoxic chemical component of the cycad seeds. In 2002, with Oliver Sacks, a literary neurologist, he claimed that the rise and fall of the fashion for eating fruit bats accounted for the emergence and decline of the neurological diseases of Guam. But further ecological studies indicated that fruit bats do not normally eat cycad seeds—indeed, the fact that a few dead ones had once gorged on them perhaps explained their demise. Although credited with seeking a more ecologically complex understanding of the problem and admired for their skills in self-promotion, Cox and Sacks faced condemnation for their lack of knowledge of cycad toxicity and failure to conduct fieldwork on Guam (Weiner 2005). Unfortunately, however, the image of bat-eating Chamorros entranced the "civilized" world almost as much as the picture of Melanesian cannibals.

Gajdusek, who frequently sought his colleague Kurland's advice on kuru, inevitably became caught up in the Guam investigations. At first Gajdusek wondered whether the neurological disorders could be transmissible. It was the early 1960s, and he was still working through the conceptual implications of scrapie. Moreover, in 1963 the Russian virologist Lev Aleksandrovich Zil'ber announced that he had successfully transmitted ALS to rhesus monkeys, provoking considerable excitement in Bethesda. A group of US scientists visited his laboratory and returned with some brain tissue, with which Gibbs and Gajdusek quickly inoculated their primates. The NIH scientists also gathered brain inoculant directly from ALS and PDC autopsies on Guam. In contrast to kuru, the results were disappointingly negative (Gibbs 1982; Gibbs and Gajdusek 1965, 1972). Although momentarily frustrated, Gajdusek was never easily daunted.

Touring Guam, Gajdusek compared its ecological setting with the settings of the other regional foci of ALS he had visited, including western New Guinea, the Kii peninsula of Japan, and Groote Eylandt, off the northern Australian coast. Cleverly, the peripatetic scientist recommended a search for features common to all these sites. At Kii, Yoshiro Yase had noticed that the soil and water were remarkably poor in zinc, magnesium, and calcium, deficiencies that might allow the buildup of aluminum in the bodies of inhabitants, especially those engaged in traditional rural activities and a subsistence lifestyle. Gajdusek and his colleagues seized on this observation and began assaying trace metals in the pathological locales and the bodies of sufferers (Gajdusek 1982; Garruto and Yase 1986). Soon they confirmed that the soil and water at all sites displayed the same composition. Sure enough, they also established that the neurofibrillary tangles in the brains of ALS and PDC victims were full of aluminum. Even more impressive, primates rendered deficient in zinc, magnesium, and calcium, and fed aluminum, developed neurological disturbances along with distinctive tangles in their brains. Gajdusek (1985) therefore speculated that trace metal imbalances might interfere with transport of neurofilaments in the axons of nerve cells, giving rise to ALS and PDC.

In studying the Guam diseases, Gajdusek never became as intimately involved with the people and the country as he had in the eastern highlands of New Guinea. His anthropological knowledge of the Chamorros remained cursory; his ecological insights derived mostly from perfunctory comparison and analogy; and his understanding of the cause of the diseases ultimately depended on transmission experiments and soil analysis. That a scientist fascinated by cultural and biological complexity so readily resorted to explanations based on relatively simple notions of contamination, whether microbial or metallic, perhaps attests to both the analytical clarity of reductionism and the difficulties of recognizing disease as configuration. In any case, the contributions of cycad toxicity and trace metal imbalance to the emergence and decline of these diseases continue to excite controversy (Friedland and Armon 2007). But it is now probably too late for the sort of social anthropology and ecological fieldwork that proved so helpful in configuring kuru in New Guinea during the early 1960s.

Viliuisk Encephalomyelitis

In 1969, as he tried desperately to foil Soviet bureaucracy and reach Yakutia, a region on the Siberian taiga home to an obscure disease called Viliuisk encephalomyelitis (VE), Gajdusek advised a Russian scientist studying the outbreak "just to quietly get a few brain biopsies and early autopsy specimens from patients ... for inoculation of either our own or his monkeys. No more is needed" (Gajdusek 1971: 28 June 1969, 34). Although Gajdusek managed to visit the local Sakha people a few times in the 1970s, it was not until travel restrictions were eased in the 1990s that his enthusiasm for solving this etiological problem was properly ignited. "This is serious and our new goal," he wrote to Gibbs back at the NIH in 1991, "to solve VE. It is as good as the kuru story!!! We must inoculate monkeys and chimpanzees *and* other animals with fresh and frozen tissue. We can have all the sera, leucocytes, CSF and autopsy tissue we want, collated as we wish."[1] With a glint in his eye, Gajdusek foresaw the same specimen rush he had once led in New Guinea and Guam; the same insistent search for blood, cerebrospinal fluid, and brains; the same death watches and fast autopsies. "Our real quest here," he wrote in his journal on September 3, 1992, "is material for further inoculation and further serology" (Gajdusek 1996: 177).

For more than a century, a fatal form of encephalomyelitis called "bokhoror" has been a plague on the few hundred thousand Sakha, a Turkic people in eastern Siberia (Goldfarb and Gajdusek 1992). Currently about five hundred people suffer from Viliuisk encephalomyelitis, and each year fifteen or so new cases appear. Usually the disease begins suddenly with fever and headache, stiffness of muscles, and slurred speech. Some patients die during the acute phase, their brains on postmortem examination showing extensive inflammation, especially of the lining, or meninges (McLean et al. 1997). Commonly, the disease becomes fluctuant or progressive, causing incoordination and speech difficulties, leading eventually to extreme muscle rigidity and dementia, and to death within six years. Some chronic panencephalitis cases can endure decades of physical impairment and cognitive deterioration. Clusters of VE occur in families and particular villages, giving rise to speculation about genetic susceptibility. Most investigators now assume VE is an infectious disease, acquired, like leprosy, only after prolonged contact with affected persons and taking years to develop (Stone 2002).

It is likely that VE was present among the Evenki in northern Siberia long before stalking the Sakha population. Cases began to proliferate in the 1930s among Sakha communities scattered along the broad Viliui River, at the end of a bloody rebellion against Stalinist rule and in the midst of famine. In the 1950s, local neurologists described an epidemic of the acute form of the disease. At one point they claimed to have isolated the responsible virus, but it proved to be a laboratory contaminant. Then some scientists from Moscow became interested. They conducted a survey of the villages, finding many other rare neurological disorders prevalent in the region. This led to a search for some genetic anomaly or predisposition. They also assayed the Sakha environment and diet, looking for toxins, trace metal deficiencies, or possible nutritional causes. Other researchers argued that VE might be an autoimmune condition. But everyone came away from Siberia baffled.

As soon as he saw VE, Gajdusek believed it was an infection. Its clinical features resembled the Parkinsonism-dementia complex of Guam, but it was clearly an independent and new disease. The flat plains, lakes, serpentine rivers, and forests of the Viliuisk area appeared similar to the country around the ALS cluster in western New Guinea, though one place was within the Arctic, and the other was tropical. The propensity to speculate on genetic causes recalled the early days of the kuru investigation. Even as he reflected on these past experiences and possible analogies, Gajdusek quickly discounted trace metal imbalances and hereditary susceptibility. "This story sounds very much like an infection," he wrote during a white night in Yakutsk in 1979, "and leprosy and other slow, long-incubation, intimate contact diseases come to mind" (Gajdusek 1996: 5 August 1979, 27). One case impressed him tremendously. Early in the 1970s, a Russian lab technician developed a neurological disorder initially diagnosed as multiple sclerosis. But she insisted that during an episode of depression she had injected herself with cerebrospinal fluid from a VE patient. When Gajdusek examined her in 1979 he became convinced she was dying from VE. Her case implied that the presumed pathogen might escape its ethnic boundaries.

Gajdusek recognized the importance of this emerging disease. "It is a new kind of infection ... resembling tuberculosis, syphilis and parasitic CNS [central nervous system] infections in epidemiology and pathology and course more than virus infections, yet it may well be a virus—and a new one, even a new kind" (Gajdusek 1996: 31 August 1979, 75). In the early 1990s the aging scientist, nearing seventy, was still declaring its significance. "That the resolution of the etiology of VE has within it the unlocking of major problems of chronic neurological disease of the CNS, I am sure, and to resolve it will be a triumph of neurobiology." Above all, "here is a detective story worthy of a real Sherlock Holmes and I enjoy being on the track once again" (Gajdusek 1996: 8 August 1991, 95, 98).

Although obsessed with experimental demonstration of the disease's communicability, Gajdusek still was aware of the need for further anthropological and ecological studies. But now he lacked the persever- ance and commitment necessary for such tasks. "It would take weeks in each village to pursue the genealogies, full details of past history and travel, full details of contacts between cases, diet, water source, and other essential epidemiological matters," he wrote (Gajdusek 1996: 8 August 1976, 37). Years after he first saw the disease, the absence of this information was galling. "Natural history of the area, the study of the biota in the lakes and the insect fauna around the people, the parasites of their domestic animals and their hunted animals, has simply not been done. Ecologically complete epidemiology remains to be done," he complained in 1991, "and most important is a completely new investigation about contact and entry of the disease into new areas on a periphery" (Gajdusek 1996: 11 August 1991, 119). Gajdusek, however, no longer possessed the temperament and physical fitness for this sort of work. Besides, he now found transmission experiments too distracting and alluring. At the end of his career he was hoping for a simple solution, an answer that would obviate long-term, intensive fieldwork. "Complex thought, which we have obviously entertained on kuru in the early days, has rarely proven true in medical research," he wrote agitatedly (Gajdusek 1996: 31 August 1992, 160).

"Attempts to isolate an etiological microbe should be more direct and dominating our approach," Gajdusek later declared (1996: 4 September 1992, 179). But all efforts to cultivate the putative microorganism have failed. Gajdusek and his colleagues waited for years to see whether inoculated primates succumbed, to no avail. The microbe, if it exists, has remained elusive. Meanwhile, bokhoror continues to extend its geographical range within Siberia (Vladimirtsev at al. 2007).

Conclusion

In 1999, Ralph M. Garruto and colleagues reviewed "natural experimental models" of human infectious disease, adducing kuru, Guam ALS, and Viliuisk encephalomyelitis. They claimed that isolated populations with "unusual genetic structures, physiological characteristics, focal endemic disease, or special circumstances" represented natural laboratories for studying "relationships among bio-behavioral, genetic and ecological processes that are involved in the development of disease." By studying health and disease in such tradition-bound enclaves, investigators might "avoid some of the confounding factors that exist in diverse modern societies" (Garruto et al. 1999: 10536). In particular, they felt that these "conceptually natural experimental models in human populations are the reverse of biological reductionism models that purport to explain living systems at all levels of organization" (p. 10536). Necessarily, the study of health and disease in small-scale, traditional societies must be "integrative and opportunistic" (p. 10537), combining "the biological, medical, and social and behavioral sciences toward the resolution of new as well as longstanding questions across disciplinary lines" (p. 10542). These pathological sentinels in the modern world thus offered opportunities to remake epidemiology in a more biologically complex and realistic fashion.

Garruto, a biological anthropologist who collaborated with Gajdusek, found the example of Viliuisk encephalomyelitis especially compelling. With his colleagues, he pointed out that further research was required to elucidate the cause of the disease, to determine how it spread, and to evaluate the risk it presented to nearby populations. He and his co-workers recommended early pathological investigation of cases, further attempts at isolating a pathogen, better characterization of genetic susceptibility, and, perhaps most strikingly, "anthropological and epidemiological studies concentrating on social and behavioral mechanisms of spread, including case control and migration studies" (Garruto et al. 1999: 10540). Garruto and colleagues might have directed attention to the anthropological investigation of kuru at this point. But evidently they found it difficult to imagine how social and cultural studies could be rendered commensurate with contemporary biological research and pathology results. Although they could provide many examples of how to enlarge the compass of infectious diseases research to include ecological and broader biological approaches, they managed only a gesture toward the incorporation of sociological analysis.

In an extensive review of the mathematical modeling of disease, Lisa Sattenspiel (1990: 268) conceded that the "weakness is that there is too little attention paid to human cultural and behavioral factors in the formulation of the [disease] models." She observed that the "majority of the models are still being developed by ecologists, parasitologists, and mathematicians, who have a tendency to focus on the biology of the infectious organism and possibly a vector species" (p. 268). As biological and ecological scenarios offered themselves up to investigators, social and cultural configurations remained opaque. Gajdusek had used recourse to archetypes of primitivism to explain the social; Burnet appealed awkwardly to sociobiology. When confronted with the social, they often defaulted to biology. "There is a crucial need," Sattenspiel concluded, "to incorporate more human elements into the modeling efforts [of mathematical ecologists]' (p. 269).

Gajdusek repeatedly recoiled from harnessing the social to the pathological, no matter how complexly configured. It was not just the distraction of transmissibility or reversion to biological training and orientation. Gajdusek initially was reluctant to accept, and thereby amplify, the role of Fore cannibalism in spreading kuru; he always resisted elaborating alleged Chamorro bat-eating in order to explain the emergence of Guam ALS. Social configurations of disease can integrate and organize behavioral patterns, political structures, and cultural assumptions; they might reveal structural inequality, institutional arrangements, disciplinary efforts, and states of exception. But they can also pathologize the social lives of particularly vulnerable people, especially those on the margins of prosperous communities and others in colonial settings. These are still the people most likely to become subject to anthropological study and to appear in sociologically configured stories of plague. Sometimes there is a certain neutrality and distance in mere microbe hunting, an appealing social disengagement, that offers protection from hasty value judgment (Farmer 1992; Sontag 2001). But in attempting to avoid generating stigma through excessively medicalized accounts of social life, we might be left with impoverished sociological understandings of disease.

Gajdusek was always close to the experience of the people he studied, aware in his personal interactions of their suffering and endurance, and sensitive to the plenitude of plague. Late in his career, in Siberia, he reflected on the perseverance of the people he encountered. "How unfortunate the patients we are seeing in their untreatable maladies," he wrote, "where we come and poke at them, disturb them, painfully draw blood from them, photograph them, all, as they know, to no avail and to no good for them. How wonderfully tolerant they are of our intrusion, ineptitude and unkindness" (Gajdusek 1996: 5 September 1992, 198). For most of his career, Gajdusek was concerned less with integrating social science with microbiology than with recognizing and respecting the fragile dignity of his research subjects as they suffered through plague. This conceptual omission may have weakened his epidemiology, but it should not blind us to his proximate understanding of the experience of calamity, with all its bewildering, antinomian, and unconstrained elements.

Notes

I am grateful for the comments of Charles Rosenberg and Mark Veitch on earlier versions of this essay and for stimulating discussions of plagues and epidemics with other participants at the Wenner-Gren symposium in Tucson. Chris Crenner helpfully secured for me a copy of Gajdusek's Viliuisk journal at short notice, and Bridget Collins provided timely research assistance.

1. Gajdusek to Gibbs, August 10, 1991, Gibbs file, D. C. Gajdusek Correspondence, ms C565, National Library of Medicine, Bethesda, MD.

Making Plagues Visible

Yellow Fever, Hookworm, and Chagas' Disease, 1900–1950

Ilana Löwy

Clues, Carlo Ginzburg proposed in his 1980 paper "Morelli, Freud and Sherlock Holmes: Clues and Scientific Method," are infinitesimal traces that make possible the comprehension of a deeper, otherwise unattainable reality. In the late nineteenth century, the rise of bacteriology led to the development of new ways of finding clues to medical mysteries and new approaches to fighting epidemics. Bacteriology was often presented as a revolutionary development in Western medicine. To an important extent, however, this discipline was an imperial science. The empire bred dangerous microbes, and their uncontrolled spread threatened imperial order. As Patrick Masson put it in 1899 in a speech at the inauguration of the London School of Tropical Medicine: "[Tropical medicine] strikes, and strikes effectively, at the root of the principal difficulty of most Colonies—disease. It will cheapen government and make it more efficient. It will encourage and cheapen commercial enterprise. It will conciliate and foster the native" (Worboys 1976: 85–86).

In the last thirty years, numerous scholars have studied the central role of colonies in the development of the "Pasteurian" disciplines. Historians have shown that key concepts and practices in these disciplines were often elaborated in the colonies or, rather, in bidirectional circulation between the metropolis and the colonies. The construction of the tropics, David Arnold proposed (1996), was an important element in the separation of Occidental culture from potentially contaminating elements. The virulence of pathogenic agents in tropical zones was seen as a faithful reflection of the violence of relations between humans and nature and among human beings in these zones (Arnold 1996). The tropics were described as a world of extremes in which the luxuriant growth degenerated quickly and led to disorder and degeneration. Western colonial intervention was legitimated by the need to regulate a chaotic and disorganized world (Livingstone 1999). Campaigns against transmissible diseases conducted in ex-colonial countries such as Brazil were similar attempts to regulate the uncontrollable universe of the tropics. There were, however, additional goals: to restore order to a muddled, uncontrollable society and to increase national cohesion (Peard 1999; Stepan 1998).

On the other hand, making transmissible diseases visible was often an ambivalent endeavor. It displayed the "backwardness" of societies that aspired to present themselves as progressive and enlightened. In parallel, however, it often enhanced the reputations of local scientists and doctors who demonstrated that they were able to master sophisticated research methods and advance scientific knowledge. In ex-colonial countries, the visualization of plagues was at the same time antithetical to modernity and a symbol of modernization.

Yellow Fever I: Making Disease Visible under Well-controlled Conditions

Yellow fever was seen as a symbol of the "malediction of the tropics." A deadly disease that massively killed newcomers to tropical countries, whether they were explorers, colonists, or soldiers, it was seen as a major threat not only to the colonial enterprise but also to newly independent Latin American countries. In the 1880s and 1890s, several researchers, among them the Mexican Manuel Carmona y Valle, the Brazilians Joao Batista Lacerda and Domingos Freire, and the Italian Giuseppe Sanarelli, each claimed to have found the "yellow fever" germ (Benchimol 1999). All of them affirmed that the putative yellow fever germ spread through direct contact, but the diffusion of yellow fever had many puzzling traits that could not be explained by such a pattern of infection.

In 1881 a Cuban physician, Carlos Finlay, proposed an alternative theory: the yellow fever agent was propagated by an insect vector, the mosquito *Stegomya faciata* (later *Aedes aegypti*) (Finlay 1881). Finlay grounded his argument in the observation of a close correlation between areas of presence of the disease and the presumed vector. In the late nineteenth century, such observations, grounded in the old-fashioned skill of the naturalist, were no longer viewed as sufficient proof of causal links between a transmissible disease and its putative etiological agent. The only truly valid etiological proof, experts believed, came from the bacteriology laboratory. For many years, Finlay tried hard to provide such a proof (Finlay 1894), but his bacteriological studies were viewed as amateurish and incompetent (Sternberg 1889). In the absence of convincing laboratory proof, Finlay's "mosquito hypothesis" was probably perceived as the amiable ramblings of a provincial doctor.

In 1899 the US Army entered Havana and faced severe yellow fever epidemics. The sanitary measures introduced by the city commander, General William Gorgas, had no effect on the epidemics. In June 1990 the US Army's medical service sent a mission to Cuba to investigate the yellow fever epidemics and propose appropriate solutions (Bean 1977, 1982; Delaporte 1992; Stepan 1978). The American experts—Walter Reed, who headed the mission, Jesse Lazear, James Caroll, and Aristides Agramonte—rapidly disqualified the bacterial hypothesis proposed by Giuseppe Sanarelli. In August the members of the Reed mission turned to the "mosquito hypothesis." This hypothesis was much more credible in 1900 than it had been in 1881, when Finlay proposed it, because it resonated with the recently uncovered mode of transmission of malaria. In addition, epidemiological studies carried out in 1898–1899 by another US Army physician, Henry Carter, in southern Mississippi made plausible the hypothesis of yellow fever transmission by a flying insect (Carter 1901).

Reed and his colleagues obtained *Stegomya* mosquitoes from Finlay and, lacking an animal model for yellow fever, decided to conduct experiments on humans. In their publications, the members of the Reed mission stressed the careful planning of these experiments (Caroll 1903). Close scrutiny of the first article published by members of Reed's mission indicates, however, that tests were conducted haphazardly during the initial phase of experimentation. The article reports three cases of an experimental yellow fever obtained by a mosquito bite, two of them in members of the Reed mission. In two of the cases (Caroll and Lazear), it was difficult to exclude another pattern of contamination, and only the third one could reasonably have been attributed to the bite of a contaminated mosquito. Moreover, five other volunteers, bitten at the same time by infected mosquitoes, remained healthy (Reed and Caroll 1901; Reed, Caroll, and Lazear 1900).

Jesse Lazear died from yellow fever. After his death and Caroll's violent illness, members of Reed's mission were persuaded that yellow fever was indeed transmitted by mosquitoes. They nevertheless needed to provide formal proof of such transmission. Volunteers were kept in strict isolation at an experimental camp in a mosquito-free area in the mountains (Columbia Barracks, in the city of Quemados, later renamed Lazear Camp), where they either submitted to bites of infected mosquitoes or were put in close contact with the belongings (clothes, sheets, kitchenware) of yellow fever patients. Some of the volunteers were US soldiers who agreed to be experimental subjects; others were new immigrants from Spain. The latter received financial compensation for participating in Camp Lazear experiments.

The human experimentation was a success. Between November 1900 and October 1901, the US experts induced fourteen cases of experimental yellow fever by mosquito bites, whereas none of the volunteers placed in close contact with objects and clothing belonging to yellow fever patients became sick. Reed and his colleagues had also shown that injection of a patient's blood into a healthy volunteer induced the disease and that a serum filtered through a porcelain filter was still infectious, a strong indication that the infectious agent was not a bacillus but a "filterable virus" (Reed, Caroll, and Agramonte 1901).

A majority of experts saw the results obtained by the Reed mission as definitive proof that yellow fever was propagated through mosquito bites. The validity of this proof relied on US experts' capacity to maintain well-controlled experimental conditions. General Gorgas (1903: 50) explained that Reed and his colleagues had "established an experimental station in the country and half a mile or more from any habitation, placed non-immunes in this camp under military control so that they could not leave it, kept them there a sufficient length of time to be certain that they had not contracted yellow fever, and then experimented upon them with the species of mosquito which, Dr. Finlay maintained, propagated yellow fever." The military surveillance of people in Camp Lazear was a central element in the success of the enterprise. US soldiers who watched over the experimental station and prevented people from leaving it guarded at the same time the quality of scientific proof. Epidemiological evidence was literarily protected by rifles and bullets.

Reed and his colleagues were lucky; none of the volunteers infected with yellow fever died from the disease (or at least, none was reported as dying from it). A Cuban doctor named Guiteras who in 1901 repeated experiments conducted by the Reed mission was less fortunate, as were his experimental subjects. Three of his eight infected volunteers died from yellow fever. Their deaths led to strong protests in Cuban newspapers against continued experiments on humans (Bean 1977, 1982; Caroll 1903). Nevertheless, experiments with human volunteers were repeated three more times between 1901 and 1904: in Vera Cruz, Mexico, and in São Paolo and Rio de Janeiro, Brazil. The Rio de Janeiro experiments (1901–1905) were conducted under the aegis of the Pasteur Institute. The French scientists—Emile Marchoux, Albert Taurelli Salimbani, and Paul Louis Simond—recruited volunteers from among new immigrants and paid them for participating in experiments on yellow fever transmission. The main thrust of these experiments was similar to those conducted by Reed's mission, and their results confirmed those obtained in Cuba: the only way to transmit yellow fever was through the bite of an infected mosquito or direct injection of patients' blood (Marchoux and Simond 1906; Marchoux, Taurelli Salimbeni, and Simond 1903).

The official publication of the results of experiments on humans conducted by the Pasteur Institute presents an image of orderly study with clearly defined experimental goals (Marchoux, Taurelli Salimbeni, and Simond 1903). The laboratory notebooks of one of the mission's scientists, Paul Louis Simond, tell a different story. They convey a strong impression of chaotic and opportunistic experimentation, conducted mainly during a single, intensive period, March–June 1902. The French scientists attempted to obtain maximal "yield" from each volunteer, submitting them to multiple and potentially confusing treatments. For example, a Portuguese immigrant, Paes, was injected on 23 April with filtered serum from a yellow fever patient. He remained healthy and on 5 May received an injection of serum from another patient, this time diluted with four parts of saline. The next day he became violently sick. The rapidity of the appearance of his symptoms made interpretation difficult: it was unclear whether the disease developed as a result of the second injection, the first, or another cause. A German immigrant, Hocheiner was injected on 30 April with twelve-day-old serum. The following day, for unspecified reasons, he received another injection of serum from a mild case of yellow fever. Nothing happened, and on 21 May he was again injected with blood from a yellow fever patient, which had been kept outside the body for eight days. Still healthy after the third injection, Hocheiner was bitten on 6 June by three infected mosquitoes, and four days later he developed a mild case of yellow fever.

According to the report of the Pasteur Institute, twenty-seven volunteers participated in the yellow fever experiments. Simond's laboratory notebook lists thirty volunteers. The "missing" cases were volunteers who died in the Petropolis camp. A German immigrant, Bordach, died in April from yellow fever inoculated through a mosquito bite. Another volunteer, an Italian immigrant named Geronimo, developed experimental yellow fever on 17 June. Two days later, perhaps during a disease-induced delirium, he left the Petropolis camp, took a train toward Rio de Janeiro, left the train in Rai de Serra, and began walking the rails with his suitcase. Railway workers retrieved him and brought him back to the station, where he died three hours later. Finally, a short note in Simond's notebook indicates that a Spanish immigrant, Soller, whose name appears several times in the experimental reports, was murdered on 3 June 1902.[1] The fates of Soller and Geronimo suggest the tensions and conflicts that existed in the Petropolis camp. This is not particularly surprising. Thirty new immigrants, all male, kept in a closed space and subjected to experiments that could kill them might have had good reasons to feel restless or even become violent. Moreover, the Pasteur Institute scientists lacked some of the advantages their colleagues from the Reed mission had. As civilians, they could not keep their volunteers under military control and impose order at the point of a gun.

Yellow Fever II: Tracing Invisible Pathogens in the Field

Yellow fever is a viral disease, and in the absence of an animal model, scientists were unable to demonstrate that people with suspicious symptoms indeed suffered from this pathology. In 1928, Adrian Stokes and colleagues successfully infected rhesus monkeys with yellow fever and then transmitted the disease from one monkey to another (Stokes, Bauer, and Hudson 1928). Their study rapidly opened the way for a better understanding of yellow fever. Max Theiler and colleagues developed a "mouse protection test," which revealed the presence of antibodies in serum—that is, of traces of past contacts with the virus (Sawyer and Lloyd 1931; Theiler 1930). In parallel, Brazilian scientists showed that people who died from yellow fever exhibited typical liver changes (de Rocha Lima 1926). The combination of the three approaches—injection of a patient's blood into monkeys, examination of the livers of people who died from a suspicious "fever," and serological surveys using the mouse neutralization test—provided a relatively accurate picture of the prevalence of yellow fever in a given area.

The collection of sera (from living people) and liver slices (from the dead) allowed epidemiological surveys to be conducted. Both methods, however, were problematic. It was not easy to convince inhabitants of poor, rural areas, devoid of medical services, to agree to give their blood for research, much less to accept regular autopsies. Nevertheless, because of strong official support from the government of Getulio Vargas, the Rockefeller Foundation (RF) experts who directed the Brazilian yellow fever service (SFA) in the 1930s successfully implemented these unpopular methods of epidemiological investigation. Vargas, brought to power in November 1930 through a peaceful putsch (the "November revolution"), aspired to construct a strong, modern Brazilian state and saw public health measures as a key means to achieve this goal. According to an agreement signed between the RF and the Brazilian government in 1930, the government provided 80 percent of SFA's budget while control of the service remained in the hands of RF experts. The agreement created a unique juridical structure: a Brazilian governmental agency directed and supervised by US citizens. It also provided full legal backing for SFA operations, including unpopular ones.

In order to map zones of yellow fever endemicity, RF experts conducted systematic serological surveys. Such surveys relied on the goodwill of the population. It was not easy to persuade all the inhabitants of a surveyed village to give blood for research. It was especially tricky to convince parents of young children to agree to blood collection, but it was important to obtain children's blood because the presence of antibodies in children was an indication that the virus was present in the area. RF researchers therefore sought the support of local authorities and, wherever possible, the Catholic Church. Judging from the number of "mice protection tests" conducted in the Rio and Bahia laboratories, the RF experts frequently were successful.[2] Sometimes they asked local doctors to collect the sera and paid them for their service, but this solution was seen as problematic because local practitioners were not considered entirely trustworthy. They were suspected, for example, of circumventing the difficulty of obtaining blood from children by labeling adult blood as that of a child. RF experts therefore often traveled to remote areas to collect blood samples themselves. Numerous, probably embellished anecdotes about these expeditions presented them as daring endeavors, confrontations of enlightened scientists with backward inhabitants of Brazil's interior. In these stories, RF experts were threatened by people who saw them as emissaries of the devil or the Antichrist who collected blood for witchcraft. As Fred Soper, the director of RF's Brazilian Bureau, put it, "we always fought the superstition of ignorant natives."[3]

Another key element of the epidemiological surveillance of yellow fever was the examination of liver tissue from people who had died of suspicious "fevers." In 1930 the RF specialists devised an instrument called the "visceroctome" that made it possible to sample cadaver liver without opening the body. The instrument could be used by nonprofessionals, so it eliminated the necessity of conducting a formal autopsy. In order to impose the practice of "visceroctomy"—the sampling of liver tissue with a visceroctome—it was necessary to promulgate a law regulating funerals, which until then had been unregulated. The new law (of 23 May 1932, articles 52–57) required an inhumation permit for burials and made private funeral sites illegal. In order to ensure the collection of liver samples from all parts of Brazil, the SFA named a "visceroctome representative" in each locality that had a cemetery (Soper, Rickard, and Crawford 1934). Persons responsible for visceroctomy services received a small sum of money for every liver sample sent to the central laboratory, and a larger sum if the sample was positive for yellow fever. Thus there was a temptation to provide liver samples from animals or from people who had not died of a sudden fever or, if a positive case was suspected, to present several samples of the same liver as if they came from different people. The RF experts therefore stressed the importance of careful control over samples sent from visceroctomy stations and diligent supervision of visceroctomy agents (Ricard 1937a).

The liver sampling was expected to be a hidden, invisible activity. The SFA promoted the construction of a special building, the *nécrotério*, in each cemetery for conducting partial autopsies. In order to prevent observation of the sampling of cadavers, the *nécrotério* was a small, windowless room with a dissection table.[4] Instructions for establishing visceroctomy posts explained that "the visceroctome should not be shown to people having no connection with the Visceroctomy Service. In most cases people do not understand the true significance of the Service and react unfavorably at the sight of the instrument. The rumors that such people spread may cause unnecessary opposition from the families concerned" (Rickard 1937b: 171).

The visceroctomist was instructed to ensure that no outsiders were present during the sampling of cadaver liver, and if the visceroctomy took place inside a private house, it should be empty, with all curtains and blinds closed. It was difficult, however, to keep visceroctomy secret. In some cases, especially when the visceroctomist wanted to punch the liver of a recently deceased child, the family forcefully resisted an act they viewed as a profanation of the body. Diaries of RF experts in Brazil report numerous violent confrontations around this practice. Five employees of the visceroctomy service were killed in such confrontations. In 1937 Wilbur Sawyer, then head of the International Health Division of the RF, learned about resistance to visceroctomy and shared his disquiet with Soper: "The continued violence which seems almost inseparable from the widespread system of visceroctomy is a matter of concern and has reached a point at which it seems there should be a modification of our program. The total experience ... brings into serious question the advisability of a method which invites such violent resistance and offends the sensibility of the public."[5]

Soper disagreed. For him, the loss of the lives of five employees was a remarkably good result if one took into account the fact that more than 100,000 liver punctures had been made in Brazil during the previous five years, many of them in regions of "extreme religious fanaticism." Moreover, he added, visceroctomy provided irrefutable proof of the presence of yellow fever in a given area. It was therefore an especially efficient means of galvanizing local authorities into action and promoting elimination of *Aedes aegypti* mosquitoes.[6] The visceroctomy posts were maintained as a central element in a dense network of devices employed to supervise Brazilian people, the potential carriers of yellow fever virus.

Hookworm: The Multiple Uses of Visible Evidence

Hookworm is a parasitic disease induced by two closely related species of intestinal worms, *Ankylostoma duodenum* and *Necator americanus.* In the late nineteenth and early twentieth centuries, physicians described the parasite's life cycle, symptoms of infection (weakness, anemia, fatigue, failure to thrive in children), method of diagnosis (search for the parasite's eggs in feces), and antihelminthic treatment (mainly thymol or extract of black fern in the early twentieth century) (Loss 1905; Stiles 1902). Hookworm is usually found in tropical and subtropical climates, and human infection is linked to poverty, the absence of latrines, and walking barefoot. Typically, an infection occurs when worms that live in contaminated soil penetrate the soles of the feet. Hookworm infection was presented as one of the reasons for the "laziness" of inhabitants of hot climates (Ettling 1981). A disease strongly correlated with dirt, pollution, and fecal contamination, the infection was also seen as a symbol of the inferiority and backwardness of native populations. Although hookworm is usually a disease of warm climates, there was one exception: mines in temperate climates (Anderson 1995). Hookworms found an ecological niche in the hot, humid microenvironments of mines, which, moreover, usually lacked privies, so the infection could propagate rapidly among workers. In the late nineteenth and early twentieth centuries, "miner's anemia" was seen as an important professional risk for miners and a serious public health threat.

The main difficulty associated with hookworm infection was not to demonstrate the presence of an infectious agent in the body—a simple feat accomplished with a microscope—but to define what its presence meant. Briefly, an antihookworm campaign can aim at eliminating either the parasite or the disease. The two goals are not identical: only people who carry a significant number of worms suffer the consequences of the infection. Those with a limited number of worms in their intestines—often the great majority of the infected— are healthy carriers who can infect others but suffer no serious harm themselves. If one wishes to eliminate the parasite, it is necessary to test everyone in an infected area and treat everyone who has hookworm eggs in his or her feces. This "parasite-oriented" approach efficiently prevents reinfection, but it forces people who feel perfectly well to accept unpleasant and occasionally dangerous therapy. The alternative is to pursue a "handicap-oriented" approach: to treat only sick people. People who suffer from the debilitating effects of hookworm infection have a direct interest in being treated and can be more easily persuaded to view antihookworm therapy as a lesser evil. If the choice is to focus on treating the sick, then the required epidemiological evidence is not merely the presence of parasite eggs in the feces but clinical signs of the disease and a quantitative evaluation of the extent of infection, which is achieved by estimating the number of eggs per gram of fecal material. Only symptomatic people are tested, and if found to be heavily infested, they receive antihelminthic therapy.

In the colonial context, the general rule was to pursue the application of the coercive parasite-oriented approach, whereas in other cases, sanitary authorities more often favored selective treatment of the sick coupled with health education.[7] The work of the Rockefeller Hookworm Commission in the US South, active in the 1910s, relied on such measures (Ettling 1981; Fosdick 1989). The same principle was applied during the intervention of RF experts in Brazil in the 1920s.[8] By contrast, the antihookworm campaign conducted in 1914–1916 by Rockefeller Foundation experts in the West Indies (Trinidad and British Guyana)— that is, in small countries under colonial rule—focused on eradicating the parasite. This campaign became the model of an "intensive method" of eradicating agents or vectors of transmissible disease. Lessons learned in the West Indies were later transposed by RF specialists to campaigns that aimed to eradicate other diseases, such as malaria and yellow fever.

The goal of the "intensive method" was to identify and treat all carriers of the parasite. The first step involved drawing a precise map of the area targeted for an eradication campaign and then collecting sample information on a number of people in each locality (Howard 1919: 20). The area was then divided into "intervention zones." Each zone was covered by an "intervention group" composed of a physician, two clerks, two "microscopists" (laboratory technicians), twelve male nurses (on horseback), and one or two manual workers. The RF experts calculated that each intervention group could provide antihelminthic treatment to approximately two thousand people; the intervention territory included roughly that number of infected people (Howard 1919: 53–55).

The next step involved conducting a census of the population in the intervention zone and then transcribing the results on specific forms. During the census, nurses distributed vials to everybody for feces samples. The nurses came back the next day to collect the fecal samples and bring them to the laboratory. People with parasite eggs were visited again by the nurses and given an antihelminthic treatment, which they swallowed in the nurse's presence. The absolute rule was that every single infected person had to be treated. Accordingly, standardized forms collected by the nurses provided limited information including people's names, their contamination status (infected or not), and the uptake of antihelminthic drug; the forms included no information about the health status of the treated people (Howard 1919: 107–108).

The RF experts claimed that the West Indian campaign was highly successful and attributed its success to the support of the British colonial administration and the mobilization of local elites. Community leaders were invited to the laboratory, where they were shown parasites and eggs and given explanations of the life cycle of the hookworm. Journalists were encouraged to write articles about the need to fight the disease. In addition, according to the RF specialists, local people were impressed by visits of "important people" (nurses on horseback) who came to their houses in order to take samples of feces and administer antihookworm therapy (Howard 1919). All these elements probably helped secure adherence to antihookworm measures. It is unclear, nevertheless, whether indeed all the worm carriers, including those who felt well, readily accepted an unpleasant treatment.

Another use of evidence was pursued against hookworm among miners in France. Albert Calmette, director of the Institut Pasteur de Lille (known mainly as the co-discoverer of antituberculosis vaccine, Bacille Calmette Guérin or BCG), was asked by mine owners to help them to control epidemics of hookworm (Löwy 2003). Calmette and his colleagues devised a persuasive method to convince miners from the Lille region to participate voluntarily in antihookworm measures.

Miners who suffered from hookworm infection (only symptomatic people were treated) were invited to spend a day in the miner's infirmary. They were put in a clean bed, made to feel pampered, and then given a dose of antihelminthic drug. When they expelled the worms, they and any other people present in the infirmary were invited to examine the parasites. The sight of fat worms bloated by ingested blood, Calmette explained, usually made a strong impression on the miners and boosted their willingness to follow hygienic regimes (Calmette and Breton 1905: 137). In that decidedly noncolonial setting—Calmette and his colleagues conducted health campaigns in close collaboration with the miners' trade unions—the public display of evidence was used to secure voluntary adherence to health measures.

Chagas' Disease: Displaying What?

Official presentations of Chagas' disease (or American trypanosomiasis) usually begin with the statement that the disease was first described in 1909 by a young Brazilian doctor, Carlos Chagas (Cox 1996). Chagas, who was sent to Lassance, Minas Gerais, to help control a malaria outbreak, was told by local people that triatomine bugs, insects frequently found in rural areas of Brazil, often bit humans during their sleep, especially in the face—hence their local name, *barbeiros* (barbers). Chagas dissected some of these insects and found that they harbored unidentified flagellated parasites. Back in Rio de Janeiro, Chagas showed that the parasites produced a disease in monkeys. He then returned to Lassance, where he found similar parasites in the blood of a child suffering from intermittent fever and enlarged lymph nodes. Chagas identified the new human parasitosis as American trypanosomiasis, showed that the infection was transmitted by infected triatomine bugs, and proposed that people who harbored American trypanosomes suffered from several chronic pathologies, among them goiter. Chagas's discovery was a double first: the description of a new nosological entity and a new parasite, and the first major contribution to tropical medicine by a Latino-American scientist. Chagas was celebrated in Brazil and abroad and in 1912 received the Schaudinn Prize for outstanding research in tropical medicine (Lewinson 1979; Romero Sa 2005).

This seemingly straightforward account of the discovery hides a much more complicated story. Initially, Chagas's finding and its international recognition were widely diffused in Brazil, but from the mid-1910s to the mid-1930s, Chagas' disease "disappeared" as a nosological entity. Numerous Latin American doctors contested Chagas's claim that he had discovered a new human disease. *Trypanozoma cruzi*, the parasite described by Chagas, could indeed infect laboratory animals, but it was unclear whether it produced the disease in humans. The symptoms attributed to infection by *T. cruzi* were variable and often found in people with other infections and parasites, and one of the main signs of the new disease reported by Chagas, goiter, was shown to be independent of infection by trypanosomes. In 1916 Chagas's interpretations of American trypanosomiasis were openly attacked at the Pan American Congress of Medicine, the first of many similar attacks. In 1922 the Brazilian Academy of Medicine appointed a commission to assess Chagas's claim that he had discovered a new nosological entity. The commission concluded in Chagas's favor, but it was a pyrrhic victory, because in parallel it classified Chagas' disease as "doubtful." As a result, the disease was omitted from the curriculums of Brazilian medical schools in the 1920s. Even though physicians occasionally observed trypanosomes in blood samples, they were unsure what the observation meant: the presence of infection was not translated into a stable sign of a disease (Benchimol and Teixeira 1993).

In 1935, the existence of a new nosological entity was supported by the description of a characteristic sign of infection by *Trypanozoma cruzi*: a typical swelling of the eye produced by a bite from the triatomine bug in the eye region.[9] The "Romania sign," named after the Argentine doctor Cecilio Romania, who first described it, made possible the first accurate description of clinical signs of infection by *T. cruzi* (Delaporte 1999). On the other hand, the Romania sign is present in only 1 to 2 percent of infected people. Systematic epidemiological surveys were necessary to determine the prevalence of Chagas' disease. Such studies, conducted in the 1950s and 1960s, revealed that this pathology was not, as Chagas himself believed, limited to a few regions in Brazil's interior but was widely diffused across Latin America (Coutinho 1999; Petraglia Kropf 2005).

The "disappearance" of Chagas' disease in Brazil was linked to local political events such as the struggle between the National Department of Health, then headed by Chagas, and the medical faculty and conflicts within the Brazilian medical profession (Coutinho and Dias 1999). It was related to the reluctance on the part of Brazilian doctors to put to the fore a disease that became a symbol of rural backwardness, poor sanitation, and mental handicap and that endangered the image of the modern, dynamic country that Brazilian elites wished to project abroad (Stepan 2001). The disappearance of Chagas' disease was also connected to Chagas's excessive—and for some erroneous—reliance on the laboratory. Chagas was able to find evidence of infection and to reproduce it in laboratory animals, but he failed to link the infection to specific clinical signs (Delaporte 2005). Finally, according to some interpretations, Chagas' disease never truly disappeared. It merely underwent numerous transformations until the diagnosis was stabilized in its present form in the late 1960s (Petraglia Kropf, Azavedo, and Ferreira 2003).

The history of Chagas' disease illustrates the difficulty of ascribing meaning to traces when it is not entirely clear what the traced object is. It also displays the specific difficulties of research on diseases that affect poor populations in developing countries. Today experts agree that the main consequence of infection with *Trypanozoma cruzi* is heart disease. Although the infection by triatomine bugs is related to poverty, usually the diagnosis of cardiac pathologies is made by specialists in well-equipped hospital settings, and it is therefore the privilege of the affluent. In order to provide epidemiological data on infection by American trypanosomiasis, it was necessary to bring the tools of the medicine of the rich to the underprivileged. Studies that established the prevalence of Chagas' disease in the Brazilian countryside were conducted by a Rio de Janeiro cardiologist, Francisco Laranja. Laranja transported electrocardiography equipment to poor rural zones and helped a medical team headed by Emmanuel Dias correlate cardiac signs with the level of antitrypanosoma antibodies in the blood (Laranja, Dias, and Nobera 1948). This costly and complicated enterprise was part of Dias's effort to persuade Brazilian health authorities that Chagas' disease was an important public health problem and to convince them to start a mass campaign to eliminate triatomine bugs (Dias 1945; Petraglia Kropf 2005). As in the case of hookworm infection, the methods chosen to display the presence of a pathology were inseparably linked with the aims of the researchers who made the evidence visible.

"Otherwise Unattainable Reality"?

Efforts to make visible an invisible agent in three "tropical plagues" show the specificity of each enterprise when it was conducted in the framework of colonial or postcolonial medicine. The methods employed to make pathogenic agents visible were very different in each case, as was the ultimate fate of the disease studied. Yellow fever is no longer a "typical" tropical plague, at least not in Latin America. The elaboration of an efficient anti–yellow fever vaccine, mosquito control, and the rapid isolation of people with the disease led to an important reduction of the number of cases of yellow fever. This is emphatically not the case for either Chagas' disease or hookworm. Nowadays it is not difficult to demonstrate an infection with *Trypanosoma cruzi*, but in the absence of a truly efficient therapy, the diagnosis of this pathology is less important than its prevention. Prevention relies above all on the elimination of its vectors, insects of the family of Triatominae. This endeavor is directly related to the improvement of living conditions in the Latin American countryside, a difficult task.[10] In the majority of Latin American countries, Chagas' disease continues to be endemic in poor, rural areas. Specialists estimate that between 16 million and 18 million people in Latin America are infected with *T. cruzi*, that approximately fifty thousand people die every year from the direct consequences of the infection, and that many others are permanently incapacitated (Kirchov 1993). Hookworm is also a "social disease." Diagnosis of the infection is simple, preventive measures have been known for at least a century, and the curative drugs employed today are more efficient and less unpleasant than those employed in the early twentieth century. Nevertheless, experts estimate that of the 740 million people today who suffer from hookworm disease, the majority live on less than $2 a day (Hotez et al. 2005).

In the 1910s, Brazilian hygienists founded the "sanitary movement," which aspired to promote general well-being through sanitation. People in the Brazilian interior, the activists of this movement affirmed, were debilitated by the parasites they harbored and therefore were indifferent, passive, and unfit to engage in productive work. The elimination of parasitic diseases such as hookworm and Chagas' disease would enable them to become efficient and energetic workers. The bright light of the microscopic field, the writer Monteiro Lobato, an enthusiastic supporter of the proposed sanitary movement, revealed the extent of the "Brazilian problem." Once the omnipresence of transmissible diseases became visible, sanitarians and politicians immediately perceived the practical solution to the problem and began to implement solutions. Epidemiological evidence, Lobato argued, was a motor of social change (quoted in Santos et al. 1991: 18). The head of the Rockefeller Foundation's International Health Division, Wilbur Sawyer, held similar views. He was persuaded that improvements in health would promptly be followed by increased production, better economic status, and fuller social development. Alas, shortly before his death in 1951 he was obliged to recognize that "the problem is much broader than health, that cannot flourish in an adverse socio-economic environment" (Sawyer 1951: 224).

In "The Adventure of the Dying Detective," Sherlock Holmes—a creation of Arthur Conan Doyle, a physician who modeled many of the methods he attributed to his detective in new diagnostic methods—pretends to be agonizing from a rare disease that exists only among workers on Sumatra plantations, in order to set a trap for a plantation owner who has murdered a relative by inoculating him with the disease.[11] The tropics, Holmes tells Watson, harbor myriad horrifying pathologies, unknown to Western doctors: "Shall I demonstrate your ignorance? What do you know, pray, of Tapanuli fever? What do you know of the black Formosa corruption?" (Conan Doyle 1982: 934). The use of germs of such a disease to kill a Londoner is presented as an abhorrent crime. By contrast, the massive number of deaths of natives on Sumatra plantations is viewed as a non-event, mentioned in passing in the story's background. Plagues that decimated the natives were often imperceptible, or rather not interesting enough to be perceived, because they were considered to belong to the natural order of things. In Conan Doyle's world, such order was disrupted only when a dishonest colonial employed tropical microorganisms to kill a white, upper-class man. In colonial and postcolonial situations, epidemiologists are not always obliged to follow infinitesimal traces to make visible a hidden reality.[12] Sometimes a willingness to look may be sufficient.

Notes

1. Paul Louis Simond, laboratory notebooks, Petropolis, Simonds Papers, Pasteur Institute Archives, Paris, file 9.

2. For example, data in Fred Soper's journal, 1932, Rockefeller Archive Center, Series 305, box 27, folder 208.

3. Notes of Lewis Hackett on yellow fever, Rockefeller Archive Center, Record Group 3.1, Series 908, box 3, folder 19.

4. Collection of SFA photographs from the 1930 archives, Casa Oswaldo Cruz, Rio de Janeiro, iconographic files, photographs series 30–63.

5. Sawyer to Soper, 6 May 1937, Rockefeller Archive Center, Record Group 1.1, Series 305, box 23, folder 182.

6. Soper to Sawyer, 12 May 1937, Rockefeller Archive Center, Record Group 1.1, Series 305, box 23, folder 182.

7. This was not an absolute rule. In Germany, the government imposed repressive measures in order to eliminate hookworm from the mines (Calmette and Breton 1905: 175–201).

8. Report on the Activities of the Rockefeller Foundation in Brazil, 1922, Rockefeller Archive Center, document RF 22.05.05.

9. Chagas thought that the parasites were transferred through bites. Today experts believe infection is diffused mainly via the insect's feces rubbed into the wound by scratching.

10. Today Chagas' disease in cities is related not only to poverty but also to contaminated blood supplies, which renders the disease more "democratic."

11. Laura Otis (1999) drew attention to the analogy between new biological and medical knowledge and the fears of dissolution of the imperial body that appear in Conan Doyle's Sherlock Holmes series.

12. For a recent example (of a man-made disaster), see Burnham et al. 2006.

Metaphors of Malaria Eradication in Cold War Mexico

Marcos Cueto

In the mid-1950s, medical experts and politicians from Washington, DC, and western Europe constructed malaria as the main plague of the developing world and launched a global campaign to eradicate the disease (Packard 2007). In this chapter I examine the motivations behind the launching of the campaign and Mexican responses to an effort at sanitation imposed from above.

The framing of malaria as a plague was instrumental in pursuing five goals. First, malaria was used to explain not only physical infirmity and economic underdevelopment but also culturally and psychologically "backward" traits of peasants, such as laziness. Second, malaria, as well as poverty, nourished conditions among the poor that encouraged them to find in communism a solution to problems of want and disease, so eradicating malaria would help in the cold war struggle against communism. Third, the fight against malaria reinforced the belief that "silver bullets," or technological solutions, would solve health problems. Fourth, the campaign against malaria would intensify the biomedicalization of rural inhabitants, because until then Western medicine was hegemonic in urban areas but not in the countryside. Finally, the propaganda linked to the campaign defined who was a modern citizen in the rural areas for the Mexican government, which in the 1950s espoused a position much like the modernization model advocated by the United States.

Sanitation from Above

An important event for launching the eradication campaign in Mexico was the 1954 malaria eradication program approved by the Pan American Sanitary Bureau, today the Pan American Health Organization (PAHO), the regional arm for the Western Hemisphere of the World Health Organization (WHO), an agency of the United Nations. The program was to be undertaken initially in Latin America and later in the rest of the world. The multilateral agency worked under the assumption that extirpating the scourge was possible because of new antimalaria drugs, which killed the malaria parasite, the plasmodium, and because of the insecticide DDT, the indoor spraying of which apparently destroyed the most dangerous species of the *Anopheles* mosquitoes that transmitted the disease. The decision to initiate the program was soon sanctioned at the annual meeting of WHO, which took place in Mexico City. Other multilateral agencies and organizations, such as UNICEF and the US State Department, then headed by the cold war warrior John Foster Dulles, firmly supported the initiative. The State Department organized a bilateral program for malaria eradication and convinced the US Congress to fund the program with several million dollars (Cueto 2007).

Under Dulles, US foreign policy, besides concentrating on bilateral military aid, paid substantial attention to international assistance to backward countries in order to decrease the possibility for the infiltration of communism, to which "needy populations" might be susceptible. There was also an economic motivation for this type of assistance. Francis O. Wilcox, the Department of State's assistant secretary of international organization affairs, explained the insufficiency of existing world trade to secure American economic well-being. It was necessary to create new markets, increase the purchasing power of people in areas where per capita income was low, and raise their standards of living so that they could participate in the world economy (Wilcox 1957). A unit of the State Department applied the concept to international health: "Good health contributes to economic progress" (International Cooperation Administration 1956: 5). It was believed that once malaria was eradicated, peasants could participate in a market economy.

The eradication campaign was fully embraced by the pro-business Mexican governments of the post-World War II period, particularly those of Adolfo Ruíz Cortínes and Adolfo Lopez Mateos, which ruled the country between 1953 and 1964. It was hoped that Mexico would set an example for the developing world. The international and Mexican political and medical leaders who designed malaria eradication in

Mexico were aware of the cold war political context in which they operated and in which they elaborated a common discourse and its metaphors.

Three recurrent metaphors characterized the campaign: military metaphors, which can be traced to prior international health interventions; metaphors relating malaria and communism; and metaphors referring to a relationship between malaria eradication and modernization. An example of the first type is the military tone of WHO and PAHO documents. In 1956 WHO announced its annual Health Day theme, "War to insects, carriers of disease," using terms such as "crusade."[1] Cold war anxieties inspired the last two kinds of metaphors. According to supporters of the campaign, malaria not only killed but "enslaved" its sufferers, causing disablement and impairment ("enslavement" was a code word applied to workers under communist regimes; Dulles 1954: 421). A number of documents suggested that the eradication of malaria would contribute to the eradication of communism.

The medical leader of malaria eradication in Latin America was Fred L. Soper, director of PAHO between 1947 and 1959, a former Rockefeller Foundation officer who had worked before in Latin America (Russell 1977; Soper 1957, 1960, 1965). A report prepared by Soper and the Argentinean Carlos Alvarado, another PAHO officer, explained the rationale for eradication. Malaria was one the main health problems in Mexico, affecting about 143 million people (36 percent of the population of the region and a third of Mexico's population), and it could be defeated with new drugs and insecticides. Soper and Alvarado responded to the growing concern over mosquito resistance to DDT. They believed that partial application of DDT, which prior to the campaign was often used inconsistently, encouraged resistance and made the campaign urgent. According to Soper, only a comprehensive campaign would eliminate malaria before resistance spread all over the region (Organización Sanitaria Panamericana 1955).

It is interesting to note the way medical leaders used political and economic arguments. Early in 1955 Soper explained the disease to UNICEF's executive board as an economic problem, using the code word "enslavement": "Malaria is a serious burden on the economy of every malarious country. It has been well said that, where malaria fails to kill it enslaves. It is an economic disease."[2] In Mexico itself, the benefits of eradication were portrayed in economic terms. A Mexican expert claimed that the campaign would increase agricultural productivity, save medical resources, reverse the depreciation of rural estates, and promote development (Vargas 1958).

American health experts portrayed the campaign in Mexico and Latin America as benefiting industrial nations because agricultural imports from malarious regions of Mexico carried additional costs due to the labor absenteeism produced by the disease.[3] In the United States, a 1957 proposal to Congress offered an argument for US aid to the eradication program. The program's backers estimated that a five- to ten-year worldwide campaign would cost $519 million. The US share of this amount would be 20 percent, or about $100 million, and the benefiting nations, WHO, UNICEF, and PAHO would pay the rest. The discussions in Congress revealed that about half the funds would be spent on insecticides and equipment produced in the United States, mainly by oil companies. As a result, the campaign would provide an indirect subsidy for these American industries.

The US State Department supported malaria eradication in Mexico as part of its cold war on communism. Officials feared that the Soviet Union might attract Mexican leaders with grants and promises of development. The department wanted to demonstrate that bilateral aid could promote orderly social progress, without a revolution. This meant the gradual elimination of extreme poverty and diseases portrayed as persistent plagues, which could be manipulated by communists to "feed false panaceas." The State Department believed that Mexicans were more "tolerant" of Marxism than Americans. There was also concern in the United States about the Soviet Union embassy's influence in Mexico and about demands made by some Mexican politicians for the nationalization of industries owned by foreigners (Cline 1981; Glennon 1987; Rabe 1988; P. H. Smith 2000).

Although the Mexican communist party did not challenge the country's political stability, the United States and the Mexican governments wanted to control the potential threat from any leftist group. They were preoccupied that communists might exploit the tradition for social justice inaugurated, if only partially fulfilled, by the Mexican Revolution of 1910. Among the influential politicians of the left was Victor Lombardo Toledano, a Mexican leader of a Confederation of Latin American Workers considered by the State Department to be a communist front organization (Rubottom 1958).

Mexican authorities were also interested in using the campaign to reinforce an emerging national health system and to extend the authority of the federal government over rural areas by providing social services. The Mexican malaria campaign began with the organization of a self-sufficient Comisión Nacional de Erradicación del Paludismo (CNEP; *paludismo* was another term in Spanish for malaria), a special government corporation within the Secretariat of Health with a great deal of money and power and many health workers. CNEP's features resonated with the military format of antimosquito campaigns of the early twentieth century and with the anxieties of the cold war. According to a magazine article, CNEP had "generals [who were] physicians and doctors in science" and "soldiers ... armed with guns that send out a spray of DDT. The enemy is mankind's most prevalent disease—malaria" (Amstrong 1958: 188). These "soldiers," the field sprayers of DDT, appeared in other documents as disciplined troops dressed in bright khaki uniforms and carrying their aluminum fumigating pumps, members "of an army of liberation, driving out disease" (Morgan 1958: 12).

Propaganda intertwined humanitarianism with stereotypes of poor rural people in developing countries. Malaria explained poverty, lethargy, resignation, and fatalism. These ideas were instrumental in constructing a racialized version of the disease. Indigenous peasants were disease carriers, and their culture was an obstacle to progress. A corollary was that US foreign aid and medical science would remove tradition, create a desire for better living standards, and promote the need to be part of a market economy. The belief that malaria was the main "drag" on development in backward countries was underlined by the *New York Times*, which explained, citing the opinions of experts, that the greatest havoc brought by the disease was the destruction of individual will: "Malariologists point out that it is common to regard people in tropical countries as indolent. 'They are not lazier than people in temperate climates,' one doctor said, 'they merely have malaria.'"[4]

CNEP's antimalaria educational unit prepared a variety of pins, radio spots, posters, and pamphlets. Its goal was to obtain the participation in the campaign of key local people—political authorities, provincial physicians, schoolteachers, priests, journalists, and administrators of rural estates.[5] The goal of the unit was to "sensitize" (*sensibilizar*) such people and gain their acceptance of DDT spraying and blood sampling (microscopic examination of blood was used as the indicator of the existence of the plasmodium), as well as to report on families who resisted having their houses sprayed.

CNEP pamphlets underscored the need for communal responsibility with titles such as "National Prosperity without Malaria" and "All [houses] must be sprayed." Posters displayed messages appealing to family and nationalist sentiments: "I am a Patriot"; "My house has already been sprayed"; "War against Malaria is for Mexico." The slogan in one publication played with cold war euphemisms: "Citizens, in your home there is a hidden enemy, paludism, destroy it!"[6] Another pamphlet with a similar message in its title—"I am a patriot, I assist the war against paludism"—resorted to war metaphors and to the citizen's obligation to "expel the enemy" from Mexican soil. The cover of yet another pamphlet gave a new meaning to the term *enemy:* it was not only the mosquito but also anyone unwilling to allow his house to be sprayed.[7] As the historian Edmund Russell (2001) observed, similar campaigns had been carried out in the United States previously, interweaving medical technology and war euphemisms.

Official nationalism harked back to the 1910 Revolution and was part of the state-building efforts of Mexican governments. Post–World War II Mexican governments promoted a unified, national popular culture as a form of political validation (Joseph and Nugent 1994). After 1940, nationalism shed its more militant and anticlerical features, typical of the 1910s and 1930s, in favor of a milder character that celebrated orderly progress and national folklore. Official nationalism emphasized the integration of ethnic groups. Indians would be "uplifted," thanks to cultural homogenization. This process would produce dynamic, individual rural citizens who felt they were part of the whole Mexican nation. For officials, nationhood, the promotion of *mestizaje* over Indian identities, and the malaria eradication campaign frequently were complementary.

CNEP tried to overcome cultural barriers by reaching out to indigenous peoples with the underlying functionalist assumption of "assisting" indigenous ethnic groups in their "transition" to modernity. An agreement toward this end was signed in 1956 between CNEP and the Instituto Nacional Indigenista, created in 1947. After the Second World War the Instituto accommodated the conservative administrations that ruled Mexico and concentrated on "instilling" modern cultural values for the "incorporation" of rural populations. The Instituto, through education and through hygiene and other social programs, aimed to change "superstitions" and "backward" lifestyles (Doremus 2001; Favre 1972; Page Pliego 2002). In a 1955 pamphlet, the Instituto explained that magical beliefs were "the main reason why no hygienic precautions are taken" by Indians, and that one of its main goals was to exchange these beliefs for scientific ideas (Instituto Nacional Indigenista 1955: 5).

Mexican educational organizations reinforced the acculturation work done by CNEP and the Instituto Nacional Indigenista. For the secretary of public education, the teaching of Spanish to Indians who were monolingual in an indigenous language was an instrument for national integration. Educational and medical activities were part of a state-supported cultural project to Westernize the rural communities through de-Indianization. The project entailed an intense but non-forcible cultural diffusion, namely, the spread of Western and biomedical cultures as the best tools to modernize rural indigenous communities and create an educated, healthy citizenry. Ultimately, its mission was to induce cultural change and to present as an inevitable trend the emergence of a single mestizo national culture—in sum, to Mexicanize the indigenous population. The governmental goals were to promote de-Indianization and accelerate the transformation of Indians into mestizos.

CNEP linked this form of nationalism to family values and women. A poster represented motherhood with the image of an indigenous woman who stated her motivations for supporting the campaign: "In Defense of my Homeland, in Defense of my Children, war on Malaria." Official propaganda also idealized the role of women as guardians of the health and welfare of their homes.[8] These messages were important in Mexico because of the Catholic tradition of glorifying mothers and the public expectation that women should fulfill a domestic role, including taking care of health problems.

Catholic traditions were also intertwined with pro-natalism. A pamphlet titled "More Mexicans, better Mexicans" emphasized a goal of the Mexican government in the campaign: to increase the economically active population. According to the pamphlet, a healthier Mexican meant a more capable citizen, a "master of his fate and therefore an exceptional man."[9] Kay Vaughan (1997) studied a similar process that had occurred before in Mexican public education: how official Mexican education linked populist strategies and pro-natalist policies for political validation.

Local Responses and Cultural Challenges

Among the fascinating educational materials from the malaria eradication campaign are the monthly bulletins from the fourteen campaign zones in Mexico.[10] They introduced the voices of local health workers in the official sanitary discourse and facilitated the creation of popular metaphors designed to adapt a state-driven campaign and locally reconstruct malaria as a plague. One persuasive gimmick used in the bulletins was to change the lyrics of popular songs and poems to link daily life with eradication activities—for example, changing the lyrics of a *corrido*, a type of ballad popular in Mexico. "Corrido a la CNEP" praised nationalism and prosperity and ended with the words "death to paludism / and long live my motherland!"[11] A poem titled "Modern

Combat" toyed with the legacy of the 1910 Revolution and the military traits of the campaign: "The squad that marches to battle / Formerly grasped the rifle… Today scientific trappings / Will win victory in combat."[12] Another poem, elaborated by a voluntary health worker from Oaxaca, picked up the theme: the sprayers were gladiators aiming to save the nation.[13]

Reception of the antimalaria campaign by provincial physicians and rural populations in Mexico was inconsistent. It followed no systematic pattern and proposed no alternative public health perspective. On the contrary, local reception was contradictory, uneven, and spontaneous. It revealed diverse and sometimes entrenched notions of health and disease that were not taken into account in metropolitan and governmental designs of malaria eradication. This created unexpected challenges for international health organizations that had to confront local cultures possessing feeble traditions of Western medicine.

One such challenge involved the cultural dimensions of different languages. CNEP used the Spanish word for malaria, *paludismo*, a French-inspired term common among medical elites who were interested not in symptoms per se but in identifying a specific clinical entity with a unique biological origin. Using a scientific name was tantamount to validating a body of technical knowledge, segregated from lay knowledge. In contrast, indigenous people used about thirty Spanish and indigenous words for malaria, such as *amarillas, calenturas, espantado, fiebre de la costa, jacaltamal, morrongo, tenahuiste, toahuiste*, and *tenahuistle* (Vargas 1965). These names reflected an understanding of illness as a series of symptoms that had lives of their own and appeared because of natural and unnatural agents.

Melding the goals of the campaign and *mestizaje*, CNEP promoted a racialized version of malaria in which being an Indian was presented as synonymous with being sick, poor, and backward. Anemia, prostration, and weariness, typical symptoms of malaria, were overemphasized to explain the traditional "apathy," "fatalism," "indolence," and even "depressive character" of rural people. This conceptualization of the disease coincided with a tradition of racial prejudice in Mexico that portrayed Indian workers as inherently dirty, lazy, and stupefied by alcohol, their reckless behavior validating exploitive working conditions (Knight 1990). In addition, for officers of CNEP, malaria eradication was a tool for the expansion of Western medicine in rural areas (Vargas and Almaraz Ugalde 1963).

CNEP criticized traditional medicine as a cultural trait of superstition that would be brushed aside by the campaign. Little attention was given to the widespread popularity of shamans and midwives and to the fact that their practices were often effective (Parsons 1931). As a result, the eradication of malaria was understood as also being the eradication of traditional and domestic healing practices and the validation of the supremacy of Western medicine. According to a Mexican health officer, the eradication campaign involved people's leaving behind atavistic lifestyles, "prejudices and superstitions ... rooted in the rural milieu" (Escobar 1963: 729).

Medical acculturation failed because it often confronted resistance from people who distrusted government officers or disliked having their houses sprayed. In addition, popular resistance was due to the initially overlooked fact that insecticides were toxic to people and their domestic animals. Some CNEP workers, most of them from urban mestizo backgrounds, linked resistance to their negative perception of the indigenous rural population. They believed peasants lived in indolence and a could-not-care-less state of mind regarding malaria eradication. The challenges of cross-cultural health care became the cornerstone of a remarkable anthropological critique against a campaign implemented from above.

During the late 1940s and the 1950s, a new subdiscipline of anthropology, called applied anthropology and latter known as medical anthropology, developed in Mexico and the United States thanks to the work of the American George Foster and the Mexican Gonzalo Aguirre Beltrán, among others (Aguirre Beltrán 1955; Foster 1969). They did not disapprove of all aspects of traditional medicine but believed it was possible to identify the positive aspects and expunge the negative ones, overcoming the mistakes of traditional medicine and making it easier to introduce Western medicine and personal hygiene in indigenous cultural settings. They also believed that anthropologists could gain the trust of peasants, facilitate better communication between health workers and indigenous people, and integrate ethnic minority groups into mainstream society (Caudhill 1953).

Early in 1951 the Institute of Inter-American Affairs of the US State Department contracted with Foster and the Smithsonian Institution for behavioral assistance in an evaluation of US bilateral health assistance in Latin America. Subsequently, the Health Advisory Committee of the Foreign Operations Administration, another unit of the State Department, included anthropologists in developing programs in "traditional" rural societies overseas. According to Foster (1976: 12), these programs were aimed at examining "the ways in which knowledge of the social, cultural and psychological factors ... influence change [to] improve health." Notable among the professionals working with Foster was Isabel Kelly, a young California anthropologist who had worked in Mexico since 1948 (González 1989; Kelly 1955, 1965).

In 1953 Kelly began to collaborate with Héctor García Manzanedo and the Mexican health secretariat on rural projects (he was an officer in the health secretariat). Kelly and García Manzanedo's work was not easy, because Mexican physicians had, since 1945, held a legal monopoly on practicing medicine, and they condemned indigenous healing practices. Shortly after the inception of the malaria eradication campaign, García Manzanedo and Kelly prepared a critical report that opposed its totalizing approach, given Mexico's indigenous diversity.[14] Their formal relationship with government institutions and the framework of applied anthropology made their criticism mild. According to the report, the government underestimated the diversity of Indian cultures. The two argued that although the campaign took technical factors into account, it overlooked an essential issue, the diversity of indigenous languages. This issue was important in southern Mexico because the many ethnic groups living in malarious areas there spoke a variety of languages and dialects. According to García Manzanedo and Kelly, although the majority of a rural population of more than 19.2 million persons spoke Spanish, 1.6 million spoke Spanish along with an indigenous language, and 795,069 people were monolingual in a native language.[15]

Initially, García Manzanedo and Kelly used language as an indicator of ethnicity ambivalently, something common among contemporary anthropologists. However, they also stressed the existence of 19.2 million rural people, most of them with some command of Spanish but part of an indigenous culture (according to a 1957 estimate, the figure 19.2 million represented more than 60 percent of the nation's population). Miguel León Portilla, a renowned Mexican anthropologist, criticized the narrowly language-based ethnic definitions used in the Mexican censuses. He believed that many people living in the countryside and urban slums should be registered as Indians because they maintained indigenous lifestyle practices such as communalism, a diet based on corn, chile, and beans, and sleeping on mats (León Portilla 1962). On the basis of these ideas, Kelly and Garcia Manzanedo went beyond a restricted linguistic indicator and suggested that even rural people with a command of Spanish would not understand the eradication campaign (León Portilla 1959).

García Manzanedo and Kelly also criticized the assumption made by the malaria eradication program that rural life was static—that people were sedentary and lived in one house. This assumption was crucial for biannual spraying operations, because it was believed that people would continue sleeping for at least a year in the same house, which held residues of the insecticide and therefore would remain free of mosquitoes. The authors of the critical report underscored that, on the contrary, human life in rural areas was dynamic, involving migration, tribal nomadism, religious pilgrimages by peasants, and the construction of temporary houses (Pampana 1963: 365). A related issue was that in some Mexican jungle areas, people were accustomed to sleeping outside during hot summers.

García Manzanedo and Kelly considered the attention CNEP gave to health education to be insufficient. They believed that few or inadequate attempts were being made to adapt scientific messages about malaria to indigenous cultures. Their report suggested increasing the number and training days of bilingual sprayers, the abilities of health educators, and the recruitment of priests and schoolteachers—who were familiar with indigenous cultures—for the eradication effort. Regarding contamination produced by insecticides, they explained their preoccupation with the fact that DDT killed not only mosquitoes but also hens, bees, and other domestic animals, something that would damage peasant families' diets, because they obtained eggs, meat, and honey from these insects and animals.

The most interesting criticism leveled by García Manzanedo and Kelly was that malaria eradication did not take into account indigenous concepts regarding blood, the body, and fevers (García, Sierra, and Balám 1999). For many indigenous communities, "fever" could be a disease in itself, and most inhabitants of rural Mexico believed that some nine types of fevers existed (Instituto Nacional Indigenista 1994). They explained malaria as the result of magical harm, eating unripe fruits, sleeping on the floor, and sudden temperature changes such as those caused by bathing in cold water after working in the sun. Fevers were treated with medicinal plants, by rubbing sick bodies with alcohol, and by drinking rue tea mixed with lime juice or strong alcoholic beverages (Fuente 1941; Madsen 1965). Another popular treatment was to "scare" the patient.

The human body itself constituted an area of conflict. According to the campaign's design, blood samples had to be obtained to confirm the presence of plasmodia. But peasants were afraid to give away their blood and resisted its withdrawal for laboratory analysis. García Manzanedo and Kelly signaled that it would not be easy to obtain blood samples from some indigenous groups and even from acculturated mestizos. For medical doctors, blood was just a liquid component of human anatomy. For peasants, blood was a nonrenewable substance. A person was permanently weakened by withdrawals of blood, and it had held mystical, religious, and historical meanings since pre-Columbian times (blood was essential in heart sacrifices for divination, preparation for war, and the "renewal" of nature). Indigenous communities in Mexico practiced bloodletting in religious offerings, and traditional healers gave blood to sufferers of anemia and malnutrition (Ingham 1984).

Blood smears were also feared in rural Mexico in the 1950s, because the loss of a vital, nonregenerative fluid was believed to be detrimental to health, to produce permanent weakness, to create sterility in men or women, and to make people prone to illnesses perceived, in rural areas, as more menacing than malaria, such as those caused by the evil eye. In addition, the intrusion of foreign objects into the body, such as the needles used for pricking fingers, was taken as a cause of sickness (Foster 1976: 14).

Blood sampling was feared, moreover, because blood could be used to cause poisoning. Drawing blood in order to obtain laboratory information played into recurrent rumors that poor people were being assessed before being destroyed. An unfounded rumor that indigenous blood was being sold to "the Americans" was consonant with the fear that prevailed in societies with acute inequalities, in which the poor harbor fear of losing their most precious goods and people to outside forces. In other cases, according to García Manzanedo and Kelly, Indians could not understand why health workers took blood from them and thereby weakened them, if they were concerned about their health. As a result, during the antimalaria campaign, some people evaded blood examination and even forbade other family members to comply.

The emphasis on blood sampling by malaria eradicators also reconfigured the process of diagnosing malaria. Before the campaign, provincial physicians had relied on clinical symptoms such as recurrent fevers to identify the disease—a less intrusive medical examination accepted by rural people. With malaria eradication, the existence of plasmodia in the blood was taken as the only evidence of malaria. Health workers magnified the menacing presence of the parasite, concealed in natives, to postulate the need to test, treat, and control symptomless persons, something difficult to grasp in an indigenous culture for which the notion of apparently "healthy" persons carrying disease was an oxymoron. Medical doctors emphasized that many infected people living in areas where malaria was endemic could have parasites in their blood but no outward symptoms, because symptoms could appear about fifteen days after the infected mosquito bite. This scientific notion was also in opposition to the popular perception of disease, which associated it with acute pain and the physical inability to work. Many lay people did not regard it possible for a person to be ill if he or she felt well or if mild symptoms did not prevent work.

García Manzanedo and Kelly's report revealed the tensions between different meanings of disease, fevers, and human blood inherent in the construction of malaria as a plague. These tensions were not resolved during the campaign. Malaria eradicators—and the few state-supported rural health services organized by the Mexican Social Security system and the health secretariat—could overcome peasant resistance, but indigenous beliefs about malaria coexisted uneasily with the policies of government health services. Although biomedicine was eventually integrated as a resource for some conditions, traditional medicine and its less complicated and expensive practices survived. As traditional healing persisted, different versions of medical pluralism developed (Fábrega and Silver 1973; Hernández Llamas 1984; Whiteford 1999).

In their report, the anthropologists confessed that they had no solution for the cultural mismatches they described. For them, it was impossible to provide a universal prescription for ethnically diverse areas. They simply indicated the campaign's lack of flexibility and expected that some changes would be made. The lack of specific advice also suggested the hegemonic position of CNEP and the limited room for alternative paths during malaria eradication. In addition, Kelly was unable to follow up on this criticism, because at the end of 1957 she left Mexico to become part of a US-sponsored anthropological project in Bolivia.

Although García Manzanedo and Kelly's recommendations were not followed, the personal impressions of a WHO officer in Mexico some years later coincided with their perspectives. The officer noticed that the "crisis" of Mexico's malaria eradication program in the so-called problem areas, where the campaign had made little progress despite the implementation of adequate technical interventions, was more intense in the territories occupied by indigenous communities, namely, in Morelos, Oaxaca, Guerrero, Michoacán, and Puebla. He even compared maps of the Indian areas and the so-called problem areas and found, to his surprise, that they were extremely similar, even "corresponding "exactly."[16]

Bugs and Rumors

A few years after the campaign began, complaints and resistance to CNEP activities appeared in some villages. Sometimes people questioned the imposition of technical interventions from outside communities and the government's scant regard for the collateral toxic effects of DDT. Some complaints concerned bedbugs, called *chinches* in Spanish. Their sudden proliferation was a major inconvenience. The blood-feeding insects are parasites on humans and domesticated animals, their bites leave inflamed, itchy red welts, and they reproduce rapidly. Villagers were convinced that the spraying teams knew about the poisonous effects of the insecticide and the proliferation of DDT-resistant bedbugs. Although the transmission of pathogens to humans by bedbugs was unlikely, people's understandable concern was that just like *Anopheles* mosquitoes, bedbugs could transmit disease. Eventually it was discovered that rural people believed DDT, known as "the dust" (*polvo*), contained *chinche* eggs and that spraying merely increased the bedbug population without beneficial effect. They feared CNEP authorities for "deceiving them" by sending a useless insecticide. Sometimes they suggested a radical change in the campaign—to eradicate bedbugs instead of *Anopheles*.[17]

A local provincial authority blamed the sprayers of DDT for wanting only to "fuck [*chingar*] the people as the government has always done."[18] His use of the strong curse verb *chingar*—which could be also translated as "to rape"—was linked to the perception of an official intervention as intolerable. CNEP resorted to the authority of the federal government in cases of open resistance. An indication of the need to persuade people to comply with malaria eradication was the emergence in the late 1960s and early 1970s of propaganda with titles that reveal a need to overcome distrust and find consent, such as "The sprayer, your friend," "Open the door of your house," and "The notifier will help you."

In some places, village dwellers believed that careless and dishonest spraying teams were diverting genuine DDT and replacing it with an inferior product.[19] The concern over bedbugs made people wash or replaster their walls after the sprayers were gone or contravene CNEP recommendations and sleep outdoors to avoid bedbug attacks. For CNEP officers, all these actions nullified the effects of the insecticide. These incidents were similar to previous indigenous rejections of sanitary campaigns, such as smallpox vaccinations, and were of the sort that commonly appear in societies marked by social inequalities. Historical studies have demonstrated the role played by rumor in unequal societies, where health measures appear to be imposed from above and are perceived by the poor as the ultimate tool used to destroy them.

Initially, CNEP had little to say with regard to bedbugs and denied a relationship between the pest and DDT. According to health officials, the insecticide did not increase the population of *chinches*—it only took them out of their hiding places, thereby giving the impression of an increased infestation. For CNEP, bedbugs could be eliminated with good sanitation, filling the fissures in walls, applying kerosene to surfaces were the bugs rested, and general house cleanliness.[20]

Years later, scientists discovered that the popular complaints were right. After a few years of DDT spraying, bedbugs developed resistance, as did other insects such as scorpions, which became a public health problem among children in rural areas. In time, bedbug infestation became a critical issue in rural Mexico's campaign, causing delays, an increase in the number of working days needed for spraying operations, and a discrediting of the whole health intervention. As a result, openly or silently, some people refused to cooperate with sprayers in tasks such as emptying houses and providing water for spraying.

Luís Vargas, a noted Mexican CNEP scientist, intervened in this issue in 1962. He launched a project to deal with bedbugs and trained entomologists to control them. The task was difficult because warm human dwellings were a suitable habitat for bedbugs, and the insects could hide in bedding and furniture. CNEP's unpreparedness in this matter was evident a few years later when the prominent malariologist Vargas described bedbugs as a serious complication only of a "public relations" nature—in other words, something that might be resolved with educational programs (Vargas 1963: 341).

Final Remarks

By the mid-1960s it was clear that little could be done against *Anopheles* resistance to insecticides. In Mexico the resistance was noticed first in Chiapas, near the Guatemalan border, in an area converted to the cultivation of pesticide-addicted commercial cotton, which helped to build up resistance among *Anopheles*. Chiapas also received immigrants from northern Guatemala, the poorest region in that Central American country (Murray 1994). By the mid-1960s, Central America had become a booming market for pesticide manufacturers and commercial cotton agriculturalists, who often used chemicals no longer allowed in industrial countries because of their toxicity. As a result, Chiapas, sections of Oaxaca, and successive parts of the country where it was hoped that malaria was ending were "lost" by malaria eradicators. Malaria reestablished itself, usually with an initial low but persistent transmission (De Zulueta and Garret-Jones 1965).

Toward the mid-1960s, the complications faced by the Mexican campaign intensified, and the enthusiasm of politicians and donors began to wane. The initial impression that "problem areas" or merely technical and administrative problems were the main causes of the campaign's shortcomings became problematic. An important factor in the campaign's lack of results was the tradition of discontinuity in public health work. When malaria declined, complacency ensued. It was difficult to persuade politicians and young health workers, who had little experience with malaria, to continue a fight for something that was no longer perceived as an emergency. Local politicians thought the threat of malaria was exaggerated to maintain a strict eradication discipline when epidemic outbreaks no longer occurred.

The 1969 World Health Assembly of WHO, which took place in Boston, reversed the goals of the malaria eradication campaign and inaugurated a period of confusion over what was the best program to control malaria (WHO 1969). A WHO resolution titled "Re-examination of the Global Strategy of Malaria Eradication" blamed the failure of malaria eradication on unforeseen socioeconomic, financial, and administrative factors and the inadequacy of basic health services in the affected countries. According to WHO malariologists based in Geneva, malaria eradication without the previous creation of rural health services was impossible, because permanent health centers should sustain antimalaria activities once the sprayers were gone.

During the 1970s and 1980s, malaria eradication went further into decline because the political context of the cold war was vanishing. Latin American intellectuals criticized "modernization," arguing that it was ethnocentric because the past of their nations did not resemble the past of the United States. These critics questioned cold war modernization models and believed that increased commercial ties with industrial nations would increase dependency (Levinson and Onis 1970; Packenham 1992; Tipps 1973). Development programs launched from capital cities were blamed for concentrating on the modern commercial areas of a country and ignoring its "backward" regions. Mexican anthropologists criticized the modernization model for its authoritarianism, questioned its assumption that Indian assimilation was desirable, observed its link with the verticality of the malaria eradication campaign, and criticized the manipulation of a "tame" version of anthropology by official programs. They also rejected the notion of a single "mestizo culture" unifying all Mexican ethnic communities and instead envisioned a pluralistic culture that would respect indigenous minorities (Bonfil 1987; Ros Romero 1992). The tragedy of the malaria eradication campaign was not only that it failed to achieve its objective but also that, by framing the disease as a plague of underdevelopment and its eradication as a tool of the cold war, and by overemphasizing silver bullets, it left in disarray and undermined other programs aimed at confronting an important rural disease.

Notes

1. "Día mundial de la Salud el 7 de abril de 1956 bajo el lema 'Guerra a los insectos portadores de enfermedades,'" Archivo Histórico de la Secretaria de Salubridad, Mexico City (hereafter AHSS), fondo Secretaría de Salubridad y Asistencia (hereafter SSA), serie Secretaria Particular, caja 33, expediente 4 (1953–1960).

2. The report of the director of the Pan American Sanitary Bureau to the UNICEF regional board is titled "Malaria Eradication in the Americas," E/ICEF/282/, and appears as Annex 2, "Excerpt from report of the UNICEF Executive Board March 1955 session," in WHO, "Malaria Eradication, proposal by the Director General, 3 May 1955," 25–26, World Health Organization Library, Geneva (hereafter WHO Library).

3. WHO, "Appraisal: The programme of the WHO for 1959–164," MHO/AD/87.59, 17 November 1959, 51, WHO Library.

4. "Doom of Malaria by '67 Envisioned," *New York Times*, 22 December 1957, 23.

5. Manuel E. Pesqueira, "A year of antimalarial activities," April 1957, in WHO Archives, series Malaria Research Collection, box WHO7.0078, folder "Mexico 1957–1958."

6. All these materials are kept at AHSS, fondo SSA, sección Comisión Nacional para la erradicación del Paludismo (hereafter CNEP).

7. *Boletín Zona VI*, CNEP, año 1, no. 2, Ciudad Valles San Luis Potosi, 15 May 1956, AHSS, fondo SSA, sección CNEP, serie Zona 6, caja 1, expediente 2.

8. These materials are kept at AHSS, fondo SSA, sección CNEP, serie Zona 6, caja 1, expediente 2.

9. "Más y mejores Mexicanos," Campaña Nacional de Erradicación del Paludismo, 1955, 1–2, AHSS, fondo SSA, sección CENP, serie Dirección, caja 1, expediente 6.

10. José Alvarez Amezqita, Secretario de Salubridad y Asistencia, "Programa de Erradicación del paludismo en México: Informe de actividades Año 1958," AHSS, fondo SSA, sección CNEP, serie Dirección, caja 44, expediente 7.

11. *El Tarasco: Boletín para el personal CNEP Zona X*, Morelia, Michoacán, AHSS, fondo SSA, sección Subsecretaría de Asistencia, caja 84, expediente 3, años 1949–1955.

12. Lid Moderna, *El Huasteco: Boletín Zonal CNEP Zona VI CD Valles San Luis Potosí VI*, July 1961, AHSS, fondo SSA, sección CNEP, serie Zona 6, caja 1, expediente 2.

13. "Himno al paludismo: Canto de fé, por E. Méndez Pérez, Auxiliar Honorario de Educación Higiénica," Oaxaca, Oaxaca, 17 September 1960, AHSS, fondo SSA, sección CNEP, serie Zona 5, caja 1, expediente 3.

14. Héctor García Manzanedo and Isabel Kelly, "Comentarios al proyecto de Campaña para la Erradicación del Paludismo en México, 1955," AHSS, fondo SSA, sección Subsecretaría de Salubridad y Asistencia, caja 49, expediente 6. A copy of the report is kept at the National Library of Medicine.

15. These figures are taken from the census of 1950, which defined ethnicity as the use of a "native tongue" and was commonly related to illiteracy. "Informes e investigaciones," AHSS, fondo SSA, sección Subsecretaría de Salubridad y Asistencia, caja 49, expediente 6.

16. In C. J. Foll, "Mexican Malaria Program (CNEP), 16 November–15 December 1962," WHO Archives, series Malaria Research Collection, box WHO 7.0079, folder México 1961–63.

17. Pablo Díaz Hernández to Juan Canales Cirilo [jefe de la Zona V CNEP], 23 August 1959, AHSS, fondo SSA, sección CNEP, serie Zona 8, caja 1, expediente 6.

18. Ibid.

19. Ibid.; "Brigada antipalúdica atacada en Oaxaca, 18 March 1957," AHSS, fondo SSA, sección CNEP, serie Zona 5, caja 1, expediente 2.

20. "¿Aumenta el Rociado los chinches?" *Boletín Zonal Mensual del CNEP Zona II*, año 2, no. 8, February 1960, 2, AHSS, fondo SSA, sección CNEP, serie Zona 1, caja 1, expediente 3.

"Steady with Custom"

Mediating HIV Prevention in the Trobriand Islands,
Papua New Guinea

Katherine Lepani

I heard a WHO statistic on the radio, coming up to World AIDS Day on December first. Every fourteen seconds a young person is infected with HIV somewhere in the world. So I am thinking, what is the Trobriand statistic? Every day? Every hour? How long will it take to wipe us out? People are scared when they hear about this disease, the death it brings, but fear does not stay with them when sex is on their minds. People put fear out of mind so they can still act free. Freedom is like a feather in Trobriand hair, our pride. It is young people's time to enjoy. So it is very hard to change our ways, very hard for us to think of fear when we are enjoying ourselves. But we need to break away from customs that put us at risk in this time of AIDS.

—Trobriand woman in her mid-forties, 8 November 2003

Biomedicine and epidemiology have made possible an understanding of HIV pathology and the way the virus damages the human immune system to the extent that infected bodies eventually die from the complications of AIDS. But these specialized fields of knowledge have been unable to prevent the persistent spread of HIV throughout the world. Three decades since the virus was first isolated and named, the magnitude of HIV represents the most serious public health issue confronting the world today. In 2007 there were an estimated 2.7 million new cases of HIV infection, 33 million people living with the virus, and 2 million AIDS deaths (UNAIDS 2008: 16). As the epigraph to this chapter suggests, the pandemic is modeled statistically like a ticking time bomb threatening to decimate even out-of-the-way places such as the Trobriand Islands, a group of small coral atolls in the Solomon Sea off the east coast of mainland Papua New Guinea (PNG), with a population of thirty thousand people.

Yet this pandemic of staggering proportions has not occurred as a singular event transcending geographic, political, and cultural boundaries. Rather, HIV infection proliferates into "multiple and overlapping epidemics" within particular social and biological contexts, "each with its own distinctive dynamics and character" (Mane and Aggleton 2001: 23). Concurrent with the global diffusion of HIV is an "epidemic of meanings" (Treichler 1999: 11), or different ways of comprehending the virus, as biomedical and epidemiological models of disease and sexuality, and the moralities these models impute, interact with local knowledge. Far greater than a microorganism, HIV looms large in the collective body, configured by discourses of risk and fear and the cultural meanings people bring to bear on experiences of sexuality, illness, and death. As a metaphor for modernity and historical transformation, the phenomenon of HIV paradoxically appeals to notions of cultural stability for mediation and response (Setel 1999). However, the rhetorical emphasis on "risk behaviors" and the depiction of "cultural practices" as causal factors in HIV transmission find ready targets in sexual practices represented by public health interventions as promiscuous, exotic, and enshrined by tradition (see Seidel and Vidal 1997; Stillwaggon 2003; see also Kelm, this volume).

The Trobriand context offers an instructive standpoint for questioning such assumptions about HIV risk and culture. In this chapter I draw on ethnographic research conducted in the Trobriands in 2001 and 2003, in which I explored the way representations of HIV and AIDS are understood through the lenses of cultural knowledge, social practice, and embodied experience. I consider the historical and contemporary tensions between converging bodies of knowledge, and the troubling contradictions between edicts of behavior change and the sustained expression of cultural values through embodied practice. Although mindful that "the way the epidemic is brought to people's attention will be the critical determinant of how they will respond to it" (Reid 1994: 1), I shift perspective to examine the way cultural knowledge is engaged to make sense of the novel and transforming phenomenon of HIV. In the Trobriands, the representation of AIDS as a looming plague from beyond the horizon, wrought by sexual excess and transgression, provides a pivotal reference for asserting cultural identity as people contemplate HIV prevention in relation to "custom" and the valued efficacy of sexual practice in maintaining social relations.

Making HIV Visible

The presence of HIV is firmly established in Papua New Guinea, the largest Pacific Island country, with a youthful population of nearly 6 million people and immense linguistic and cultural diversity. Diagnosed cases of HIV have increased annually by 30 percent since 1997. In 2008 the national prevalence was projected at 2 percent, with an estimated 60,000 people living with HIV. The cumulative total of notified cases of HIV since the first reported case in 1987 was 18,484 in December 2006, and cases have been reported in rural and urban areas in all nineteen provinces (National AIDS Council Secretariat 2008: 17–19). The provision of voluntary counseling and testing services and antiretroviral therapies remains limited throughout the country, especially in rural areas.[1]

Although a comprehensive national program for responding to HIV has been in place for more than a decade, dramatic rhetoric about waging a battle against the "killer disease" has set the overriding tone of communication. Militaristic metaphors, which feature in the global discourse on HIV (Treichler 1999: 31–32), have found popular expression in PNG as well, including tropes about the "AIDS war" and awareness posters that depict traditionally clad warriors bearing shields in the shape of condoms. Awareness information modeled on epidemiological "risk groups" and amplified by an amalgamation of Christian and traditional cosmological beliefs has intensified moralistic responses in which fear, shame, and blame are persistent expressions (Hammar 2007).

In a context of limited primary health services and unavailability of HIV voluntary counseling and testing facilities, estimations of the number of Trobrianders affected by HIV remain speculative. There are several anecdotal reports of people returning home to the Trobriands after testing positive for HIV in urban centers. In some instances, AIDS is perceived as the probable cause of death if the deceased suffered prolonged, degenerative illness after traveling or residing outside the islands. Speculations are based as well on the numbers of coffins sent home for burial from other parts of the country. In 2001, the district health center on the main island of Kiriwina reported the first confirmed case of HIV based on antibody testing conducted by the central government laboratory in Port Moresby. The health extension officer

(HEO) requested the test when the patient failed to respond to drug treatment for diagnosed tuberculosis. The HEO called this the "first home-grown case" because the patient had never traveled outside of the Trobriands (T. Elliot, HEO, personal communication, 2003). Only seventeen years old, the female patient died at home in the village within six months of confirmed diagnosis. A further confirmed case in 2004 involved a pregnant woman in her early twenties, diagnosed during routine prenatal testing while residing in Port Moresby. The baby died at three months of age, and the young woman died a month later after returning home to the Trobriands to bury her baby.

Despite the indeterminacy of HIV prevalence in the Trobriand population, the discursive presence of the epidemic is immediately apparent. The islands are inundated with the paraphernalia of the national awareness campaign—caps, T-shirts, posters, stickers. The ubiquitous hallmark of the campaign—billboards and signs in the national colors of red, black, and yellow, bearing the message "Protect yourself from AIDS: Don't have sex, be faithful, or always use a condom"—appears at the entrance of the government office in Losuia, the district headquarters on Kiriwina. Talk about HIV and AIDS has gained prominence through various structured awareness activities as well as the informal exchange of information. As Trobrianders contemplate the presence of HIV in their midst, fear about the unseen and unknown qualities of the elusive virus is commonly expressed: "When we got the awareness, we are all afraid of AIDS, so we are asking, do you have any ideas to help us see this thing, to help us with our feeling about AIDS, to help us understand about AIDS so we won't be afraid?" (Trobriand woman in her mid-fifties, 19 September 2003).

This supplicatory question, directed to me during a group discussion, is an example of how perfunctory "awareness" about HIV typically invokes fear of AIDS without supporting conceptual connections between viral transmission and the manifestation of illness. Importantly, it underscores the need for sustained communication, once initial information is imparted, to enable the ongoing synthesis of different forms of knowledge. The woman's question also reveals how the transformative response to new information is embodied and internalized, a provocative reminder of the significance of emotional understandings in the production of knowledge. Moreover, the question confronted me with the ethics of ethnographic engagement and the obligation to answer questions and not simply ask them.

The woman's question arose when we were talking about *sovasova*, the illness caused by breach of the Trobriand incest taboo, when members of the same matrilineal clan have sexual relations (Lepani 2007). The discussants were explaining to me how clear signs and symptoms—weight loss, nausea, and malaise—herald the onset of illness and how affected people use herbal and magical treatments to successfully manage *sovasova*. They were also reflecting on the sexual practice that causes *sovasova* and how people can avoid the illness altogether by simply not having sex with a fellow clan member. Nonetheless, the cultural resources available for treatment allow a breach of the taboo to be a safe possibility, albeit socially undesirable. Our ensuing discussion teased out broad comparisons between *sovasova* and HIV, demonstrating how cultural models of disease etiology provide interpretative frames for making sense of new phenomena (see Farmer 1990). Then the discussion came up against an unresolved tension regarding treatment, and that was when the woman interposed her question. In the Trobriands, received information about HIV and AIDS has typically carried the misleading message "No treatment, no cure," which instills fear of the "killer disease" with the tacit intention of promoting prevention through behavior change. The message is antithetical to Trobriand models of medicine and also contradicts popular notions of biomedicine, which is commonly perceived to have a diagnostic regimen of drug treatment for every known disease.

How did I answer the request for help in seeing the ominous yet invisible virus so that fear might be transformed through insight? My immediate response was a hesitant pause. Overwhelmed by the ethical quandary, which confronted me many times during my research, I began rehearsing in my mind a battery of my own unanswered questions. How can HIV awareness complement cultural constructions of illness to better enable prevention? How can awareness shift from a preoccupation with AIDS symptoms—uncannily similar to Trobriand constructions of *sovasova* as well as the familiar infectious diseases tuberculosis, pneumonia, and malaria—and focus on sexual practice and HIV prevention? And most pressing, how do I ethically explain that in fact there *are* treatments for HIV-infected people, but antiretroviral drug therapies are not readily accessible in PNG, where the national health system struggles to provide the rudiments of primary health care? Such an admission brings into sharp relief the inequities of access to knowledge as well as resources. The admission also feeds another kind of fear, the anxiety of knowing that resources are not yet in place to deal with an impending epidemic, as was candidly expressed to me by the district health workers. The global disparities in resource distribution that impede local capacities to effectively respond to HIV intensify the ambiguities and contradictions that pervade HIV communication (see Farmer 1999). Once again I found myself trying to balance information about HIV with contextual reality by responding with what might have seemed circuitous logic. Reflection on sexual practice makes the virus visible and helps deflect fear. Once the virus is conceptually visible, then possibilities for prevention become viable. Our discussion was recharged with more talk about *sovasova*, notions of risk, sexual liaisons, infidelities, and ambivalent feelings about condom use.

The puzzle of HIV visibility requires reflection on susceptibility to inform preventive action. Community-based HIV awareness activities in the Trobriands typically rehearse the standard epidemiological check-list of sexual risk behaviors: early onset of sexual activity, multiple and concurrent sexual partners, high prevalence of sexually transmitted infections (STIs), and low levels of condom use. Less often do such exercises move out from the model of risk behavior to consider the "biological synergism" between HIV and other pathogens and social conditions (Singer and Clair 2003: 428; see also Singer, this volume), including immunity compromised by endemic malaria, high rates of pneumonia and other respiratory infections, increased cases of tuber-culosis across all ages, and limited infrastructure and resources for the provision of comprehensive health services. These factors are com-pounded by increased mobility between the Trobriands and urban centers, intensified commercial trade networks through maritime travel, limited income earning opportunities in the local economy, and greater population pressure on a finite resource base. Yet many Trobrianders more readily identify aspects of "custom" that might facilitate viral transmission: the sexual freedom of young unmarried men and women; the period of abstinence during pregnancy and lactation, when women acknowledge that their husbands are likely to have other sexual partners; the mobility of exchange relations, including the traditional Kula trade ring, which hold opportunities for expanding sexual networks; and Milamala, the annual season of yam harvest festivities, when ancestral spirits return to the world of the living and sexuality is celebrated.

Indeed, Milamala has come to epitomize the risk of cultural practice for HIV in the Trobriands. In recent years, harvest festivities have assumed a commercial dimension in order to attract tourists. Organized by local businesses, the district government, and host villages, the annual Milamala Festival receives funding from provincial tourism grants. During the festival period, the subject of HIV enters more frequently into conversations as people speculate on the heightened levels of sexual activity, especially during *karibom*, an all-night dance promenade.

Likewise, the effusive *tapiokwa* dance, performed in costumed splendor as harvested yams are ceremoniously carried from the gardens to yam storage houses in the villages, is emblematic of perceived cultural risk. With thrusting pelvises and the ribald chanting of the word *mweki* (literally, "to visit"), a poetic synonym for *kayta*, or sexual intercourse, *tapiokwa* is regarded as the signature dance of the Trobriands, performed for tourists and visitors to the islands and imitated by other Papua New Guineans at cultural festivals and community events throughout the country. Repeated calls in PNG to regulate or ban cultural practices perceived as promoting sexual promiscuity and contributing to HIV risk include a call from a member of parliament to blacklist *tapiokwa* (*Post Courier*, 7 August 2006).

The emphasis in HIV discourse on sexual promiscuity easily overlays perduring representations of Trobriand sexuality as exotic and excessive and the Trobriands as a place where "chastity is an unknown virtue," as the legendary anthropologist Bronislaw Malinowski claimed (1922: 53). Malinowski's classic ethnography of the Trobriands, *The Sexual Life of Savages*, titillated European imaginings when it was first published in 1929, and popular retellings soon located the Trobriands in an idealized place of primordial desire—the "Islands of Love." This eroticized geography continues to be inscribed today in journalistic accounts and tourism promotion (Senft 1998), influencing contemporary perceptions of Trobriand sexuality. When I asked Trobrianders what "Islands of Love" signified to them, the answer almost invariably was, "Trobriands is a sharing and caring place." Perhaps this is a rehearsed counter to the imposed reputation of sexual extravagance, or a rote platitude imbued in part by Christianity and biblical scriptures. Or perhaps it expresses the cultural ethos of reciprocity and *bobwailila*, which means love, gift, generosity, or contribution. In whatever ways Trobrianders interpret this representation, the label has now entered into the national discourse on HIV and is used to describe the perceived environment of risk in the Trobriands (Dekuku and Anang 2003; Elliot, Kitau, and Pantumari 2006).

While I was walking with a group of friends on the crowded main street in Losuia during the 2003 inaugural Milamala Festival, all of us admiring the hundreds of young people dressed for dancing in traditional finery, a middle-aged woman spontaneously remarked to me, "While we are promoting our culture, we are promoting the spread of the AIDS virus." This perceptive observation is not a mere indictment of so-called risky cultural practices in the "Islands of Love" but reflects a more complex understanding of the contextual factors that influence HIV transmission. During the conversation that followed this remark, the broader context of risk was described: increased mobility involving tourists, visiting government officials, and public servants; cross-generational partnering of young women with older men, whose longer sexual histories hold greater potential for exposure to HIV and other STIs; the sudden influx of cash, which encourages transactional sexual activity; and the failure of leaders and festival organizers to adequately address HIV prevention in the context of harvest festivities and to ensure the wide availability of condoms. Yet "culture," as the embodied expression of place identity, carries the burden of culpability for viral transmission.

Fidelity to Culture

> In the Trobs, "steady" is sticking to our community life style. Both boys and girls have multiple partners; we are steady with custom.
>
> —Clement Moseturi, health worker, 23 October 2003

In spite of the ready indictment of cultural practices for HIV transmission, the specter of AIDS as a deadly disease wrought by sexual excess and transgression is not easily accommodated by Trobriand models of sexuality and disease. Talking about HIV prevention through reflective evaluation is fraught with contradictions when practices defined by cultural values are held against a morally inflected discourse that frames sexuality in terms of risk, promiscuity, and the imperative for behavior change (see Boyce et al. 2007). Trobriand mediations of HIV invert prevention messages with irony, offering new interpretations that are cognizant of cultural vulnerability. Mediations reflect a struggle between fear and desire and the attempt to reconcile behaviors attributed to HIV risk with sexual practices that are life-affirming and valued for regenerating the social relations of exchange between people of different clans (Lepani 2008).

Sexuality as a pleasurable expression of Trobriand sociality is especially important for young people. The commencement of sexual activity signifies viable physical and social development, a prerequisite for growth into healthy, strong, adult women and men. Although there are rules and restrictions about whom one can have sex with and where encounters can take place, young Trobrianders enjoy considerable sexual freedom before marriage, based on a protocol of mutual respect and consent, rehearsing their future roles as married adults by forging alliances that will sustain the relations of social reproduction. *Kubukwabuya*, the collective term for unmarried male and female youths, also means "freedom," a reference to a life stage that embodies the autonomy to act on desire, to attract the desire of others, and to engage freely in sexual liaisons in the quest for a compatible marriage partner.

The sexual mobility enjoyed by Trobriand youths is signified by the gendered terms *ulatile* and *kapugula*, male and female, respectively, which refer to the collective activity of going out at night to look for sexual partners, ideally expanding the reach of desire beyond the familiarity of one's village peer group. Nothing quite exceeds the heightened sense of expectation and intrigue that embellishes young people's nocturnal mobility. Their night-time activity offers protection from the potential harm of *yoyowa*, or malevolent witches, who also claim the hours of darkness for their pursuits, as well as disoriented and restless *kosi*, the ghosts of the recently deceased. The life-affirming enterprise of *kubukwabuya* is the antithesis of disease and an antidote to the destruction and death embodied by supernatural beings.

Kubukwabuya sexual networks are intricately woven into the Trobriand social landscape, the village being the central axis. Young people normally commence their sexual activity in early puberty within the familiar social boundaries of their village *tubwa*, or age cohort. Sexual networks then radiate outward on the basis of traditional affiliations between villages as well as friendships established by preceding age groups. In one group discussion, an older woman explained, "Young ones go out at night to other villages. Because they are young, boys and girls are free to make their own choice, where they go out and how they attract each other and mix themselves up in a group. That's their freedom. Different girls from different villages, different boys from different villages" (4 November 2003). In another discussion, an older man explained, "It's how villages go together and have an understanding. We have to be careful in making arrangements to show our respect, otherwise it's like stealing." A young boy added, "Our thinking is this, if there is space in there for us, we can have it. If the space is covered up, no vacancies, then we will look elsewhere" (10 October 2003).

That Trobrianders conceptualize their sexual networks spatially rather than numerically is indicated by informal accounts from local volunteers who worked as interviewers for a behavioral surveillance survey conducted by the PNG Institute of Medical Research in 2002. The volunteers observed that respondents tended to answer the standard question about how many sexual partners they had had in the past week by recalling the names of villages where their partners were from and the locations where encounters took place. Numbers were associated with the equal pairing of *tubwa* group members rather than with individual tallies of partners. Such conceptualizations reveal how sexual agency and embodied practice are affectively influenced by associations of place identity, relationality, and collectivity, in sharp contrast to the perspectives of behavioral surveillance models, which view the individual as an autonomous and bounded unit (Gordon 1988) and sexual acts as an independent, quantifiable variable disembodied from cultural meanings and the realities of lived experience (Clatts 1995).

The Trobriand word *bidubadu*, or "plenty," is commonly used to describe the level of sexual activity among young people, evoking the plenitude of *kubukwabuya* freedom and mobility. *Bidubadu* indicates how young people's search for the "right partner" typically entails an extended period of multiple and concurrent partnering before the transition to adulthood and marriage. Importantly, the notion does not imply promiscuity or indiscriminate excess. Young people represent their sexual freedom as a process of decision making that involves careful discernment and studied selection, not careless abandon. Sexual agency is also influenced by *kwaiwaga*, or love magic, a cultural construct so potent that it ultimately defines the embodied experience of sexual desire, seduction, and consummation and the acquiescence of autonomy to fidelity. Both males and females use *kwaiwaga* to demonstrate their power to seduce and attract potential partners and to cause "love" to overcome the chosen partner, thus making visible their own agency in another person's embodied desires. The use of *kwaiwaga* is the primary means to secure fidelity and pave the way for the bond of marriage. In this way, the efficacy of *kwaiwaga* shifts the pleasures of intimate sociality from the domain of mutual desire into full public view, where sexual alliances serve the larger social networks within which they operate (Weiner 1988: 71).

As a medium for exercising control over the agency of others, *kwaiwaga* bolsters confidence in sexual pursuits while diminishing the uncertainty of outcome. The notion of "risk" in linking multiple sexual partnering to disease exposure has little salience in this cultural configuration. Neither does the breach of *sovasova*, which is conceptualized as a sexually transmitted disease, correspond to taking a chance with an unknown outcome (Lepani 2007). The Trobriand concepts that most closely approximate "risk" are *katuigaki*, meaning a flippant disregard of warning, and *besobeso* (literally, "this way and that way"), meaning a random carelessness or displaced action contrary to social conventions. Although both words are used to describe sexual practice that does not conform to the protocol of mutual desire and collective endeavor, the consequence of such action is not associated with disease.

Although being "steady with custom" is associated with HIV vulnerability, perceptions of HIV risk are also expressed in terms of external difference associated with intrusions from beyond familiar boundaries. The following statement by a middle-aged Trobriand man involved in HIV awareness activities reveals how notions of cultural identity and attachment to place provide a sense of resilience and immunity to novel pathogens:

> Whenever we mention about wearing condoms, or sticking to one sexual partner, or not having sex, then everybody starts laughing. Because, you know, they tell us, this AIDS you are talking about, we know nothing about it, it doesn't come here. This AIDS is only for *dimdims* [white foreigners]. We natives, we don't have this AIDS business. We only know that we stay around in our village and if *bwagau* [sorcery] comes then we die. We would never know if somebody dies because of AIDS. You see? The idea is that AIDS is just a foreign word … a *dimdim* sickness only. (10 October 2003)

The tension between cultural risk and cultural resiliency reflects the deeper history of encounters with introduced diseases able to penetrate place identity, the imagined boundaries of protection, and the ensuing interactions between different models of disease etiology.

Surveillance and the Cartography of Risk

> Can you imagine the "Islands of Love" with no people on them? That's what it will be like, ten, twenty years' time from now.
>
> —Ethel Jacob, community leader, 23 September 2003

The arrival of HIV in the island landscape is but the latest wave of exogenous pathogens and models of disease to interact with Trobriand ways of knowing and being. Indeed, when first coined during the early colonial period, the expression "Islands of Love" represented an illusory contrast to the realities of introduced sexually transmitted diseases. The Trobriand word *pokesa*, derived from the English word "pox" to signify syphilis, genital ulcers, and, more generally, any ulcerous sore on the body, is testament to the new diseases associated with the arrival of *dimdim* foreigners in the late nineteenth and early twentieth centuries and the medical interventions that followed. Concern about the demise of the population, which numbered approximately 10,000 people in 1905, prompted colonial officials to embark on a mission to eradicate the "baneful diseases" of syphilis and gonorrhea (Black 1957: 233–234). Although cognizant of the foreign origin of the new diseases, colonial officials and Christian missionaries sought to reverse their devastating effects on fertility and mortality by regulating and reforming what they perceived as undisciplined and immoral native bodies (Reed 1997). Women in particular were viewed as unbridled, licentious, and irresponsible from an early age, requiring moral supervision to promote monogamy "as the sexual norm, the only legitimate avenue for satiating desires, preventing venereal disease, and raising the birth rate" (Reed 1997: 71).

The medical interventions were dogmatic and confrontational, engendering dread rather than confidence in the new system of diagnostic and treatment procedures based on Western models of disease etiology (Hughes 1997). Upon taking up his appointment in 1905 as general medical officer and assistant resident magistrate in the Trobriands, Raynor Bellamy was in charge of the newly built "lock" hospital, so called because of the colonial government's legal power to confine infected patients. According to Bellamy, Trobrianders had no prior knowledge of how STIs spread, and his patients were "incredulous" when he instructed them on the mode of transmission (Black 1957: 234). In 1906 Bellamy estimated that about 10 percent of the population, including children, showed symptoms of STIs, and in 1908 he commenced a program of systematic examination and treatment of every man, woman, and child (Black 1957: 234). Reports suggest that Bellamy quickly gained the confidence of Trobrianders "beyond his most sanguine expectations" and that people began to come voluntarily for treatment (Black 1957: 234). Bellamy's regimented approach, which involved punishment of absconders, is credited with reducing the incidence of infection from 5.22 percent in 1908 to 1.37 percent in 1915 (Black 1957: 234). Reporting on vital statistics for the years 1919 to 1926, Bellamy confidently confirmed that STI cases were reduced to less than 1 percent and no longer affected birth and death rates, but that two "pandemic waves of influenza," in 1921 and 1925, were responsible for a population decline (Bellamy 1990: 299–300).

Medical interventions to control STIs in the Trobriands continued under successive colonial authorities. In 1939 a medical team arrived in the islands to conduct a further survey and reported no difficulty in gathering 5,400 people for examinations, a feat credited to the effectiveness of Bellamy's years of service. The team remarked that "the occasion was accepted as a gala event" (Black 1957: 236). My research questions prompted no personal or collective memories about such surveillance events, apart from the occasional humorous recounting of a scenario in which people ran into the bush when they heard that the medical patrol was coming to their village. By contrast, nowadays young children's squeals of delight greet the blaring siren of the health center ambulance, making its rounds on immunization patrols (the supply of petrol and vaccines permitting). In whatever ways previous generations collectively responded to colonial patrols that involved population-wide examinations in search of diseased genitals, the effects of these historical interactions have been absorbed into current understandings of disease etiology and approaches to treatment. Indeed, the interventionist approach to STIs in colonial PNG set the precedence for attitudes in the era of AIDS, particularly the sentiment frequently expressed throughout PNG that the only way to control the spread of HIV is to lock up those who are positive (Hughes 1997: 244).

Sitting in the STI testing laboratory at Losuia district health center in 2003, I searched for a residual presence of the colonial period but found only the predictable air of resignation that seems to hang over many rural health centers in PNG. The facility's chronic lack of maintenance and refurbishment betrayed the genealogy of clinical medical practice in the Trobriands, particularly the recent past of the 1960s and 1970s, when the center thrived as a surgical hospital under the directorship of a resident medical officer. People continue to refer to the center as the "hospital," as though it were still a bastion of colonial and missionary presence or a promise of development under the newly independent nation-state. But expectations have diminished along with standards of health service delivery, decentralized under state reforms in the mid-1990s, and the disintegrating infrastructure, plagued by constant disruptions to the supply of water and electricity because the pipes are broken or the generator has yet again run out of fuel. The disheveled state and scattered contents of the laboratory room accentuate the paucity of available supplies and equipment. The mold and dust on the walls and shelves suggest an acquiescence to neglect that says something about local capacity and function. But the general disarray goes far beyond localized laxity; it speaks strongly of indifference and marginalization not only from provincial and national levels but from the global centers of power that condemn out-of-the-way places to mediocrity, even failure.

In 2003, Clement Moseturi was officially the laboratory technician but had worked at the health center for many years in several capacities. In recent years he had looked after communicable diseases and was on the nursing roster in the wards, because of the number of tuberculosis patients and the chronic shortage of personnel. Clement was adept at drawing posters. One of his posters on the wall in the TB ward showed a bone-thin patient with an outstretched hand, ready to receive the daily dose of drug therapy. The handwritten text, in both English and Trobriands, described the elements of DOTS, the "directly observed therapy" short-course strategy for TB treatment. Another of his posters, taped to the wall of the outpatient clinic, depicted various situations in the Trobriands identified as susceptible to HIV transmission—"harvest festivities, when people gather for lovemaking, on the road, the place full of coconuts." On the day of my visit, Clement was working on a new poster about the risk of HIV transmission during Milamala. As he drew, I asked him to explain the STI record book and what it revealed about the situation in the Trobriands. He told me:

> We do STI testing—gonorrhea, syphilis… We don't do HIV testing; there's no facility due to power problems. There are a great number of people suffering with gonorrhea. We do contact tracing and bring patients in for review. We supply the patient with contact cards to give to their partners. However many they need, we give them, but it is not effective. We need to physically follow up, go out to the villages, talk to the people directly and not expect them to come to us. There is embarrassment and shame to come here with the card. In many cases, people say their contact was a "market spin," they met on the road, or the partner is from far away, so it is hard to follow up. No names are exchanged between the partners, maybe only place names, so the person can tell us only this village or that village. With our system it is impossible to determine patterns in STI prevalence. We have to assume that every village, every area has an STI problem. You'll see from the book that villages close to town and the guest lodge are the most commonly infected areas, especially on the female side. But maybe it's just that they come to the clinic for treatment because they are close by. Men from outer areas are more mobile than women, so infection is taken back to the villages that way. We cannot specify which group, which village is most infected unless we take a survey. We presume HIV is already here. One positive case has been seen. It is already spreading but it is not yet known. People don't see it yet. (23 October 2003)

Clement's acknowledgment of the ineffective approach and reach of available clinical services, and his mention of the need for a survey to map STI prevalence, can be understood in relation to both the seeming historical efficacy of medical patrols in controlling STIs before the age of antibiotics and the penchant for epidemiological surveillance in the age of AIDS. From a service delivery point of view, his descriptive assessment also reflects uneasy questions about the provision of HIV voluntary counseling and testing and their integration with existing sexual and reproductive health services. Clement's remark that HIV is already spreading but not yet known, because of its invisibility, underscores the importance of symptoms in Trobriand models of disease. Moreover, it accentuates the clinical difference between diagnosing STIs that manifest in recognizable and visible symptoms and testing for evidence of the invisible virus. Clement's observations invite further consideration of methodologies of counting and accounting for, and ways of imagining and responding to, the presence of disease in a population.

"A Mixture of Ideas": Pluralistic Understandings of Disease

A comparative analysis of *sovasova*, *pokesa*, and HIV reveals the interaction between different models of meaning in Trobriand articulations of disease causality, prevention, and treatment, and it raises important questions about the efficacy of medical pluralism for HIV prevention (Lepani 2007). Describing the diagnosis and treatment of *sovasova* and *pokesa*, the HEO at the health center told me in December 2003 that disease symptoms "can be treated with a mixture of ideas" combining traditional and modern medicine. His explanation is indicative of pluralistic understandings of illness and the way the complementary application of different prevention and treatment therapies assists in obtaining desired outcomes. Indeed, it can be argued that pluralism reflects a conceptual preference for models of reciprocity in understanding health and disease, a preference that emanates from the core Trobriand value of mutual difference in achieving collective well-being.

Complementary approaches to prevention and treatment are particularly salient when models of meaning incorporate the powerful explanatory constructs of witchcraft and sorcery. In Trobriand cosmology, supernatural agency holds an etiological link to all illness, misfortune, and death, whether perceived as the immediate or the underlying cause (Malinowski 1929: 137, 192; Weiner 1988: 39–41). Causes of illness and death are understood in moral terms wherein malicious acts of witchcraft and sorcery represent the ultimate threat to sustaining the relations of social reproduction. Protective magic is used to bolster resistance, and treatment regimes assume paramount importance in the struggle to restore social balance. Although symptoms are evidence of social disorder, the restoration of bodily and social well-being requires more than merely symptomatic treatment; it demands treatment for the underlying cause. Fundamental to healing is the need to name the source of the illness and make it visible through an evaluative process that employs magic, prayer, herbal medicines, and clinical treatments in various combinations to achieve remedial effect. The etiological explanation that physical suffering is rooted in social relationships shifts focus away from the sick person as independently responsible for the condition and promotes the mobilization of social resources to defuse the effects of illness and restore equilibrium, not only in the patient's body but in the collective body (Weiner 1976: 86; see also Scheper-Hughes and Lock 1987: 7, 15; Lindenbaum, this volume).

The dual cause and consequence of *sovasova* represents an anomaly in the Trobriand model of disease etiology. Although *sovasova* threatens moral order by undermining the relations of difference that ensure clan vitality and social reproduction, the cause of illness remains a question of internal agency and is not attributed to external forces, even if breach of the proscription makes one more vulnerable to supernatural exploits. By contrast, malevolent magic is perceived as the underlying cause of *pokesa*, despite the recognized link between sexual activity and ulcerous symptoms. Given the analogy Trobrianders draw between *sovasova* and AIDS, it is uncertain whether or not AIDS will be attributed to witchcraft as the experience of living with HIV becomes more pronounced.[2] Because *sovasova* stands outside the paradigm of witchcraft and sorcery, it offers a compelling conceptual approach for mediating HIV. Yet it also holds an unsettling bridge to the question of treatment, empowering confidence in the ability to manage and control the potential impact of AIDS (Lepani 2007).

The following statement by a traditional healer pinpoints the explanatory power of malevolent magic as the underlying cause of disease and links AIDS etiology to the ongoing moral struggle against witchcraft and sorcery (see Ashforth 2002: 129). The man's reference to Africa suggests a perceived correlation, in the context of the global geography of AIDS, between HIV prevalence and places where the fundamental theory of disease causation attributes disease to supernatural powers:

Every sickness should have a treatment and a cause. People want to know what causes sickness. For HIV, in our terms, our understanding, the belief from custom, from our parents, it will be seen to be caused by *bwagau*, not by sexual activity. For example, like malaria. We know the parasite comes from the anopheles mosquito, but how does the malaria get into the mosquito? Who put the malaria into the mosquito? We think that the spell of *bwagau* or *yoyowa* put the sickness in there. The mosquito is just the carrier. So there is always a reason underneath the sickness. For AIDS, the thinking will be the same. The natives of Africa, some of them have very strong *bwagau* there. AIDS does not just come out by itself, it is not automatic. It was put there in the first place by magic. (20 October 2003)

The dynamic interplay between colonial medicine, contemporary health services, and traditional regimes for defining and responding to disease creates the context in which HIV is spreading in the Trobriands and will undoubtedly influence people's evolving interpretations, their experiences of living with the virus, and the effectiveness of treatment and palliative care. Commenting on medical pluralism with particular reference to PNG, Lindenbaum (1991: 177) wrote that the successful provision of culturally appropriate health services "is achieved not by manicuring Western medical categories to fit local conceptions, but by broadly appreciating indigenous definitions of the desirable paths to take in order to achieve control of destiny in illness and health." Pluralistic and reciprocal approaches to HIV communication recognize the way interactions between divergent models of meaning shape new understandings. The facilitation of dialogical mediations between indigenous models of disease and representations of HIV is critical for producing knowledge that will enable prevention.

Rather than deploying militaristic metaphors about waging a battle against the impending doom of AIDS and conceptualizing sexuality and cultural practice in terms of risk—and HIV as a plague of promiscuity—a different tempo and tone of knowledge making are needed. Making sense of HIV involves personal and collective reflection on cultural meanings and lived experiences of sexuality and disease. When people obtain a confident understanding of the invisible virus in relation to cultural knowledge, the capacity to imagine and realize prevention, including the use of condoms for protection, becomes more viable. Ethnographic research has an important contribution to make in facilitating the interchange between bodies of knowledge and illuminating entry points for epidemiological interventions. In the Trobriands, as elsewhere, the path forward should not forge a divide between cultural practices and HIV prevention—between freedom and fear—but instead focus on how culture can be effectively engaged.

Notes

I extend my appreciation and respect to the many Trobrianders who made this research possible. I am especially indebted to my research collaborators, Diana Lepani Siyotama, Florence Mokolava, Ethel Jacob, and the late Asi Toyola, for their commitment to the project and their invaluable advice and support. I gratefully acknowledge scholarship support from the Gender Relations Centre, Australian National University, and a research grant from the PNG National AIDS Council. I thank the Wenner-Gren Foundation for the opportunity to participate in the plagues symposium and for the constructive comments and suggestions generously offered by the other participants.

1. Financial and technical support for expanding HIV testing and treatment services is provided through international donors including the Australian Agency for International Development, the Global Fund for AIDS, TB and Malaria, and the Clinton Foundation HIV/AIDS Initiative.

2. See Haley 2008 and Hammar 2007 for ethnographic examples from other places in PNG where deaths attributed to AIDS are believed ultimately to be the result of witchcraft and sorcery. See Ashforth 2002 for the way the witchcraft paradigm of disease complicates the social and political context of HIV in South Africa.

eighteen

Explaining Kuru

Three Ways to Think about an Epidemic

Shirley Lindenbaum

In this essay I explore the ways in which three sets of actors explained kuru, the devastating disease that once threatened the survival of the Fore, a population in the eastern highlands of Papua New Guinea. Since 1957, when Vincent Zigas and Carleton Gajdusek first encountered the disease, medical investigators, anthropologists, and the Fore have all contributed their ideas about the cause of the epidemic, presenting explanatory frameworks that reflect their cultural and historical assumptions about disease causation, their different relationships with the object of study, and their relationships with one another. I focus my discussion mainly on the years 1961 to 1999, the period for which I have field data.

I also explore a second theme, one that engaged participants at the Tucson conference: the different meanings associated with the words *epidemic* and *plague*. A general sense emerged that *epidemic* is associated with counting, imposing order on events, and introducing the authority of numbers. *Plague*, it seems, does a different kind of social work, suggesting suffering and carrying with it a moral load.

Medical accounts, in general, portrayed kuru as an epidemic, describing the epidemiological, clinical, and pathological dimensions of the disease. Anthropologists had a foot in both camps, adopting the language of medicine but conveying also Fore beliefs and experiences. Without using the terms *epidemic* and *plague*, the Fore, too, spoke of kuru as both a demographic and a social disaster. The topic of cannibalism, the key to the transmission of the infectious agent, was addressed in different ways by the three sets of actors.

The Medical Assessment of Kuru

The first published reports of kuru (Gajdusek and Zigas 1957; Zigas and Gajdusek 1959) provided a clinical description of the disease and its patterns of occurrence. Kuru was described as an almost invariably fatal, acute, progressive, degenerative disease of the central nervous system, said to be restricted to members of the Fore cultural and linguistic group and their immediate tribal neighbors, with whom they intermarried. The victims were predominantly women and adolescents of both sexes. Adult men were rarely victims, and no cases had been found in children under four or five years of age. One percent of the Fore population was thought to be affected. Cases removed from the Fore environment did not recover. A framework for future clinical and epidemiological research was thus quickly established.

By 2005, continued surveillance of the population by the Institute of Medical Research in Papua New Guinea allowed its director, Michael Alpers (2005), to report a waning epidemic during the period 1987–1995, although the clinical features and duration of the disease were unchanged, averaging about twelve months from onset to death. With the cessation of cannibalism by 1960, the transmission of kuru had stopped, and by 1995 the incubation period had reached at least thirty-five years. With no kuru death in 2005 and only one in 2007, the epidemic appears to be coming to an end.

Summarizing etiological hypotheses a few years after his 1959 report, Gajdusek suggested that "infectious, toxic, deficiency, or hypersensitivity factors may operate with genetic dependence" (Gajdusek 1963: 164). Nonetheless, he observed, "we are investing our maximum effort ... in an attempt to discover a virus aetiology" (p. 159). As Warwick Anderson (this volume) notes, the mantle of ethnographer and geographer that Gajdusek adopted on first encountering the disease had already shifted to that of microbe hunter. For the remainder of the 1960s and during the early 1970s he continued to provide an abundance of medical hypotheses: infectious etiology, possible plant toxins, metallic poisoning (Reid and Gajdusek 1969; Sorenson and Gajdusek 1969), and a return to an earlier supposition that the genetic constitution of the kuru-affected populations could not be dismissed (Plato and Gajdusek 1972). Cannibalism was discounted or given low priority, perhaps because Gajdusek's 1957 data on Fore cannibalism were inaccurate (Lindenbaum 1982) or because he thought the idea was too exotic (Anderson 2008: 169; Glasse and Lindenbaum 1992; Rhodes 1997: 103).

In 1976, when Gajdusek was awarded the Nobel Prize in medicine, his acceptance speech drew attention to his contribution to "recognition of a new group of viruses possessing unconventional physical and chemical properties and biological behavior far different from those of any other group of microorganisms" (Gajdusek 1977: 943). While he spoke in detail about this "exciting frontier in microbiology," he briefly addressed the topic of cannibalism. Citing two papers he had published in 1973 and 1977, and overlooking earlier anthropological reports and publications, especially two papers concerning the role of cannibalism in the transmission of kuru (Alpers 1968; Mathews, Glasse, and Lindenbaum 1968), Gajdusek offered the fanciful suggestion that the sole route of transmission of the virus was the Fore's rubbing themselves with body substances from the deceased during mortuary ceremonies, a practice the Fore deny (Alpers 2005), or their obtaining it through cuts and scratches acquired during dissection of the corpse.

In his important history of kuru research, Warwick Anderson (2008) addressed the complexity of Gajdusek's reluctance to adopt the cannibalism hypothesis. He also considers the question in his chapter in this volume, drawing on Charles Rosenberg's notion of two styles of reasoning historically employed to account for epidemic disease: configuration and contamination. Before physicians had any knowledge of specific infectious agents, medical explanations are said to have favored configuration, which is "holistic and emphasizes system, interconnection, and balance, while the contamination theme foregrounds a particular disordering element. The configurational style of explanation is interactive, contextual, and often environmental; the emphasis on contamination, reductionist and monocausal" (Rosenberg 1992a: 295). Anderson suggests that in his quest for the microbe, Gajdusek moved away from the more encompassing perspectives of anthropology and social epidemiology toward a laboratory-oriented, contamination style of thought.

Anderson's analysis illuminates the nature of the contrast between medical and anthropological modes of enquiry, a distinction addressed by Bakhtin in his discussion of what he called the "exact" and the human sciences (Bakhtin 1986: 159–172). The exact sciences are monologic because they are concerned with objects of knowledge; the human sciences are necessarily dialogic, because they are concerned with other subjects (Dentith 1995: 20). "Monologue is finalized and deaf to the other's response, does not expect it and does not acknowledge in it any decisive force... It closes down the represented world and represented persons" (Bakhtin 1984: 293). Gajdusek's private concern for the human dimensions of the epidemic remained constant, but his pursuit of the elusive infectious agent led him to follow a scientific path that "to some degree materializes all reality"(Bakhtin 1984: 293). As Anderson's historical account suggests, Gajdusek's collection of brains and body fluids became progressively detached from its social origins as the specimens traveled from his bush laboratory to distant research institutes. Body parts, which the Fore considered to be part of the person, were turning into objects of knowledge.

Anthropology and a Foot in Both Camps

Robert Glasse and I began our anthropological study of the disease in 1961 with a grant from the University of Adelaide provided by John Bennett, one of the first to propose a genetic hypothesis for kuru (Bennett, Rhodes, and Robson 1959). Bennett had asked that we study kinship, hoping this would provide data to confirm the theory. We learned Fore kin terms, drew genealogical charts, observed kinship in action, and began to understand something of Fore domestic and political relations (S. Glasse 1964; Glasse and Lindenbaum 1969, 1976, 1980; Lindenbaum 1971). Bennett had requested that we document Fore "pedigrees," a clue to the problem that lay ahead. It soon became apparent that many of the kuru victims were not closely related biologically but were kin in a nonbiological sense.

Data we gathered in 1962 from the Fore indicated that kuru had spread slowly through Fore villages within living memory, and its progress through Fore territory followed a specific, traceable route (Glasse 1962a, 1962b). This finding was again at odds with a purely genetic model, which implied that kuru must have been of remote evolutionary origin and ought to have been in epidemiological equilibrium. As John Mathews (1971: 99) observed later, kuru was too common and too fatal to be a purely genetic disorder unless the hypothetical kuru gene was maintained at high frequency by a mechanism of balanced polymorphism, for which there was no evidence. Our genealogies, which also recorded causes of death, confirmed Fore assertions that the disease was not of great historical depth. Kuru deaths clustered in the generations of young people and their parents and were extremely rare in the next ascending generation. Moreover, the Fore could name for us and for later investigators those who had died of kuru and those who had participated in the consumption of the deceased person. This made it possible to construct a coherent account of the appearance of the disease some four to twenty years after the ingestion of cooked human tissues containing the transmissible agent (Mathews, Glasse, and Lindenbaum 1968).

Genetics had provided an entry for a dialogue with medical science, but we soon measured our ethnographic findings alongside epidemiological data. Taking a historical approach toward cultural beliefs and practices, we gathered detailed information about cannibalism in 1961 and 1962 and continued to do so in 1963, as described in a report to John Gunther, the director of public health for Papua New Guinea and the source of our grant money for the second year of research (Glasse and Glasse 1963). We drew attention to the extensive data we had concerning the possibility of an association between the consumption of the dead and the spread of kuru. Our thoughts about the relationship between kuru and cannibalism derived from data concerning Fore rules for the consumption of human flesh, which seemed to fit the epidemiological evidence available to us at that time.

By the 1960s, cannibalism had been suppressed under pressure from the government and missions, but the Fore spoke openly about recent mortuary practices. All body parts were eaten except the gall bladder, which was considered too bitter, and not all bodies were eaten. The Fore did not eat those who had died of dysentery, leprosy, and sometimes yaws, but kuru victims were viewed favorably. Most significantly, not all Fore were cannibals. Cannibalism occurred more frequently among adult men in the North Fore than in the South Fore, where men rarely ate human flesh, and those who did said they avoided eating the bodies of women. Small children residing in houses with their mothers ate what their mothers gave them. Initiated youths moved to the men's house at about age ten, leaving behind the world of immaturity, femininity, and cannibalism. Consumption of human flesh was thus limited largely to adult women, children of both sexes, and a few adult men, matching the epidemiology of kuru in the early 1960s. In addition, cannibalism was reported to be customary in the north until the late 1940s. By the 1950s, when the anthropologists Ronald and Catherine Berndt undertook fieldwork in the north, they reported that cannibalism had ceased in the northern region but was still practiced surreptitiously in the south (Berndt 1962: 269–290), something the South Fore later confirmed. This again matched the epidemiological findings in the 1960s, providing a compelling set of associations. In the South Fore, the area with the highest incidence of kuru, cannibalism had continued longer than it had in the north.

Although we had no satisfactory model for explaining how the disease might be transmitted, we often spoke about kuru and cannibalism to those who visited us in the field. Our findings received little, often skeptical attention from the scientific community (see Glasse and Lindenbaum

1992) until the anthropological and medical stories came together in 1966, when chimpanzees injected with brain material from victims of the disease exhibited a clinical syndrome akin to kuru (Gajdusek, Gibbs, and Alpers 1966). This gave credence to the cannibalism hypothesis, and following reports that both kuru and Creutzfeld-Jakob disease (CJD) were transmissible, Alpers and Rail (1971) suggested that kuru, like CJD, had begun as a single sporadic mutation and that kuru had spread throughout the population as the result of cannibalism. In the following years, as the consumption of the dead was abandoned, kuru disappeared among children, and the age of those afflicted with the disease also rose. Evaluating epidemiological and ethnographic data, anthropology had provided a compelling set of associations, accepted by the "exact sciences," albeit only after laboratory experimentation settled on the notion of an infectious agent. This allowed medical investigators to talk authoritatively about the disease in terms of causation.

Fore Explanations for Kuru

The Fore, too, had been on a quest to establish the cause of kuru and interrupt the toll of sickness and death.[1] When the Fore first encountered kuru in the 1930s, they called it *negi nagi*, a term meaning "foolish person," because the afflicted women seemed to laugh immoderately and had loose control of their limbs. When it was apparent that the victims were dying, the Fore concluded that sorcerers were at work, a sociomedical diagnosis that sent them on a different course of therapeutic and preventive activities.

In the 1960s, at the height of the epidemic in the south, the South Fore responded first by taking ambulant victims of the disease on curing pilgrimages, the most spectacular of which took place at Uvai, among the neighboring Gimi people, west of the Yani River. Between April and August 1961 more than seventy patients walked for two days to reach a self-proclaimed Gimi curer whose treatment consisted of indigenous therapies—bloodletting, the ingestion of medicinal leaves and barks, and the identification of the location where the guilty sorcerer could be found. The curer had often visited the distant government station at Okapa, and the large structures he built at Uvai to house the patients and their relatives resembled the colonial hospital. He also recruited assistants to help provide therapy, in imitation of the "doctor boys" used by the colonial administration to provide health care in the Okapa hospital.

Fore curers closer to home named the person they considered responsible for a victim's illness. Sometimes the sick women revealed the identity of their aggressor, saying it came to them in a dream. Once detected, the sorcerer might be persuaded to remove the sorcery bundle, a parcel of bark, leaves, and a "power-imbued" stone, which, with a fragment associated with the victim (hair clippings, food scraps, excrement, a piece of clothing), he had buried in muddy ground. As the bundle rotted, the victim's health was said to deteriorate. Groups of men carrying bows and arrows met for sorcery discussions, hoping to deflect further aggression, and waterholes were guarded throughout the night. To prevent the theft of food scraps to be used for sorcery, paths were rerouted to ensure that travelers bypassed certain hamlets where the incidence of the disease was known to be high. Divination tests to reveal the sorcerers' identities gave rise to new tensions as accusations showed that men living in close proximity harbored mutual suspicions. By the year's end, the women who had returned from the Gimi pilgrimage were beginning to die. To the often-expressed fear of extinction through the loss of women's reproductive power was now added a fear of internal disruption so great that the Fore said social life was in danger.

Between 1957 and 1977 some twenty-five hundred people in a population of fourteen thousand died from kuru, most of them women in their reproductive years, and most of them in the south. The South Fore population declined until 1961 (Mathews 1971: 2). Concerned about the shortage of wives, the Fore understood that their survival was threatened. This was the setting in which the South Fore began to hold public meetings to denounce acts of sorcery, speak about past animosities, and reveal the concealed thoughts that they said gave rise to acts of aggression. In one community after another, from the beginning of November 1962 to the middle of March 1963, hostile groups gathered to discuss the emergency (Lindenbaum 1979: 79–99), replicating meetings they knew had been held by the North Fore in 1957. The South Fore were aware that the disease had once been more severe in the north, and they attributed its decline there to the meetings in which the North Fore had denounced sorcerers and burned sorcery paraphernalia.

The Meetings of 1957 and 1962 in North and South

In 1957 and 1962 the Fore were testing in public their own bases of knowledge, but they also had other audiences in mind. By the early

1950s the North Fore had begun to experience the intrusive presence of outsiders and to become acquainted with other ways of behaving and viewing the world. In 1954 the colonial administration established a patrol post at Okapa. The first government-appointed village leaders (Luluais and Tultuls) were selected in 1955, and work started on the Okapa-to-Kainantu road. In 1956 the first plane landed at the Tarabo airstrip in neighboring Keiagana territory. A government primary school at Okapa enrolled its first students in 1957, and in the same year, a number of investigators arrived to study kuru. Lucy Hamilton Reid began to examine Fore diet, documenting and weighing the food eaten by individuals in sample North Fore households (Reid and Gajdusek 1969). The medical team built a hospital to provide local health care, and Gajdusek began his intensive studies of the disease. The Fore were rapidly becoming exposed to new sources of knowledge and enveloped in a new set of social relations.

In 1950 the Lutheran church established a mission base nearby at Tarabo (Mathews 1971: 58), and native evangelists soon began to fan out among the Fore, issuing directives enjoining them to change their ways. With little supervision, and with the support of native police, the evangelists proposed changing behaviors said to be uncongenial to Christianity—not necessarily the same behaviors singled out by the European missionaries of their parental church. Haircutting and wearing cotton clothing were encouraged, but the use of pig fat to oil hair and anoint newborn babies was discouraged or prohibited, as were the seclusion of women during menstruation, separate eating and sleeping quarters for women and men, and the performance of sacred rituals and ceremonies. Sorcery, cannibalism, and garden burial were also prohibited. Responding to this dizzying array of proclamations and new experiences, and demoralized by the severity of kuru mortality, which by 1957 had reached epidemic proportions, the North Fore held the antisorcery meetings that in retrospect seemed so effective. Belief in the efficacy of sorcery was enhanced by the North Fore's interactions with native police, who also believed in the power of sorcerers, as well as with missionaries, whose condemnation of the practice had the same effect (Berndt 1962: 382–329).

By the 1960s a similar conjunction of forces had occurred in the South Fore. In 1957 John James, an American missionary, commenced his activities at Purosa, under the auspices of the World Missions, Incorporated. He was joined in 1961 and 1962 by two women missionaries in two nearby settlements. The presence of outsiders with new objects and other ideas about the world appears to have greatly impressed the

South Fore. One year after James's arrival, the patrol officer, Jack Baker, reported talk of cargo cult activity at Purosa, centered largely on Fore expectations of what would follow baptism. A similar reaction occurred when James extended his activities to the South Fore settlements at Aga-Yagusa (Mathews 1971: 57).

With the South Fore population in decline, Fore orators called on their audiences to replicate the earlier success in the north. A notable aspect of the South Fore meetings was the degree to which the colonial presence had an effect on thought and behavior. The recently appointed Luluais and Tultuls called on their local constituents and others in the region to attend the meetings they sponsored. These leaders were the main speakers at most events. Conditioned by a sense of government oversight, they talked about the responsibility that had been thrust upon them when they received their brass badges of office. At one meeting the Kamila Luluai announced:

> We brassmen accept the authority of whitemen, but the kanakas [ordinary natives] don't have good thoughts.[2] They are killing our women.[3] We Luluais and Tultuls like you whitemen. We tell people that in the past we didn't have brass, and now we must follow the orders of the kiap [the colonial government officer], yet the kanakas continue to kill our women. My wife just died of kuru. She was a good woman, like a man, as tall as me, and I am filled with sorrow. When will the kanakas adopt good ways? We brassmen can talk to the kiap and then all the men can be taken off to a "place nothing," leaving the women and children behind. I can talk to the kiap tomorrow and ask him to send us away to this remote place where we can suffer and give up these old ways. Then we can return and see if kuru has finished or not.

Robert Glasse and I were present at most of these meetings. Our Fore research assistants provided simultaneous translation into Melanesian Pidgin and provided reports of meetings we were unable to attend. As in 1957, when the Fore spoke in public they now had several audiences in mind—fellow residents, the colonial administration, and ourselves. The Fore had at times considered us to be a favorable conduit to the *kiap*.

The threat of banishment proposed by the Luluai derived its force from the regime's access to an armed police force and its ability to jail those who disobeyed the new laws. Government patrols, though infrequent, caused a ripple of anxiety as the official parties camped for several days in selected communities, where they carried out a census, identified people with leprosy to send for treatment at a distant government hospital, and adjudicated disputes that local groups had been unable to resolve.

A key theme of the South Fore meetings concerned things hidden and things revealed. Sorcery, like warfare, was considered a form of assault, but one carried out in secret. *Kio'ena*, the Fore word for sorcery, means "the hidden thing," and much of the oratory gained its sense of truth from public confession. Men of the senior generation spoke of their attempts to "work kuru." At Ivaki, they said they had talked and talked until their bellies pained. They now called on men to raise their right, poison-working hands as a sign that they would not be used again for kuru. They asked men from Umasa, Oulesa, and Oriesa, places where they knew the incidence of kuru was high, to do the same. Luluais and Tultuls could observe these raised hands, and if women still came down with kuru, they could talk about it again. They agreed with a speaker who said that during initiation their fathers had warned them not to tell others when one of their own kin group had made a kuru bundle. This was what they were doing now—keeping their knowledge hidden. One speaker suggested that if the men were photographed, the film would reveal sorcerers holding the kuru bundle in their right hands. (Gajdusek had passed through the area taking photographs in 1957, and we also had a camera in 1961.) By 1970, following greater interaction with kuru investigators, the ophthalmoscope was thought to be more powerful than divination for revealing sociomedical evidence.

Some Fore present at the meetings in the 1960s drew on a rhetoric of shame to persuade men to change their ways. The Purosa Luluai, a greatly respected wartime leader, described the humiliation felt by an older generation tarred by accusations of sorcery and the sense that his generation was no longer respected as a source of authoritative knowledge: "You young men think kuru is an old thing, but you are wrong. It is new. Our children laugh at us and mockingly call us old men. They admire the government, and they like to have good clothes and buy things from stores. Our children call us 'kuru men,' and we are ashamed. We must stop making kuru now!"

Women attending the meetings were a solemn audience. When they participated, they also spoke of shame in ways that appealed to men's sense of morality and appeared to embarrass them. Aware of the demographic dimensions of the epidemic, the Fore drew on the emotive language of plagues. The Tultul from the neighboring Awa people said, "We men living on the other side of the Lamari River are good people. You Fore are no good... Why don't you stop making kuru? Will you finish off all your women before you do? Where do you think you will then find wives? This fashion you are following is no good. We Awa visit your meetings and hear you say you will stop making kuru, but new cases are still arising. We are fed up with you."

Sickness or Sorcery?

The Fore had confronted a multitude of new objects and technologies and a new regime of power and knowledge that had different conceptions of how to live in the world, the most challenging aspect of which now concerned how to explain kuru. The central issue being debated in the 1960s concerned whether kuru was a form of "sickness" or a result of sorcery. Knowledge that the *kiap* and kuru investigators considered kuru to be "sickness" provided the counterpoint for all the discussions about disease causation. The Fore had experienced epidemics in the recent past, the illnesses referred to as *ai'yena* ("sickness"), not *kio'ena* (sorcery). Old people could recall two measles epidemics: "one when I was initiated, which was severe," said one elderly man, "and one more recently when the road to Purosa was built, which affected only a few people."[4] Mumps and dysentery, also called "sickness," had arrived "when the planes flew overhead"—a reference to 1943, during the Second World War—and the illnesses "came down the road from the north, from the government station at Moke."

The Fore were not distinguishing between sickness and sorcery on the basis of an understanding of germ theory and biological concepts of disease causation. Ailments identified as sickness were said to come down the road like winds, were often curable by Western medicine, and did not elicit moral talk, because they were not considered to result from human aggression. Sicknesses, then, were what we might call epidemics. Sorcery-caused conditions, on the other hand, were usually fatal and resulted from the malicious activities of humans using secretly guarded technologies. They came closer to our definition of plagues.

When the Fore discussed kuru, however, they used the Pidgin terms *sik kuru* and *sik malaria*, the latter a concept introduced by the *kiap* and medical investigators to explain by analogy how they believed kuru had come about. Like malaria, kuru was pictured as a sort of insect in the blood. Many people were acquainted with malaria. A few young men had seen the disease when they worked in coastal areas, and they understood that mosquitoes were the cause. At that time mosquitoes were absent in the Fore region, but many people were aware that populations living farther south and at lower elevations were troubled by both mosquitoes and malaria. In time, *sik malaria* came to mean the disease malaria, but it was also used as a generic term for other forms of "sickness" considered treatable and not thought to be caused by sorcery.[5]

Some Fore were uncomfortable with this explanation. They observed that people were often bitten by insects when they spent time in the bush, and the nonfatal ailments they suffered there were said to have been caused by *masalai* (bush spirits). The Wanitabe Luluai observed, "The two of us [he and the Kamila Luluai] have worked hard to find the cause of kuru. We have traveled around and around looking in 'ples masalai' [spirit places] to find the insect that bites us, but we have been unable to find it. Moreover, men, not women, spend time in the bush, and men are not coming down with the disease. Men are the ones making kuru."

This describes accurately the epidemiological patterns of the 1960s. People who held this view thought that the *kiap* and kuru investigators were making an error. Like epidemiologists, the Fore had always observed the age and gender of victims of the epidemic:

"People say there are two roads to kuru. One that it is sik malaria, and the other that men work it, and tell us so," said the Wanitabe Tultul. "Here is what I think. If it was sik malaria some men would get it too, and so would tiny girls who still drink their mothers' breastmilk, or those who are just beginning to walk. But it is young women and middle-aged women, those with three or four children, who get it, so I think men are making kuru.

The mosquito analogy thus challenged Fore conceptions of the origin of kuru and its mode of transmission. The meetings provided a venue for restating their authoritative narrative about the history of kuru: the first observed cases among the Fore; its origin at Uwami, north of Fore territory, where the "poison" was purchased by men wishing to harm an opponent; and the subsequent trading of knowledge and technology, each link explained in terms of the purchasers' intent to execute "payback" killings for earlier offenses. This account depicted the progress of kuru over a period of years from Uwami through the North Fore to the South Fore, a rendering in Fore terms of the epidemiological path of the infectious agent that medical and anthropological research later confirmed (Mathews, Glasse, and Lindenbaum 1968).

The meetings also elicited tangled tales of reciprocal attacks and the acceptance of bribes to "buy the hand to kill someone living close by." Wrestling with conflicting explanations, the Fore reaffirmed their worldview and drew upon their understanding of the nature of social relationships and the reciprocal obligations of kinship, co-residence, and losses that required retaliation. Aware that the colonial government held different views about the cause of disease, as well as about the legitimacy of fighting with spears and sorcery, they examined their ways of thinking about the world, but an alternative analysis was literally "unthinkable." The epidemic provided sorry evidence that sorcery worked and that the normal restraints of "warfare" had been disregarded. Fore orators drew attention to both numbers and ethics, speaking in the language of both epidemics and plagues. The Fore were keen observers of the associations among person, place, and time, and their observations were in many ways as exact as those of epidemiologists. When they shifted from association to explanation, however, the Fore fused categories that medical science and anthropology kept separate.

For four and a half months the Fore expressed their anxieties and concerns in a ceremonial setting and an increasingly conventionalized format. Speakers reviewed the history of political alliances and animosities, noting that past warfare had concentrated on enemies, people in other places. Now, "we are killing people in our own lines [kin and co-residents]." This tendency toward "endosorcery" could be accounted for by changing behaviors. With the end of warfare, it was "easier for enemies to come to our houses to take away food and body scraps to kill our women," an analysis that typically matched epidemiological observations with historical experience.

The days passed, and speakers had come at the problem from every direction. Angry men should kill just one man, destroy his dog, or cut down his banana trees. One thing was enough. In February 1963, a government census patrol came through the South Fore. Particular attention was given to providing an accurate count of kuru deaths in the past year and the names of any new cases. Following the census at Wanitabe, it became apparent that three new cases had gone unreported. In the preceding weeks, many people were aware that new cases had arisen even as they pledged an end to sorcery. The threat to call upon the *kiap* to take men into exile was already being reconsidered. Concerned that they might be punished when the *kiap* learned about new cases, the Luluais suggested that kuru must now be considered "sickness." Later conversations with both Luluais provided no indication that they believed this to be the case.[6]

The question of whether the epidemic was caused by sorcerers, so often addressed at the kuru meetings, arose again in the 1990s. By then kuru was becoming rare, the political and social order had changed

(Papua New Guinea had been an independent nation for more than fifteen years), and the debate began to absorb new thoughts, to reflect new experiences and social relations, and to incorporate new ways of talking about kuru.

The 1990s

By 1991, when I returned after an absence of some twenty years, the Fore population had undergone a spectacular recovery. My updated genealogies now recorded many families with seven or eight living children, whose names often reflected their parents' membership in one of two missions, Seventh-Day Adventist and Open Bible, the latter an American Pentecostal organization that had arrived in the Wanitabe area in the early 1970s. In 1982 the Open Bible mission had opened a clinic, providing health care for pregnant women and vaccinations for childhood diseases. By the 1990s, in addition to two mission families, a mission nurse worked at the clinic, which was now a government health center.[7] The Fore men's house no longer existed. Emulating white residential arrangements, and encouraged by the missions, most Fore now lived in nuclear family households. Assured by the missionaries that the ghosts of the dead would not harm them, the Fore buried deceased relatives no longer in abandoned gardens but often in well-tended graves beside the house.[8]

Christian religion now permeated all aspects of daily life. Saturdays were days of prayer and no work for Seventh-Day Adventists, as Sundays were for Open Bible adherents. The pace of secular life had also changed. The school bell clanged at seven o'clock on weekday mornings, calling children to the nearby Community School, which was staffed mostly by teachers from other regions of Papua New Guinea.[9] Local markets, said to have begun in 1981, were held on two days each week. Young women and men paraded self-consciously back and forth in small groups, fashioning a new space for courtship. Unlike women in their fifties and sixties, who were still haunted by the fear that kuru would reappear, young people with little memory of the peak years of the epidemic dropped biscuit wrappings (new items of consumption and potential sorcery items) near the marketplace and on local paths.

The marketplace also provided an audience to whom the newly elected local leaders could address local issues. With independence in 1975, the old *kiap* was no more, and the Luluais and Tultuls had been replaced by elected local councilors and committee men, although the provincial and national governments were not a strong presence. The sense of government oversight that had clouded people's thoughts and actions in the 1960s had been replaced by an awareness that a desirable future depended on gaining access to a distant political and economic system.

A key to a different financial future had been provided in 1957 when the colonial government introduced coffee as a cash crop. The Fore planted coffee trees on their own land and, when the first crop matured in the 1960s, used the money to buy highly prized items such as steel axes, spades, cloth, and knives (Sorenson 1976: 230). In 1969 the government purchased some Fore land for coffee plantations and, by 1990, when the first crop on the plantations matured, began to pay the Fore to pick coffee and process the seeds for market. By 1991, at the half-year mark, the government corporation had already distributed 90,000 kina.

Money was now flowing along old and new pathways. Brideprice at Purosa, which in the 1960s consisted of shells, small amounts of colonial money, and locally produced items (bark cloaks, string bags, sugarcane, and vegetables), had by 1991 risen to 1,500 kina for an un-educated bride or a poor worker, 2,000 for a good worker, and 3,500 to 5,000 for a (rare) high school teacher.[10] Death payments had also ballooned. A mortuary payment at Waisa in 1991 drew in 12,000 kina, 85 boxes of frozen lamb parts, and piles of clothing and blankets. Local items consisted only of 42 pigs, 12 chickens (stolen from the Open Bible chicken coop), sugarcane, and vegetables. The coffin was purchased in Goroka for 300 kina, and an Open Bible pastor presided over the ceremony. Huge compensation claims were now paid for people injured or killed in road accidents.[11] An Open Bible pastor described this use of money as "a false economy." Money should be invested to make more money, he said, not spent on consumer "parties"—a reference to the Pidgin term *pati*, which was applied to such ceremonial food exchanges.

People described their sense of change as a feeling of living in different eras: the time of fighting and the time of markets. In the past, men stood guard while women worked in the gardens. Now, men planted some market crops, and women prepared bigger gardens. "In the past we only thought about growing food to eat. Now we think about food for the market"—a structural view of historical change that might be described as configurational.

New social forms and behaviors pivoted around money. The Open Bible mission promoted women's savings clubs, which the mission hoped would not be used for "parties." The reciprocities underpinning Fore economic and social life were discouraged, though not forbidden.

Nevertheless, the Christian message was "Give freely, and don't expect a return. Free gifts are gifts to the Lord." The Open Bible missionaries and Seventh-Day Adventists both introduced tithing. As in labor camps elsewhere in the world, men formed a ring to pool wages, and the designated recipient was free to use the sum for personal use. Men gambled on local rugby games, women on women's basketball. Some men spent their days playing "Lucky," a card game said to be a recent addiction among young people who were not mission adherents. Sex for money was reported in the marketplaces at Purosa and Okapa, and bandits now held up vehicles traveling local roads. Access to money appeared to be encouraging the intensified circulation of wealth, not forming a significant basis of capital accumulation (Maclean 1982).[12]

Wage labor provided an additional source of income for Fore who worked elsewhere in Papua New Guinea. In the 1960s a small number of Fore had chosen to work with medical investigators, and some with Robert Glasse and me.[13] By the 1990s this generation was well positioned to recall the epidemic and to provide their views about why it was coming to an end. Almost all had lost their mothers and many sisters to kuru. They saw themselves as "men in the middle," standing between the elders who had stayed at home, spoke no Pidgin, and held different values and their own, better-educated children, who would experience a different future. Most had little formal schooling, and some had grown to maturity during a time when youths were not initiated. By the 1990s the revived ceremonies indoctrinated initiates with new kinds of knowledge. Gone were the painful nose piercing, the hoaxes, the sleep deprivation, and the lessons about warfare, hunting, shell money, and appropriate gifts to matrikin. Initiates were now drilled about the value of schooling, church attendance, growing coffee, starting a business, and making money in order to look after the family. Schoolteachers reinforced these messages.

As elsewhere in Papua New Guinea, a more individualized, self-owning person is said to be emerging among the Fore in the context of conversion to Christianity, commodity consumption, and wage labor (Robbins 2004). Yet individuals remain embedded in long-practiced reciprocal obligations (Wardlow 2006). "Men in the middle" were in a position to reflect on these changes and to provide their views about why the kuru epidemic appeared to be ending.

The Explanations of Three "Men in the Middle"

I have chosen three "men in the middle" from the Wanitabe area—"K," "N," and "O"—to illustrate the ways in which some Fore now speak about the epidemic. Men in the middle from Waisa, several hours' walk from Wanitabe, would provide an interesting comparison. Waisa, long an outpost for kuru investigation, has since 1996 become the center for prion research among the Fore, resulting in more intense interactions with scientific investigators. Kuru, like bovine spongiform encephalopathy (BSE) and variant Creutzfeldt-Jakob disease (vCJD) are now considered to be acquired forms of prion disease.[14]

By the 1990s, K's sorcery beliefs concerning kuru were intact, N was ambivalent about the cause of the epidemic, and O said he now thought, and hoped, that kuru was indeed a form of "sickness." Though all three adhered to the most widespread view—that they belonged to a generation not schooled in kuru sorcery (signaling the end of an ability to cause the disease)—they offered additional explanations for the end of kuru that reflected their different life experiences since the 1960s and the new sets of social relations within which their knowledge was produced.

K had worked as a research assistant for Robert and me and had attended the kuru meetings of the 1960s. Now elected as a local councilor, he considered himself to be a leader and facilitator of the new political and commercial order. Like the *kiaps* of yesteryear, he had the authority to conduct local court cases and expect some compliance. K told his story in heroic mode: "I told people I had outlawed kuru sorcery. I spoke strongly about this. I was instrumental also in introducing markets here. And I said that if people had any problems, they should come to us, the councillors and committee men. They listened to me and stopped making sorcery. And as you see, there are now plenty of men and women here."

N was also a research assistant in the 1960s. Following our departure in 1963, he had signed on as an assistant to a number of medical investigators. He observed medical examinations and assisted in collecting blood and urine samples and in gaining family permission for autopsies. His association with kuru research lasted until 1977, and he worked with me again for short periods during the 1990s. Between 1964 and 1967 he accompanied government medical patrols that he said gave people "two injections to kill the germs that came in the blood," which he thought were responsible for ending kuru. N appears to have been describing the public health patrols that used BCG vaccine to prevent tuberculosis and benzathine penicillin injections against yaws.[15] Like K, he drew on his own experiences and social relationships with outsiders, as well as the knowledge and authority they harvested (for a time he was also an elected councilor). In his view, kuru had now joined the list of ailments eradicated by Western medicine.[16]

O was born in 1962 and was too young to have attended the kuru meetings. Unlike K and N, he had completed primary school. Often present when N spoke about kuru, he provided a different personal account:

> My strongest thoughts are that it is not men who are doing this, because if men did it they could transfer this knowledge to their brothers and children... These people could then train the Amoras [an adjacent community], and then another houseline and another, and it would spread across the eastern highlands and on to other provinces. But it stops inside our district, so I think it is a sickness that comes along from time to time when people died of kuru and people ate them.
>
> My mother and father both died of kuru, so I thought I would get it, too. But I didn't, and I have six children and none of them are getting this 'sickness.'... So I think I am lucky that whitemen came at this time and gave injections, otherwise I would have had kuru and died. I have a strong hope that it was the injections that conquered it.

O said he had changed his thoughts about kuru following a conversation we had in 1991. I had just given him a photograph of his mother when she was pregnant with him. I had known his mother well, and this was a bond in our long friendship. "You told me my mother had died of kuru," he said. "I don't remember her. So I am a child of two people with kuru in the blood." (I had also told him that I thought kuru was transmitted by eating people who had died of the disease.) "I thought at first that my father had 'sick malaria,' but then his body began to shake and he had to walk about with a stick, and there came a time when he fell down and couldn't walk any more and he just stopped in the house... I looked after him... I was a small boy. My mother and father had died of kuru and I was very confused."

I asked if he had ever thought that a kuru sorcerer had killed his father, and he replied,

> No, it came from eating people... Here's an example. I eat plenty of green vegetables and good *habus* [meat], and this good food produces blood. So this first man ate someone, and this produced the "sickness" inside the blood, and he sleeps with his wife, and his semen [considered to be transformed blood] goes into the mother, and she gives birth to the child, and the "sickness" goes into the baby. This is what I think... I think that my father's father ate someone and he gave it to my father, and he gave it to my mother, and I thought I would get it too.

O's concept of nutrition and bodily substance, blended with Fore and Western ideas about disease transmission, does not reflect the scientific understanding of kuru transmission. O's explanation depends on an original act of human consumption by an adult male (historical accounts favor an original female consumer). This is followed by vertical transmission from a male ancestor and the sexual transfer of body substances to his mother (neither mode of transmission has been demonstrated). He thought also that his mother had not eaten human flesh (the scientific explanation for acquiring kuru). He believed that he and his children had been protected from kuru by the intervention of Western medicine (also unfounded). He said that the (Seventh-Day Adventist) church had not influenced his thinking about sorcery or cannibalism. "They tell us that the gospel says we can't kill people, steal women, or speak untruths. What I have told you about kuru, these are my thoughts." O's recent adoption of cannibalism as an explanation for kuru, central to anthropological and medical explanations, finds little room in most Fore accounts. When raised, it is expressed with uncertainty.[17]

These three men in the middle, like most other adult Fore men and women, also shared the modernist mantra that the end of the epidemic could be attributed to a break with the past brought about by the adoption of Christianity, markets, and the education of children. Kuru sorcerers were said to have found more profitable avenues for their activities. When they gave their own, more considered accounts, however, the ideas of all three "middlemen" reflected individual life experiences as well as the new social relations within which their knowledge was produced.[18] K's intervention as a new political actor had brought an end to kuru sorcery; N's key role in medical work had contributed to the eradication of the disease; and O's few years of schooling, his close association with N and me, and the disturbing experience of caring for his sick father had provided him with a different fundament of knowledge and experience. O provided perhaps the most complex account, but all three reflect an array of simultaneously held explanations that derived from old and new sources of knowledge, local concepts of physiological inheritance, keen epidemiological observations, and personal experience. Theories of disease causation provided a catchment for changing understandings about the nature of existence.

Three Speech Genres

The Fore have been much affected by the powerful discourses of others. Colonial words were compelling until self-government in 1975, when the Fore began to provide their own authoritative political statements. Religious messages have remained intact, inserted into a cosmology that had no similar concept of a supreme being. Western medical beliefs, however, are still being tested, and no single explanatory position has yet emerged. Moreover, the "sickness" versus sorcery debate concerns only kuru. No one believes that sorcery in general is a thing of the past. The exchange economy, resilient in the context of new sources of money and prestige, still binds the Fore to the reciprocities and social forms that underwrite their moral understanding of the universe and a sorcery-based theory of disease causation.

Like Carleton Gajdusek, the legion of investigators in research institutes around the world present their findings to fellow scientists in a predominantly monological format.[19] As both a natural science and a humanistic discipline, anthropology mediates between human biology and ecology, on the one hand, and the study of human understanding, on the other (Wolf 1974: 13). In their communications with medical investigators and the Fore, anthropologists speak in double dialogical mode, engaging with two socially and historically grounded languages that themselves contain multiple voices. Fore disease explanations, neither simply monological nor dialogical, contain elements of both but differ from the discourses of medicine and anthropology. Calling upon information recognized by both the exact and the human sciences (clinical description, epidemiological observation, and an assessment of human behavior), and responding to the influential words of outsiders, the Fore present their findings as a fusion of subjects, not as separate domains of experience. For them, kuru was simultaneously an epidemic and a plague. We arrive at the fullest cultural, historical, and scientific understanding of the disease when we combine all three styles of explanation.

Notes

1. I compare here the written accounts of the "exact" and human sciences with the oral arguments of the Fore. Bakhtin distinguished between spoken (primary) and written (secondary) speech genres but considered them both

historical and social in nature, forms of communication or utterances that exist between people who occupy particular places in a network of social relationships (Dentith 1995: 39).

2. *Kanaka* is a Pidgin word often used in the early 1960s but now viewed as derogatory.

3. Luluais and Tultuls lost more wives than other men because they had the status, networks, and resources to marry again and thus to suffer more loss.

4. The Okapa-Purosa road was built between 1955 and 1957.

5. There is no neat correlation between Western and Fore illness categories. Fore etiological beliefs fall into two categories: maladies caused by sorcerers and ailments caused by less malign forces such as nature spirits (*masalai*) inhabiting spirit places and ghosts of the recently dead. Calamities ascribed to sorcery involve life-threatening conditions (such as kuru) that endanger the survival of women, who ensure social survival. Less malign forces cause illness among adults and sickness and death among children. Influenced by missionaries, the Fore no longer pay much attention to ghosts of the dead.

6. The Kamila Luluai asserted, as did the man I later refer to as "K" in the 1990s, that his oratory decrying sorcery had been instrumental in directing the sorcerers' attention to other activities.

7. The ceremony to protect the health of small children, observed in the 1960s, was no longer held.

8. In the 1960s the Fore had said that angry ghosts punished the living for small property infringements, causing small ailments (nausea, weakness, fainting). Missionaries were less successful in defusing fear of *masalai* (bush spirits), thought to cause nonthreatening illnesses. *Masalai*, however, when referred to as "Satan," appear to have lost much of their ambiguous, trickster-like features.

9. The primary school began informally in 1967. By the 1990s, plans were under way for a high school.

10. In 1991, 1 kina equaled US$1.10.

11. Ivaki demanded and received 10,000 kina from Purosa when one of its team members was injured in a rugby tackle. The government coffee corporation helped Purosa pay the claim, and donors were still working to pay off this debt. In the past, the Fore gave compensation payments to war allies, not to those they injured or killed.

12. Maclean argued that gambling had intensified the circulation of money and was the antithesis of investment, and that this applied also to bridewealth, death payments, and the burgeoning system of compensation payments.

13. The medical investigators were Gajdusek, Alpers, Hornabrook, and Mathews.

14. The epidemics of kuru and BSE both result from the amplification of the prion agent following intraspecies recycling (endocannibalism) of the infectious prion among humans and cattle, respectively. Research on kuru has contributed to understanding and controlling the epidemics of BSE in the United Kingdom and elsewhere, as well as its human counterpart, variant Creutzfeldt-Jakob disease. Incubation periods for kuru of more than fifty years following oral transmission, associated with strong dependence on host genetics, provide a powerful basis for exploring the wider implications of kuru for other human diseases. Although Bennett's earlier genetic hypothesis no longer holds, a genetic theory has been rescued to explain some differences in incubation period (see Collinge et al. 2006; Mathews 2008).

15. Michael Alpers, personal communication, 2006. Alpers, a kuru investigator, was not part of these government census and health patrols.

16. Medicine did not in fact find a cure for kuru. The epidemic ended following the Fore's abandonment of the practice of consuming deceased kin.

17. This was still true in July and August 2008, when I made a short return visit to the South Fore.

18. Wardlow (2002) makes a similar "sociology of knowledge" argument to explain Huli women's changing beliefs about the etiology of sexually transmitted disease.

19. Michael Alpers and John Mathews are exceptions. Both have continued to take account of the environmental and social aspects of the disease.

References

Abu-Raddad, L. J., P. Patnaik, and J. G. Kublin. 2006. Dual infection with HIV and malaria fuels the spread of both diseases in sub-Saharan Africa. *Science* 314 (5805): 1603–1606.

Achterberg, Jerusha T. 2009. Computational models frame new and outstanding biological questions of *Mycobacterium tuberculosis*. Working paper 93, Center for Statistics and the Social Sciences, University of Washington.

Ackerknecht, Erwin H. 1948. Anticontagionism between 1821 and 1867. *Bulletin of the History of Medicine* 22: 562–593.

Afkhami, Amir. 2003. Compromised constitutions: The Iranian experience with the 1918 influenza pandemic. *Bulletin of the History of Medicine* 77 (2): 367–392.

Agramonte, A. 1906. Notas clínicas sobre una epidemia reciente de dengue. *Revista de Medicina y Cirugía* 11 (12): 222–226.

Aguilera, Solis, and Ana Vanessa Plasencia. 2005. Culturally appropriate HIV/AIDS and substance abuse prevention programs for urban native youth. *Journal of Psychoactive Drugs* 37 (3): 299–304.

Aguirre Beltran, Gonzalo. 1955. *Programas de salud en la situación intercultural*. Mexico City: Instituto Indigenista Interamericano.

Ahmad, O. B., A. D. Lopez, and M. Inoue. 2000. The decline in child mortality: A reappraisal. *Bulletin of the World Health Organization* 78 (10): 1175–1191.

Ahmed, F. U., C. B. Mahmood, J. D. Sharma, S. M. Hoque, and R. Zaman. 2001. Dengue and dengue haemorrhagic fever in children during the 2000 outbreak n Chittagong, Bangladesh. *Dengue Bulletin* 25: 33–39.

AIDS Alert. 2001. Are Native Americans the next brush fire in the HVI epidemic? *AIDS Alert* 2001: 27–28.

AIDS Policy and Law. 2003. Native Americans enter HIV spotlight at national conference. *AIDS Policy and Law* 8 (2): 9.

Alexander, D. J. 2000. A review of avian influenza in different bird species. *Veterinary Microbiology* 74 (1–2): 3–13.

Almond, Douglas. 2006. Is the 1918 influenza pandemic over? Long-term effects of *in utero* influenza exposure in the post-1940 U.S. population. *Journal of Political Economy* 114 (4): 672–712.

Alpers, Michael P. 1968. Kuru: Implications of its transmissibility for the interpretation of its changing epidemiologic pattern. In *The Central Nervous System,* edited by O. T. Bailey and D. E. Smith, 234–251. Baltimore, MD: Williams and Wilkins.

———. 2005. The epidemiology of kuru in the period 1987 to 1995. *Communicable Disease Intelligence* 29 (4): 391–399.

———, and L. Rail. 1971. Kuru and Creutzfeldt-Jakob disease: Clinical and aetiological aspects. *Proceedings of the Australian Association of Neurology* 8: 7–15.

American Journal of Public Health. 1915. Public health work among the Indians. *American Journal of Public Health* 5: 271.

Ammon, Catherine E. 2001. The 1918 Spanish flu epidemic in Geneva, Switzerland. *International Congress Series* 1219: 163–168.

Amstrong, O. K. 1958. All out attack on malaria. *Readers Digest,* July, 188–191.

Anderson, A. 2008. Mark of shame: Social stigma, tuberculosis and Asian immigrants to New Zealand. In *Multiplying and dividing: Tuberculosis in Canada and Aotearoa New Zealand,* edited by J. Littleton, J. Park, A. Herring, and T. Farmer, 196–204. Research in Anthropology and Linguistics, e series. Auckland: Anthropology Department, University of Auckland.

Anderson, C. R., W. G. Downs, and A. E. Hill. 1956. Isolation of dengue virus from a human being in Trinidad. *Science* 124: 224–225.

Anderson, Margo J. 1988. *The American census: A social history.* New Haven, CT: Yale University Press.

Anderson, Roy M., and Robert M. May. 1979. Population biology of infectious diseases. *Nature* 280: 361–370.

———. 1991. *Infectious diseases of humans: Dynamics and control.* Oxford: Oxford University Press.

Anderson, Warwick. 1995. Excremental colonialism: Public health and the poetics of pollution. *Critical Inquiry* 21: 640–669.

———. 2004a. *Colonial pathologies: American tropical medicine, race, and hygiene in the Philippines.* Durham, NC: Duke University Press.

———. 2004b. Natural histories of infectious disease: Ecological vision in twentieth-century biomedical science. *Osiris* 19: 39–61.

———. 2008. *The collectors of lost souls: Turning whitemen into kuru scientists.* Baltimore, MD: Johns Hopkins University Press.

Anderton, Douglas L., and Susan Hautaniemi Leonard. 2004. Grammars of death: An analysis of nineteenth-century literal causes of death from the age of miasmas to germ theory. *Social Science History* 28 (1): 111–143.

Andreev, E. M. 1982. The method of components in the analysis of length of life. *Vestnik Statistiki* 9: 32–47.

Angotti, T. 1995. The Latin American metropolis and the growth of inequality. *NACLA Report on the Americas* 28: 13–18.

Anonymous. 1990. Dengue hemorrhagic fever in Venezuela. *Epidemiological Bulletin of the Pan American Health Organization* 11: 7–9.

Arboleda, M. 1995. Social attitudes and sexual variance in Lima. In *Latin American male homosexualities*, edited by S. O. Murray, 100–110. Albuquerque: University of New Mexico Press.

Armelagos, George. 1990. Health and disease in prehistoric populations in transition. In *Disease in populations in transition*, edited by A. C. Swedlund and G. Armelagos, 127–144. New York: Bergin and Garvey.

———, Kathleen Barnes, and James Lin. 1996. Disease in human evolution: The re-emergence of infectious disease in the third epidemiological transition. *National Museum of Natural History Bulletin for Teachers* 18 (3): 1–6.

———, and K. N. Harper. 2005. Genomics at the origins of agriculture, part 2. *Evolutionary Anthropology* 14 (3): 109–121.

Arms Family Papers. Box 4, F7, Pocumtuck Valley Memorial Association Library, Deerfield, MA.

Arnold, David. 1996. *The problem of nature: Environment, culture and European expansion.* Oxford: Oxford University Press.

Arriaga, E. 1984. Measuring and explaining the change in life expectancies. *Demography* 21: 83–96.

Ashforth, Adam. 2002. An epidemic of witchcraft? The implications of AIDS for the post-apartheid state. *African Studies* 61 (1): 121–143.

Ashman, Jill J., David Perez-Jimenez, and Katherine Marconi. 2004. Health and support service utilization patterns of American Indians and Alaska Natives diagnosed with HIV/AIDS. *AIDS Education and Prevention* 16 (3): 238–249.

Associated Press. 2006. Final figure for August shows no drop in violent deaths in Baghdad. September 7. http://accuweather.ap.org/preserver/tmp/PLS/157.252/233.12–291980010/iconnA21TC/apiconnA21TC_Final_f_206437.

Azambuja, Maria Inês Reinert. 2004. Spanish flu and early 20th-century expansion of a coronary heart disease-prone subpopulation. *Texas Heart Institute Journal* 31 (1): 14–21.

———, and Bruce B. Duncan. 2002. Similarities in mortality patterns from influenza in the first half of the 20th century and the rise and fall of ischemic heart disease in the United States: A new hypothesis concerning the coronary heart disease epidemic. *Cadernos de Saúde Pública* 18 (3): 557–566.

Baer, Hans A. 2007. *Global warming, human society and critical anthropology: A research agenda.* Melbourne, Australia: University of Melbourne Press.

———, Merrill Singer, and Ida Susser. 2003. *Medical anthropology and the world system.* 2nd ed. Westport, CT: Bergin and Garvey.

Bailey, Norman T. J. 1975. *The mathematical theory of infectious diseases and its applications.* 2nd ed. London: Griffin.

Bakhtin, M. M. 1981. *The dialogic imagination: Four essays.* Translated by C. Emerson and M. Holquist. Austin: University of Texas Press.

———. 1984. *Problems of Dostoevsky's poetics.* Minneapolis: University of Minnesota Press.

———. 1986. *Speech genres and other late essays.* Translated by Vern W. McGhee. Austin: University of Texas Press.

Baldwin, J. A. 1996. Developing culturally sensitive HIV/AIDS and substance abuse prevention curriculum for Native American youth. *Journal of School Health* 66 (9): 322–327.

———. 2000. Alcohol as a risk factor for HIV transmission among American Indian and Alaskan Native drug users. *American Indian and Alaska Native Mental Health Research* 9 (1): 1–16.

Barber, Katrine. 2005. *Death of Celilo Falls.* Seattle: University of Washington Press.

Barman, Jean. 2005. Aboriginal women on the streets of Victoria: Rethinking transgressive sexuality during the colonial encounter. In *Contact zones: Aboriginal and settler women in Canada's colonial past,* edited by K. Pickles and M. Rutherdale, 205–228. Vancouver: University of British Columbia Press.

Barnes, David S. 1995. *The making of a social disease: Tuberculosis in nineteenth-century France.* Berkeley: University of California Press.

Barrett, R., C. Kuzawa, T. McDade, and G. Armelagos. 1998. Emerging and re-emerging infectious diseases: The third epidemiological transition. *Annual Review of Anthropology* 27: 247–271.

Barrett, Ron, and Peter J. Brown. 2008. Stigma in the time of influenza: Social and institutional responses to pandemic emergencies. *Journal of Infectious Disease* 197 (Supplement 1): S34–37.

Barry, John M. 2004. *The great influenza: The epic story of the deadliest plague in history.* New York: Viking Adult.

Barua, D. 1992. History of cholera. In *Cholera,* edited by D. Barua and W. B. Grenough, 1–36. New York: Plenum Medical Book Company.

Bashford, A. 2004. *Imperial hygiene.* New York: Palgrave Macmillan.

BBC (British Broadcasting Corporation). 2005. Avian flu found in parrot in UK. Electronic document, http://news.bbc.co.uk/1/hi/uk/4365956. stm.

BBC News. 2004. Iraq death toll "soared post-war." October 29. http://news.bbc.co.uk/go/pr/fr/-/2/hi/middle_east/3962969.stm.

Bean, William B. 1977. Walter Reed and the ordeal of human experiments. *Bulletin of the History of Medicine* 60 (1): 75–92.

———. 1982. *Walter Reed: A biography.* Charlottesville: University of Virginia Press.

Bellamy, R. L. 1990. Trobriand vital statistics in 1926. In *A history of medicine in Papua New Guinea: Vignettes of an earlier period,* edited by Sir B. G. Burton-Bradley, 299–310. Kingsgrove, NSW: Australasian Medical Publishing.

Belshe, Robert. 2005. Origins of pandemic influenza: Lesson from the 1918 virus. *New England Journal of Medicine* 353 (21): 2209–2211.

Benchimol, Jaime. 1999. *Dos microbios os mosquitos: Febre amarela e revolucao pasteuriana no Brasil.* Rio de Janeiro: Editora de Universitade Federal Fluminense.

———, and Luis Antonio Teixeira. 1993. *Cobras, largatos e outros bichos: Uma historia comparada dos institutos, Oswaldo Cruz e Butantan.* Rio de Janeiro: Editora Fiocruz.

Bennett, J. H., F. A. Rhodes, and H. N. Robson. 1959. A possible genetic basis for kuru. *American Journal of Human Genetics* 11: 169–187.

Benson, Todd. 1999. Blinded by science: American Indians, the Office of Indian Affairs, and the federal campaign against trachoma, 1924–1927. *American Indian Culture and Research Journal* 23 (3): 119–142.

Berkelman, Ruth L., and Phyllis Freeman. 2004. Emerging infections and the CDC response. In *Emerging illnesses and society: Negotiating the public health agenda,* edited by R. M. Packard, P. J. Brown, R. L. Berkelman, and H. Frumkin, 350–387. Baltimore, MD: Johns Hopkins University Press.

Bernal, D. 1828. *Memoria sobre la epidemia que ha sufrido esta ciudad, nombrado vulgarmente el dengue.* Havana: Oficina del Gobierno y Capitanía General.

Berndt, R. M. 1962. *Excess and restraint: Social control among a New Guinea mountain people.* Chicago: University of Chicago Press.

Berridge, Virginia, and Philip Strong. 1992. AIDS and the relevance of history. *Social History of Medicine* 5 (1): 130–138.

Bertolli, Jeanne, A. D. McNaughton, Michael Campsmith, Lisa M. Lee, Richard Leman, Ralph Bryan, and James W. Buehler. 2004. Surveillance systems monitoring HIV/AIDS and HIV risk behaviors among

American Indians and Alaskan Natives. *AIDS Education and Prevention* 16 (3): 218–237.

Birchenall, Javier A. 2007a. Economic development and the escape from high mortality. *World Development* 35 (4): 543–568.

———. 2007b. Escaping high mortality. *Journal of Economic Growth* 12 (4): 351–387.

Bisbal, Marcelino. 1994. *La mirada comunicacional.* Caracas: Alfadil.

Bisset, J. 2002. Uso correcto de insecticidas: Control de la resistencia. *Revista Cubana de Medicina Tropical* 54: 202–219.

Black, Robert H. 1957. Dr. Bellamy of Papua. *Medical Journal of Australia* 2: 189–197, 232–238, 279–284.

Bonfil, Guillermo. 1987. *México profundo: Una civilización negada.* Mexico City: Secretaría de Educación Pública.

Boni, M. F., J. R. Gog, V. Andreasen, and F. B. Christiansen. 2004. Influenza drift and epidemic size: The race between generating and escaping immunity. *Theoretical Population Biology* 65 (2): 179–191.

Borgundvaag, Bjug, Howard Ovens, Brian Goldman, Michael Schull, Tim Rutledge, Kathy Boutis, Sharon Walmsley, Allison McGeer, Anita Rachlis, and Carolyn Farquarson. 2004. SARS outbreak in the greater Toronto area: The emergency department experience. *Canadian Medical Association Journal* 171 (11): 1342–1344.

Bourdieu, Pierre. 1991. *Language and symbolic power.* Translated by G. Raymond and M. Adamson. Cambridge, MA: Harvard University Press.

Boyce, P., M. Huang Soo Lee, C. Jenkins, S. Mohamed, C. Overs, V. Paiva, E. Reid, M. Tan, and P. Aggleton. 2007. Putting sexuality (back) into HIV/AIDS: Issues, theory and practice. *Global Public Health* 2 (1): 1–34.

Bradley, D. J. 1993. Environmental and health problems of developing countries. In *1993 Environmental Change and Human Health,* 234–246. Ciba Foundation Symposium 175. Chichester, UK: Ciba Foundation.

Brandt, Lilian. 1903. Social aspects of tuberculosis. *Annals of the American Academy of Political and Social Science* 21: 65–76.

Bravo, J. R., M. G. Guzmán, and G. P. Kouri. 1987. Why dengue haemorrhagic fever in Cuba? Individual risk factors for dengue haemorrhagic fever/dengue shock syndrome (DHF/DSS). *Transactions of the Royal Society of Tropical Medicine and Hygiene* 81: 816–820.

Briggs, Charles L. 2003. Why nation-states can't teach people to be healthy: Power and pragmatic miscalculation in public discourses on health. *Medical Anthropology Quarterly* 17 (3): 287–321.

———. 2005. Communicability, racial discourse, and disease. *Annual Review of Anthropology* 34: 269–291.

————. 2007. Anthropology, interviewing, and communicability in contemporary society. *Current Anthropology* 48 (4): 551–580.

————, and Daniel C. Hallin. 2007. Biocommunicability: The neoliberal subject and its contradictions in news coverage of health issues. *Social Text* 25 (4): 43–66.

————, and Daniel C. Hallin. n.d. Health reporting as political reporting: Biocommunicability and the public sphere. *Journalism: Theory, Practice, and Criticism.* In press.

————, with Clara Mantini-Briggs. 2003. *Stories in the time of cholera: Racial profiling during a medical nightmare.* Berkeley: University of California Press.

British Columbia Ministry of Health, Vital Statistics Branch. 1945. *Causes of death.* Sessional Papers. Victoria, BC: Queen's Printer.

Brookes, B. 2006. Health education film and the Maori: Tuberculosis and the Maori people of the Wairoa District (1952). *Health and History* 8 (2): 45–68.

Brown, David. 2006. Study claims Iraq's "excess" death toll has reached 655,000. *Washington Post,* 11 October, A12.

Brown Family Papers. Pocumtuck Valley Memorial Association Library, Deerfield, MA.

Brundage, J. F. 2006. Interactions between influenza and bacterial respiratory pathogens: Implications for pandemic preparedness. *Lancet Infectious Diseases* 6 (5): 303.

————, and G. D. Shanks. 2008. Deaths from bacterial pneumonia during 1918–19 influenza pandemic. *Emerging Infectious Disease* 14 (8): 1193–1199.

Bryder, L. 1991a. Tuberculosis in New Zealand. In *History of tuberculosis in Australia, New Zealand and Papua New Guinea,* edited by A. J. Proust, 79–89. Canberra: Brolga Press.

————. 1991b. Tuberculosis and the Maori, 1900–1960. In *The impact of the past upon the present: Second national conference of the Australian Society of the History of Medicine, Perth, July 1991,* edited by P. Winterton and D. Gurry, 191–194. Perth: Australian Society of the History of Medicine.

————. 1996. A health resort for consumptives: Tuberculosis and immigration to New Zealand, 1880–1940. *Medical History* 40: 453–471.

Buckley, H., and N. Tayles. 2000. Subadult health in prehistoric Tonga, Polynesia. *American Journal of Physical Anthropology* 113: 481–505.

Budrys, Grace. 2003. *Unequal health: How inequality contributes to health or illness.* Lanham, MD: Rowan and Littlefield.

Buikstra, Jane E. 1984. The lower Illinois River region: A prehistoric context for the study of ancient diet and health. In *Paleopathology at the origins of agriculture*, edited by M. Cohen and G. Armelagos, 215–234. New York: Academic Press.

Bullock, S. L., T. Myers, L. M. Calzavara, R. Cockerill, and V. W. Marshall. 1993. Major socio-cultural factors and HIV among First Nations people: Results of the Ontario AIDS and health lifestyle survey. Abstract. *International Conference on AIDS* 9: 934 (abstract no. PO-D33-4296).

———, T. Myers, L. M. Calzavara, R. Cockerill, V. W. Marshall, and A. Burchill. 1996. Unprotected intercourse and the meanings ascribed to sex by Aboriginal people living on-reserve in Ontario, Canada. Abstract. *International Conference on AIDS* 11: 50 (abstract no. Mo.D.483).

Burke, D. S., A. Nisalak, D. E. Johnson, and R. M. Scott. 1988. A prospective study of dengue infections in Bangkok. *American Journal of Tropical Medicine and Hygiene* 38: 172–180.

Burnet, F. Macfarlane. 1940. *Biological aspects of infectious disease.* Cambridge: Cambridge University Press.

———, and E. Clark. 1942. *Influenza.* London: Macmillan.

Burnham, Gilbert, Ryiadh Lafta, Shannon Doody, and Les Roberts. 2006. Mortality after the 2003 invasion of Iraq: A cross-sectional cluster sample survey. *Lancet* 368 (9545): 1421–1428.

Burns, Herbert A. 1932. Tuberculosis in the Indian. *American Review of Tuberculosis* 26 (July–December): 498–506.

Butterfield, K. 2006. Tuberculosis in the Pacific? Research portfolio, University of Auckland.

Buve, A., M. Caraël, R. J. Hayes, B. Auvert, B. Ferry, N. J. Robinson, S. Anagonou, et al. 2001. Multicentre study on factors determining differences in rate of spread of HIV in sub-Saharan Africa: Methods and prevalence of HIV infection. *Aids* 15 (Supplement 4): S5–14.

Cáceres, Carlos F., and Oscar G. Jiménez. 1999. Fletes in Parque Kennedy: Sexual cultures among young men who sell sex to other men in Lima. In *Men who sell sex: International perspectives on male prostitution and HIV/AIDS*, edited by P. Aggleton, 179–194. Philadelphia: Temple University Press.

———, and Ana Maria Rosasco. 1999. The margin has many sides: Diversity among gay and homosexually active men in Lima. *Culture, Health and Sexuality* 1 (3): 261–275.

Calmette, Albert, and Michel Breton. 1905. *L'Ankylostomiase, une maladie sociale, (anémie des mineurs): Biologie, clinique, traitement, prophylaxie.* Paris: Masson et Cia.

Calzavara, L., A. N. Burchell, T. Myers, S. L. Bullock, M. Escobar, and R. Cockerill. 1998. Condom use among Aboriginal people in Ontario, Canada. *International Journal of STD and AIDS* 9: 272–279.

Camargo, S. 1967. History of *Aedes aegypti* eradication in the Americas. *Bulletin of the World Health Organization* 36: 602–603.

Camus, A. 1947. *La peste*. Paris: Gallimard. Published in English as *The plague*, New York: Modern Library, 1948.

Canadian Public Health Journal. 1941. Tuberculosis in the Indian population. *Canadian Public Health Journal* 32 (1): 38–39.

Carlson, E. 2006. Ages of origin and destination for a difference in life expectancy. *Demographic Research* 14: 217–236.

Caroll, James. 1903. The etiology of yellow fever. *Journal of the American Medical Association*, 23 May. Reprinted in *Yellow fever: Compilation of various publications*, edited by M. Owen, 175–185. Washington, DC: Government Printing Office, 1911.

Carrier, Joseph M. 1976. Cultural factors affecting urban Mexican male homosexuality. *Archives of Sexual Behavior* 5: 103–124.

———. 1995. *De los otros: Intimacy and homosexuality among Mexican men*. New York: Columbia University Press.

Carrillo, Héctor. 2002. *The night is young: Sexuality in Mexico in the time of AIDS. Worlds of desire.* Chicago: University of Chicago Press.

Carter, T. Henry. 1901. A note on the spread of yellow fever in houses, extrinsic incubation. *Medical Record* 59 (24): 937–939.

Castro, A., and P. Farmer. 2005. Understanding and addressing AIDS-related stigma: From anthropological theory to clinical practice in Haiti. *American Journal of Public Health* 95 (1): 53–59.

Caudhill, William. 1953. Applied anthropology in medicine. In *Anthropology today,* edited by A. L. Kroeber, 771–806. Chicago: University of Chicago Press.

CBS News. 2002. Global warming may spread diseases. 20 June. Electronic document, www.cbsnews.com/stories/2002/06/20/tech/main512920.shtml.

CDC (Centers for Disease Control and Prevention). 2002. About the *Emerging Infectious Diseases* journal. Electronic document, www.cdc.gov/ncidod/eid/about/background.htm.

———. 2003. Fact sheet: Dengue and dengue hemorrhagic fever. 10 November. Atlanta: CDC.

———. 2005. AIDS public information data set, 2001, www.cdc.gov/hiv/softward/apids.htm.

———. 2007. *Dengue fever.* Atlanta: CDC.

Chadwick, Douglas. 1993. Seeking meanings. *Defenders Magazine.* Electronic document, www.defenders.org/bio-bi02.html.

————. 2003. Pacific suite. *National Geographic* 203 (2): 104–127.

Chan, Alex. 2004. HIV-positive injection drug users who leave the hospital against medical advice: The mitigating role of methadone and social support. *Journal of Acquired Immune Deficiency Syndrome* 35 (1): 56–59.

Chan, J., C. Ng, Y. Chan, T. Mok, W. Who, S. Lee, S. Chu, W. Law, M. Lee, and P. Li. 2003. Short-term outcome and risk factors for adverse clinical outcomes in adults with severe acute respiratory syndrome (SARS). *Thorax* 58 (8): 686–689.

Chan, M. C. W., C. Y. Cheung, W. H. Chui, S. W. Tsao, J. M. Nicholls, Y. O. Chan, R. W. Y. Chan, et al. 2005. Proinflammatory cytokine responses induced by influenza A (H5N1) viruses in primary human alveolar and bronchial epithelial cells. *Respiratory Research* 6 (135): n.p. Electronic document.

Chandavarkar, Rajnarayan. 1992. Plague panic and epidemic politics in India, 1896–1914. In *Epidemics and ideas: Essays on the historical perception of pestilence,* edited by T. Ranger and P. Slack, 203–240. Cambridge: Cambridge University Press.

Chanyapate, Chanida, and Isabelle Delforge. 2004. The politics of bird flu in Thailand. Electronic document, http://focusweb.org/content/index2.php?option=com_content&do_pdf=1&id=273.

Chatterjee, R. 2007. Portrait of a killer. *ScienceNow Daily News* (American Association for the Advancement of Science). Electronic document, http://sciencenow.sciencemag.org/cgi/content/full/2007/117/2.

Chen, J. M., J. W. Chen, J. Dai, and Y. Sun. 2007. A survey of human cases of H5N1 avian influenza reported by the WHO before June 2006 for infection control. *American Journal of Infection Control* 35: 351–53.

Chen, Kwang-Ming, ed. 2004. *The mysterious diseases of Guam.* Agana, Guam: Richard F. Taitano Micronesian Area Research Center, University of Guam.

Cheung, C., L. Poon, A. Lau, W. Luk, Y. Lau, K. Shortridge, S. Gordon, Y. Guan, and J. Peiris. 2002. Induction of proinflammatory cytokines in human macrophages by influenza A (H5N1) viruses: A mechanism for the unusual severity of human disease? *Lancet* 360 (9348): 1831–1837.

Chiang, C. 1984. The life table and its applications. Malabar: Krieger Publishing.

Chowell, G., C. E. Ammon, N. W. Hengartner, and J. M. Hyman. 2006a. Estimation of the reproductive number of the Spanish flu epidemic in Geneva, Switzerland. *Vaccine* 24 (44–46): 6747–6750.

———, C. E. Ammon, N. W. Hengartner, and J. M. Hyman. 2006b. Transmission dynamics of the great influenza pandemic of 1918 in Geneva, Switzerland: Assessing the effects of hypothetical interventions. *Journal of Theoretical Biology* 241 (2): 193–204.

Chungue, E., V. Deubel, O. Cassar, M. Laille, and P. M. Martin. 1993. Molecular epidemiology of dengue 3 viruses and genetic relatedness among dengue 3 strains isolated from patients with mild or severe form of dengue fever in French Polynesia. *Journal of General Virology* 74 (12): 2765–2770.

Clark, Samuel J. 2006. Demographic impacts of the HIV epidemic and consequences of population-wide treatment of HIV for the elderly: Results from microsimulation. In *Aging in Sub-Saharan Africa: Recommendations for furthering research,* edited by B. Cohen and J. A. Menken, 92–116. Washington, DC: National Academies Press.

Clarke, Juanne N. 2005. Canadian Aboriginal people's experiences with HIV/AIDS as portrayed in selected English language Aborignal media (1996–2000). *Social Science & Medicine* 60: 2169–2180.

Clatts, Michael. 1995. Disembodied acts: On the perverse use of sexual categories in the study of high-risk behavior. In *Culture and sexual risk: Anthropological perspectives on AIDS,* edited by H. Ten Brummelhuis and G. Herdt, 241–256. Amsterdam: Gordon and Breach.

Cline, Howard F. 1981. *Mexico: Revolution to evolution, 1940–1960.* Westport, CT: Greenwood Press.

Cockburn, T. A. 1971. Infectious disease in ancient populations. *Current Anthropology* 12 (1): 45–62.

Coffee, M., M. N. Lurie, and G. P. Garnett. 2007. Modelling the impact of migration on the HIV epidemic in South Africa. *Aids* 21 (3): 343–350.

Cohen, Mitchel. 1998. Resurgent and emergent disease in a changing world. *British Medical Bulletin* 54: 523–532.

Cohen, M. N., and G. J. Armelagos. 1984. *Paleopathology at the origins of agriculture.* New York: Academic Press.

Cohn, Samuel K., Jr. 2002. *The black death transformed: Disease and culture in early Renaissance Europe.* Cambridge: Cambridge University Press.

Collier, Richard. 1996 [1974]. *The plague of the Spanish lady: The influenza pandemic of 1918–1919.* London: Alison and Busby.

Collinge, John, Jerome Whitfield, Edward McKintosh, John Beck, Simon Mead, Dafydd J. Thomas, and Michael P. Alpers. 2006. Kuru in the twenty-first century: An acquired human prion disease with very long incubation periods. *Lancet* 367: 2068–2074.

Colwell, R. 1996. Global climate and infectious disease: The cholera paradigm. *Science* 274: 2025–2031.

Comaroff, John, and Jean Comaroff. 1991. *Of revelation and revolution: The dialectic of modernity on a South African frontier.* Chicago: University of Chicago Press.

Conan Doyle, Arthur. 1894. The adventure of Silver Blaze. In *The Memoirs of Sherlock Holmes.* London: G. Newnes.

———. 1982. The adventure of the dying detective. In *The Penguin complete Sherlock Holmes,* 932–941. Hammondsworth, UK: Penguin.

Condran, Gretchen A. 1995. Changing patterns of epidemic disease in New York City. In *Hives of sickness: Public health and epidemics in New York City,* edited by D. Rosner, 27–41. New Brunswick, NJ: Rutgers University Press.

Connors M. M., V. Catan, I. Escolano, and S. Brown. 1992. Ethnic, cultural, and subcultural influences on HIV risk behavior: A model to help explain differences in rates of HIV infection among intravenous drug users by ethnic group in the US. Abstract. *International Conference on AIDS* 8: C301 (abstract no. PoC 4339).

Conway, G. 1992. HIV infection in American Indians and Alaskan Natives: Surveys in the Indian Health Service. *Journal of Acquired Immune Deficiency Syndromes* 5: 803–809.

Cooper, S., and D. Coxe. 2005. *An investor's guide to avian flu.* Toronto: BMO Nesbitt Burns Research.

Corbett, E. L., C. J. Watt, N. Walker, and D. Maher. 2003. The growing burden of tuberculosis: Global trends and interactions with the HIV epidemic. *Archives of Internal Medicine* 163 (9): 1009–1021.

County of San Diego. 2004a. First possible human case of West Nile virus reported. 6 July 2004. San Diego, CA: County of San Diego Health and Human Services Agency.

———. 2004b. State Dept. of Health Services says it is not West Nile virus. 7 July 2004. San Diego, CA: County of San Diego Health and Human Services Agency.

County of San Diego Board of Supervisors. 2004. *San Diego County child and family health and well-being: Report card 2004.* San Diego, CA: County of San Diego Health and Human Services Agency.

Coutinho, Marilla. 1999. Ninety years of Chagas' disease: A success story at the periphery. *Social Studies of Science* 29 (4): 519–549.

———, and Joao Carlos Pinta Dias. 1999. The rise and fall of Chagas' disease. *Perspectives on Science* 7: 447–485.

Cox, F. E. G. 1996. New World trypanosomiasis. In *The Wellcome Trust illustrated history of tropical diseases,* by F. E. G. Cox, 193–205. London: Wellcome Trust.

Cox, N. J., and K. Subbarao. 2000. Global epidemiology of influenza: Past and present. *Annual Review of Medicine* 51: 407–421.

Cox, Paul Alan, and Oliver W. Sacks. 2002. Cycad neurotoxins, consumption of flying foxes, and ALS-PDC disease in Guam. *Neurology* 58: 956–959.

Craib, Kevin J. P., Patricia M. Spittal, Evan Wood, Nancy Laliberte, Robert S. Hogg, Kathy Li, Katherine Heath, Mark W. Tyndall, Michael V. O'Shaughnessy, and Martin T. Schechter. 2003. Risk factors for elevated HIV incidence among Aboriginal drug users in Vancouver. *Canadian Medical Association Journal* 168 (2): 19–24.

Creighton, Charles. 1891. *A history of epidemics in Britain,* vol. 1, *From* A.D. *664 to the extinction of plague.* Cambridge: Cambridge University Press.

Crimp, Douglas, and Adam Roston. 1990. *AIDS demographics.* Seattle: Bay Press.

Crosby, Alfred W. 1972. *The Columbian exchange: Biological and cultural consequences of 1492.* Westport, CT: Greenwood.

———. 1989. *America's forgotten pandemic: The influenza of 1918.* Cambridge: Cambridge University Press. Originally published 1976 as *Epidemic and peace, 1918.*

———. 2003. *America's forgotten pandemic: The influenza of 1918.* 2nd ed. Cambridge: Cambridge University Press.

Cross, Eleanor, and Kenneth Hyams. 1996. The potential effect of global warming on the geographic and seasonal distribution of *Phlebotomus papatasi* in Southwest Asia. *Environmental Health Perspectives* 104: 724–727.

Crown, Margie, K. Duncan, M. Hurrell, R. Ootoova, R. Tremblay, and S. Yazdanmehr. 1993. Making HIV prevention work in the North. *Canadian Journal of Public Health* 84 (Supplement 1): S55–S58.

Cruz, R. 2002. Estrategías para el control del dengue y del *Aedes aegypti* en las Américas. *Revista Cubana de Medicina Tropical* 54: 189–201.

Cueto, Marcos. 2007. *Cold war, deadly fevers: Malaria eradication in Mexico, 1954–1971.* Baltimore, MD: Johns Hopkins University Press.

Cummings, D. A., R. A. Irizarry, N. E. Huang, T. P. Endy, A. Nisalak, K. Ungchusak, and D. S. Burke. 2004. Travelling waves in the occurrence of dengue haemorrhagic fever in Thailand. *Nature* 427: 344–347.

Daley, Daryl J., and J. M. Gani. 1999. *Epidemic modelling: An introduction.* Cambridge: Cambridge University Press.

Daniel, Thomas M. 1997. *Captain of death: The story of tuberculosis.* Rochester, NY: University of Rochester Press.

Dantes, H., J. Koopman, C. Addy, and M. E. A. Zárate. 1988. Dengue epidemics on the Pacific Coast of Mexico. *International Journal of Epidemiology* 17: 178–186.

Daragahi, Borzou. 2006. Iraq disputes war dead count; Officials call 600,000 far too high, while last month's Baghdad tally is put at more than 2,660. *Los Angeles Times*, 12 October, A4.

Dardagan, Hamit, John Sloboda, and Josh Dougherty. 2006. Reality checks: Some responses to the latest *Lancet* estimates. Press release no. 14, 16 October. *Iraq Body Count*, www.iraqbodycount.org/press/pr14.php.

Das, D., M. Baker, and L. Calder. 2006. Tuberculosis epidemiology in New Zealand, 1995–2004. *New Zealand Medical Journal* 119: U2249.

———, M. Baker, K. Venugopal, and S. McAllister. 2006. Why the tuberculosis rate is not falling in New Zealand. *New Zealand Medical Journal* 119: U2248.

Davis, M. 2005. *The monster at our door: The global threat of avian flu.* New York: Henry Holt.

Dawkins, K. 1996. The interaction of ethnicity, sociocultural factors and gender in clinical psychopharmacology. *Psychopharmacology Bulletin* 32 (2): 283–289.

Dawson, Peter. 2001. The relocation of Aboriginal people in Canada. PhD dissertation, York University, Toronto.

Dean, Hazel D., C. Brooke Steele, Anna J. Satcher, and Allyn K. Nakashima. 2005. HIV/AIDS among minority races and ethnicities in the United States, 1999–2003. *Journal of the National Medical Association* 97 (7): 5S–12S.

Decock, S., C. Verslype, and J. Fevery. 2007. Hepatitis C and insulin resistance: Mutual interactions. A review. *Acta Clinica Belgica* 62 (2): 111–119.

Dekuku, R. Chris, and Joseph Anang. 2003. Attempts at gaining some understanding of the possible factors that promote HIV/AIDS spread in Papua New Guinea. *Papua New Guinea Journal of Agriculture, Forestry and Fisheries* 46 (1–2): 31–39.

Delaporte, François. 1992. *Histoire de la fièvre jaune.* Paris: Payot.

———. 1999. *La maladie de Chagas: Histoire d'un féau continental.* Paris: Payot.

———. 2005. Chagas today. *Parassitologia* 47: 319–327.

Deloria, Philip. 2004. *Indians in unexpected places.* Lincoln: University of Nebraska Press.

Denny, Clark, D. Holtzman, and N. Cobb. 2003. Surveillance for health behaviors of American Indians and Alaskan Natives: Findings from behavioral risk factor surveillance system, 1997–2000. *Morbidity and Mortality Weekly Report, Surveillance Summaries* (Centers for Disease Control) 52 (SS-7): 5.

Dentith, Simon. 1995. *Bakhtinian thought*. New York: Routledge.

Department of Health. 1952. *TB among the Maori* (film). Wellington, New Zealand: Department of Health.

de Rocha Lima, Henrique. 1926. O diagnostico post mortem de febre amarella. *Folha Medica* 7: 169–172.

Deubel, V., R. M. Nogueira, M. T. Drouet, H. Zeller, J. M. Reynes, and D. Q. Ha. 1993. Direct sequencing of genomic cDNA fragments amplified by the polymerase chain reaction for molecular epidemiology of dengue-2 viruses. *Archives of Virology* 129: 197–210.

DeWitte, Sharon N., and James W. Wood. 2008. Selectivity of black death mortality with respect to preexisting health. *Proceedings of the National Academy of Sciences USA* 105 (5): 1436–1441.

De Zulueta, J., and C. Garret-Jones. 1965. An investigation of the persistence of malaria transmission in México. *American Journal of Tropical Medicine and Hygiene* 14 (1): 63–77.

Diamond, Catherine, A. Davidson, F. Sorvillo, and S. Buskin. 2001. HIV-infected American Indians/Alaska Natives in the western United States. *Ethnicity and Disease* 11: 633–643.

Diamond, Jared M. 1966. Zoological classification system of a primitive people. *Science* 151: 1102–1104.

Dias, Emmanuel. 1945. *Um ensaio de profilaxi de moléstia de Chagas*. Rio de Janeiro: Impresa Nacional.

Dickason, Olive Patricia. 1997. *Canada's First Nations: A history of founding peoples from the earliest times*. 2nd ed. Toronto: Oxford University Press.

Diekmann, O., and J. A. P. Heesterbeek. 2000. *Mathematical epidemiology of infectious diseases: Model building, analysis, and interpretation*. Chichester, UK: John Wiley.

DiLiberti, J. H., and C. R. Jackson. 1999. Long-term trends in childhood infectious disease mortality rates. *American Journal of Public Health* 89 (12): 1883.

Dinh, P., H. Long, N. Tien, N. Hien, L. Mai, L. Phong, L. Tan, N. Nguyen, P. Tu, and N. Phuong. 2006. Risk factors for human infection with avian influenza A H5N1, Vietnam, 2004. *Emerging Infectious Diseases* 12 (12): 1841–1847.

Doll, Richard. 1987. Major epidemics of the 20th century: From coronary thrombosis to AIDS. *Journal of the Royal Statistical Society, Series A* 150 (4): 373–395.

Dolman, Claude E., and Richard J. Wolfe. 2003. *Suppressing the diseases of animals and man: Theobald Smith, microbiologist*. Boston: Boston Medical Library.

Dominici, F., A. McDermott, S. L. Zeger, and J. M. Samet. 2003. Response to Dr. Smith: Timescale-dependent mortality effects of air polution. *American Journal of Epidemiology* 157: 1071–1073.

Doremus, Anne. 2001. Indigenism, mestizaje and national identity in México during the 1940s and 1950s. *Mexican Studies/Estudios Mexicanos* 17 (2): 375–402.

Dormandy, Thomas. 1999. *The white death: A history of tuberculosis.* New York: New York University Press.

Douglas, M. 1992. *Risk and blame: Essays in cultural theory.* London: Routledge.

Dow, D. A. 1999. *Maori health and government policy 1840–1940.* Wellington, New Zealand: Victoria University Press.

Dressler, William, and J. Bindon. 2000. The health consequences of cultural consonance: Cultural dimensions of lifestyle, social support, and blood pressure in an African American community. *American Anthropologist* 102 (2): 244–260.

Du Bois, M. J., P. Brassard, and C. Smeja. 1996. Survey of Montreal's Aboriginal population's knowledge, attitudes and behaviour regarding HIV/AIDS. *Canadian Journal of Public Health* 87 (1): 37–39.

Dubos, René. 1980 [1965]. *Man adapting.* Enlarged ed. New Haven, CT: Yale University Press.

———, and J. Dubos. 1952. *The white plague: Tuberculosis, man and society.* Boston: Little Brown.

Duffin, Jaclyn. 2005. *Lovers and livers: Disease concepts in history.* Toronto: University of Toronto Press.

Dulles, John F. 1954. Intervention of international communism in the Americas. *Department of State Bulletin* 30: 419–426.

Dunsford, D. 2008. The bright light of action and hope: Illuminating the complexity of tuberculosis in New Zealand in the 1940s. In *Multiplying and dividing: Tuberculosis in Canada and Aotearoa New Zealand,* edited by J. Littleton, J. Park, A. Herring, and T. Farmer, 179–186. Research in Anthropology and Linguistics, e series. Auckland: Anthropology Department, University of Auckland.

Duran, Bonnie, and Katrina Waters. 2004. HIV/AIDS prevention in "Indian country": Current practice, indigenist etiology models, and postcolonial approaches to change. *AIDS Education and Prevention* 16 (3): 187–201.

Duster, Troy. 2003. Buried alive: The concept of race in science. In *Genetic nature/culture: Anthropology and science beyond the two-culture divide,* edited by A. Goodman, D. Heath, and M. S. Lindee, 258–277. Berkeley: University of California Press.

Dye, Christopher, Suzanne Scheele, Paul Dolin, Vikram Pathania, and Mario C. Raviglione. 1999. Global burden of tuberculosis: Estimated incidence, prevalence, and mortality by country. *Journal of the American Medical Association* 282 (7): 677–686.

Ebi, Kristie, Rosalie Woodruff, Alexander von Hildebrand, and Carlos Corvalan. 2007. Climate-change-related health impacts in the Hindu Kush–Himalayas. *EcoHealth* 4 (3): 264–270.

Echeverri, Beatriz. 2003. Spanish influenza seen from Spain. In *The Spanish influenza pandemic of 1918–1919: New perspectives*, edited by H. Phillips and D. Killingray, 173–190. London: Routledge.

Ehrenkranz, N. J., A. K. Ventura, R. R. Cuadrado, W. L. Pond, and J. E. Porter. 1971. Pandemic dengue in Caribbean countries and the southern United States: Past, present, and potential problems. *New England Journal of Medicine* 285: 1460–1469.

Elliot, Tirah, Russel Kitau, and Joachim Pantumari. 2006. Abstract: Why sexually transmitted infections are high in Trobriand Islands. Paper presented at the eighteenth annual conference of the Australia Society for HIV Medicine, Melbourne, 11–14 October.

Elperin, Juliet. 2005. Scientists link global warming, disease. *Hartford Courant*, 17 November, 2.

Epstein, Helen. 2007. *The invisible cure: Africa, the West, and the fight against AIDS*. New York: Farrar, Straus and Giroux.

Epstein, Paul. 2005. Climate change and human health. *New England Journal of Medicine* 353: 1433–1436.

———. 2007. Chikunguny fever resurgence and global warming. *American Journal of Tropical Medicine and Hygiene* 76 (3): 403–404.

———, E. Chivian, and K. Frith. 2003. Emerging diseases threaten conservation. *Environmental Health Perspectives* 111 (10): A506.

———, and Evan Mills. 2005. *Climate change futures: Health, ecological and economic dimensions*. Cambridge, MA: Center for Health and the Global Environment, Harvard Medical School.

———, and Christine Rogers. 2004. *Inside the greenhouse: The impacts of CO_2 and climate change on public health in the inner city*. Cambridge, MA: Center for Health and the Global Environment, Harvard Medical School.

Escobar, C. Sergio. 1963. La erradicación del paludismo: Producto del esfuerzo conjunto nacional. *Salud Pública de México* 5: 727–731.

Estrada, A. L., J. R. Erickson, S. Stevens, and M. Fernandez. 1990. HIV risk behaviors among Native American IVDUs. Abstract. *International Conference on AIDS* 6: 270 (abstract no. F.C.757).

Ettling, John. 1981. *The germ of laziness: Rockefeller philanthropy and public health in the new South.* Cambridge, MA: Harvard University Press.

Evans, R. J. 1987. *Death in Hamburg: Society and politics in the cholera years 1830–1910.* Oxford: Clarendon Press.

Fabrega, Horacio, and Daniel Silver. 1973. *Illness and shamanistic curing in Zinacatán.* Stanford, CA: Stanford University Press.

Fagan, Brian. 2004. *The long summer: How climate changed civilization.* New York: Basic Books.

Fanning, Patricia J. 2008. The good, the bad and the immigrant: The 1918 influenza epidemic in a representative community. Paper presented at the Social Science History meetings, October, Miami, FL.

FAO (Food and Agriculture Organization of the United Nations). 2007. *The global strategy for prevention and control of H5N1 highly pathogenic avian influenza.* Rome: FAO.

Farmer, Paul. 1990. Sending sickness: Sorcery, politics, and changing concepts of AIDS in rural Haiti. *Medical Anthropology Quarterly,* n.s., 4 (1): 6–27.

———. 1992. *AIDS and accusation: Haiti and the geography of blame.* Berkeley: University of California Press.

———. 1999. *Infections and inequalities: The modern plagues.* Berkeley: University of California Press.

Favre, Henri. 1972. *Cambio y continuidad entre los Mayas de México.* Mexico City: Siglo XXI.

Fenner, Frank J., and F. N. Ratcliffe. 1965. *Myxomatosis.* Cambridge: Cambridge University Press.

Ferrie, Joseph P., and Werner Troesken. 2005. Water and Chicago's mortality transition, 1850–1925. *Explorations in Economic History* 45 (1): 1–16.

Finlay, Carlos. 1881. El mosquito hypoteticamente considerado como agente de transmisión de la la febra amarilla. *Annales de la Academia de Ciencias Médicas, Físicas y Naturales de la Habana* 28: 147–164. Reprinted in *Trabajos selectos,* by C. J. Finlay, 27–43. Havana: Secretaría de Sanidad y Beneficiencia, 1912.

———. 1894. Yellow fever: Immunity, modes of propagation, mosquito theory. *Comptes Rendus du Huitième Congrès International d'Hygiène et de Demographie, Budapest.* Reprinted in *Trabajos selectos,* by C. J. Finlay, 264–268. Havana: Secretaría de Sanidad y Beneficiencia, 1912.

Finn, C. 2006. The Maori problem? A political ecology of tuberculosis among Maori in Aotearoa/New Zealand between 1918 and 1945. Master's thesis, University of Auckland.

Fiske, Joanne. 2006. Political status of Native Indian women: Contradictory implications of Canadian state policy. In *In the days of our grandmothers: A reader in Aboriginal women's history in Canada*, edited by M.-E. Kelm and L. Townsend, 336–366. Toronto: University of Toronto Press.

Fixico, Donald L. 1986. *Termination and relocation: Federal Indian policy, 1945–1960*. Albuquerque: University of New Mexico Press.

———. 2006. *Daily life of Native Americans in the twentieth century*. Westport, CT: Greenwood.

Fleck, Ludwig. 1935. *Genesis and development of a scientific fact*. Chicago: University of Chicago Press.

Flexner, Simon. 1922. Experimental epidemiology. *Journal of Experimental Medicine* 36: 9–14.

Forget, G., and J. Lebel. 2001. An ecosystem approach to human health. *International Journal of Occupational and Environmental Health* 7 (Suppl. 2): S3–S36.

Fosdick, Raymond B. 1989. *The history of the Rockefeller Foundation*. New Brunswick, NJ: Transaction.

Foster, George M. 1969. *Applied anthropology*. Boston: Little, Brown.

———. 1976. Medical anthropology and international health planning. *Medical Anthropology Newsletter* 7 (3): 12–18.

Foster, John Bellamy. 2000. *Marx's ecology: Materialism and nature*. New York: Monthly Review Press.

Fox, Webster L. 1927. Trachoma among the North American Indians. *Hygeia* (February): 84–86.

Frank, Steven. 2003. Canada. *Time* magazine online edition, www.time.com/time/magazine/article/0,9171,447173,00.html?iid=chix-sphere.

Franks, Peter, Peter Muennig, Erica Lubetkin, and Haomiao Jia. 2006. The burden of disease associated with being African-American in the United States and the contribution of socio-economic status. *Social Science & Medicine* 62: 2469–2478.

Freudenberg, N., M. Fahs, S. Galea, and A. Greenberg. 2006. The impact of New York City's 1975 fiscal crisis on the tuberculosis, HIV, and homicide syndemic. *American Journal of Public Health* 96 (3): 424–434.

Friedland, R. P., and C. Armon. 2007. Tales of Pacific tangles: Cycad exposure and Guamanian neurodegenerative diseases. *Neurology* 68: 1759–1761.

Frohlich, Katherine, Nancy Ross, and Chantelle Richmond. 2006. Health disparities in Canada today: Some evidence and a theoretical framework. *Health Policy* 79: 132–143.

Frost, Wade Hampton. 1919. The epidemiology of influenza. *Public Health Reports* 34 (33): 1823–1835.

———. 1939. The age selection of mortality from tuberculosis in successive decades. *American Journal of Hygiene*, volume 30, section A (3): 91–96.

Fuente, Julio de la. 1941. Creencias indígenas sobre la onchocercosis, el paludismo y otras enfermedades. *América Indígena* 1 (1): 43–46.

Fuller-Higginson Papers. Agnes Higginson Fuller diary. Pocumtuck Valley Memorial Association Library, Deerfield, MA.

Gajdusek, D. Carleton. 1963. Kuru. *Transactions of the Royal Society of Tropical Medicine and Hygiene* 57 (3): 151–169.

———. 1971. *Journal of expeditions to the Soviet Union, Africa, the Islands of Madagascar, la Réunion and Mauritius, Indonesia, and to East and West New Guinea, Australia and Guam . . .*, 1 June 1969–3 March 1970. Bethesda, MD: National Institute of Neurological Diseases and Stroke.

———. 1977. Unconventional viruses and the origin and disappearance of kuru. *Science* 197 (4307): 943–960.

———. 1982. Foci of motor neuron diseases in high incidence in isolated populations of East Asia and western Pacific. In *Human Motor Neuron Disease,* edited by L. P. Rowland, 363–393. London: Pitman Books.

———. 1985. Interference with axonal transport of neurofilaments as the common etiology and pathogenesis of neurofibrillary tangles, ALS, PDC, and many other degenerations of the central nervous system: A series of hypotheses. *New England Journal of Medicine* 312: 714–719.

———. 1989. Cycad toxicity is not the cause of high incidence ALS/PDC on Guam, Kii peninsula of Japan, or in West New Guinea. In *ALS: Concepts in pathogenesis and etiology*, edited by A. J. Hudson, 317–324. Toronto: University of Toronto Press.

———. 1996. *Viliuisk encephalomyelitis: Journals of unrequited quests for etiology, 1976, 1979, 1991, 1992, 1993.* Bethesda, MD: National Institute of Neurological Diseases and Stroke.

———, C. J. Gibbs, and M. P. Alpers. 1966. Experimental transmission of a kuru-like syndrome to chimpanzees. *Nature* 209: 794–796.

———, and V. Zigas. 1957. Degenerative disease of the central nervous system in New Guinea. *New England Journal of Medicine* 257: 974–978.

Galdston, Iago, ed. 1954. *Beyond the germ theory: The roles of deprivation and stress in health and disease.* New York: New York Academy of Medicine.

Galishoff, Stuart. 1969. Newark and the great influenza pandemic of 1918. *Bulletin of the History of Medicine* 43 (3): 246–258.

Gambaryan, A., A. Tuzikov, G. Pazynina, N. Bovin, A. Balish, and A. Klimov. 2006. Evolution of the receptor binding phenotype of influenza A (H5) viruses. *Virology* 344 (2): 432–438.

Gandhi, N. R., A. Moll, A. Sturm, R. Pawinski, T. Govender, U. Laloo, K. Zeller, J. Andrews, and G. Friedland. 2006. Extensively drug-resistant tuberculosis as a cause of death in patients co-infected with tuberculosis and HIV in a rural area of South Africa. *Lancet* 368 (9547): 1575–1580.

García, Hernán, Antonio Sierra, and Gilberto Balám. 1999. *Wind in the blood: Maya healing and Chinese medicine.* Berkeley, CA: North Atlantic Books.

Garfield, Richard M. 2005. Nightingale in Iraq. *American Journal of Nursing* 105: 69–72.

———, and Alfred I. Neugut. 1991. Epidemiologic analysis of warfare: A historical review. *Journal of the American Medical Association* 266: 688–692.

Garmaise, David. 2003a. Commons committee recommends significant increase in funding for AIDS strategy. *Canadian HIV/AIDS Policy and Law Review* 8 (2): 24–25.

———. 2003b. Many people in marginalized communities are not accessing antiretroviral therapy: BC study. *Canadian HIV/AIDS Policy and Law Review* 8 (3): 27–28.

Garrison Quartermaster's Office. 1862. Gibraltar, 20 June. National Archives, Gibraltar.

Garruto, Ralph M., D. C. Gajdusek, and K. M. Chen. 1981. ALS and PDC among Filipino migrants to Guam. *Annals of Neurology* 10: 341–350.

———, M. A. Little, G. D. James, and D. E. Brown. 1999. Natural experimental models: The global search for biomedical paradigms among traditional, modernizing, and modern populations. *Proceedings of the National Academy of Sciences USA* 96: 10536–10543.

———, R. Yanagihara, and D. C. Gajdusck. 1985. Disappearance of high-incidence ALS and PDC on Guam. *Neurology* 35: 193–198.

———, and Yoshiro Yase. 1986. Neurodegenerative disorders in the western Pacific: The search for mechanisms of pathogenesis. *Trends in Neuroscience* 9: 368–374.

Gauthier-Clerc, M., C. Lebarbenchon, and F. Thomas. 2007. Recent expansion of highly pathogenic avian influenza H5N1: A critical review. *Ibis* 149 (2): 202–214.

Geger, Michael. 2006. *Bird flu: A virus of our own hatching.* New York: Lantern Books.

Gershman, J., and A. Irwin. 1999. Getting a grip on the global economy. In *Dying for growth: Global inequality and the health of the poor,* edited by J. Y. Kim, J. Millen, J. Gershman, and A. Irwin, 11–43. Monroe, ME: Common Courage Press.

Gibbons, R. V., and D. W. Vaughn. 2002. Dengue: An escalating problem. *British Medical Journal* 324: 1563–1566.

Gibbs, C. J., Jr. 1982. An update on long-term in vivo studies designed to identify a virus as the cause of ALS, PDC, and PD. *Advances in Neurology* 56: 343–353.

————, and D. C. Gajdusek. 1965. Attempts to demonstrate a transmissible agent in kuru, ALS, and other subacute and chronic progressive nervous system degenerations of man. In *Slow, latent, and temperate virus infections,* edited by D. C. Gajdusek, C. J. Gibbs Jr., and M. Alpers, 39–48. Washington, DC: National Institute of Neurological Diseases and Blindness.

————, and D. C. Gajdusek. 1972. ALS, PD, and ALS/PDC on Guam: A review and summary of attempts to determine infection as etiology. *Journal of Clinical Pathology* 25 (Supplement 6): 132–140.

Gibbs, M. J., and A. J. Gibbs. 2006. Was the 1918 pandemic caused by a bird flu? *Nature* 440 (9): E8.

Giere, Ronald N. 1999. *Science without laws: Science and its conceptual foundations.* Chicago: University of Chicago Press.

Gilbert, A. 1994. *The Latin American city.* London: Latin American Bureau.

Giles, Jim. 2006. Iraqi death toll withstands scrutiny. *Nature,* 19 October, 728–729.

Gilley, Brian Joseph, and John Hawk Co-Cke. 2005. Cultural investment: Providing opportunities to reduce risky behavior among gay American Indian males. *Journal of Psychoactive Drugs* 37 (3): 293–298.

Gilman, Sander. 1988. *Disease and representation: Images of illness from madness to AIDS.* Ithaca, NY: Cornell University Press.

Giménez, Lulú, and Angela Hernández. 1988. *Estructura de los medios de diffusión en Venezuela.* Caracas: Universidad Católica Andrés Bello.

Ginzburg, Carlo. 1980. Morelli, Freud and Sherlock Holmes: Clues and scientific method. *History Workshop* 9: 5–36.

Glantz, Stanton A., John Slade, Lisa A. Bero, Peter Hanauer, and Deborah E. Barnes, eds. 1998. *The cigarette papers.* Berkeley: University of California Press.

Glass, R. I., and R. E. Black. 1992. The epidemiology of cholera. In *Cholera,* edited by D. Barua and W. B. Greenough, 129–154. New York: Plenum Medical Book Company.

Glasse, Robert M. 1962a. The spread of kuru among the Fore. Mimeograph. New Guinea Department of Public Health. Reissued 1963, Bethesda, MD: National Institutes of Health.

———. 1962b. Cannibalism in the kuru region. Mimeograph. Papua New Guinea Department of Public Health. Reissued 1963, Bethesda, MD: National Institutes of Health.

———, and Shirley Glasse. 1963. Report to the director of public health of fieldwork by R. M. and S. Glasse. November 1962–April 1963. Archives of the Papua New Guinea Department of Public Health.

———, and Shirley Lindenbaum. 1969. South Fore politics. *Anthropological Forum* 2. Reprinted in *Politics in New Guinea: Traditional and in the context of change. Some anthropological perspectives,* edited by R. M. Berndt and P. Lawrence, 362–377. Perth: University of Western Australia Press, 1971.

———, and Shirley Lindenbaum. 1976. Kuru at Wanitabe. In *Essays on kuru,* edited by R. W. Hornabrook, 8–52. Farringdon, UK: E. W. Classey.

———, and Shirley Lindenbaum. 1980. South Fore kinship. In *Blood and semen: Kinship systems of highland New Guinea,* edited by V. Carroll, 441–462. Ann Arbor: University of Michigan Press.

———, and Shirley Lindenbaum. 1992. Fieldwork in the South Fore: The process of ethnographic enquiry. In *Prion diseases of humans and animals,* edited by S. Prusiner, J. Collinge, J. Powell, and B. Anderton, 77–91. London: Ellis Horwood.

Glasse, Shirley. 1964. The social effects of kuru. *Papua New Guinea Medical Journal* 7: 36–47.

Glennon, John P., ed. 1987. *Foreign relations of the United States, 1955–1957: American republics; Multilateral; Mexico; Caribbean.* Washington, DC: Government Printing Office.

Goffman, Erving. 1981. *Forms of talk.* Philadelphia: University of Pennsylvania Press.

Goldberg, Myla. 2005. *Wickett's remedy.* New York: Anchor Books.

Goldfarb, Lev G., and D. C. Gajdusek. 1992. Viliuisk encephalomyelitis in the Iakut people of Siberia. *Brain* 115: 961–978.

Goldman, N., and G. Lord. 1986. A new look at entropy and the life table. *Demography* 23: 275–282.

Golubovsky, M. D. 1980. Mutational process and microevolution. *Genetica* 52–53: 139–149.

Goodreau, Steven M. 2006. Assessing the effects of human mixing patterns on human immunodeficiency virus-1 interhost phylogenetics through social network simulation. *Genetics* 172 (4): 2033–2045.

———, L. P. Goicochea, and J. Sanchez. 2005. Sexual role and transmission of HIV Type 1 among men who have sex with men, in Peru. *Journal of Infectious Diseases* 191 (Supplement 1): S147–158.

González, Yólotl, ed. 1989. *Homenaje a Isabel Kelly.* Mexico City: Instituto Nacional de Antropología e Historia.

Gordon, Deborah R. 1988. Tenacious assumptions in Western medicine. In *Biomedicine examined,* edited by M. Lock and D. Gordon, 19–56. London: Kluwer Academic.

Gore Gillon, G. 1901. A factor in open-air treatment. *New Zealand Medical Journal* 2: 1.

Gorgas, William C. 1903. Recent experience of the United States Army with regard to sanitation of yellow fever in the tropics. *Journal of Tropical Medicine* 6: 49–52.

GRAIN. 2006. *Fowl play: The poultry industry's central role in the bird flu crisis.* GRAIN Briefing, February 2006. Electronic document, www.grain.org/briefings/?id=194.

Gratz, N. 1999. Emerging and resurging vector-borne diseases. *Annual Review of Entomology* 44: 51–75.

Gray, G., and D. Ropeik. 2002. Dealing with the dangers of fear: The role of risk communication. *Health Affairs* 21 (6): 106–116.

Greaves, T. 2005. Water struggles of indigenous North America. In *Globalization, water and health,* edited by L. Whiteford and S. Whiteford, 153–184. Santa Fe, NM: School of American Research Press.

Green, D. 1997. *Faces of Latin America.* London: Latin American Bureau.

Green, M. S., T. Swartz, E. Mayshar, B. Lev, A. Leventhal, and P. E. Salter. 2002. When is an epidemic an epidemic? *Israel Medical Association Journal* 4: 3–6.

Greenwood, Major. 1919. The epidemiological point of view. *British Medical Journal* 2: 405–407.

Grigsby, J. S. 1991. Paths for future population aging. *Gerontologist* 31 (2): 195–203.

Grmek, Mirko D. 1969. Préliminaires d'une étude historique des maladies. *Annales: Économies, Sociétés, Civilisations* 24 (6): 1473–1483.

———. 1990. *History of AIDS: Emergence and origins of a modern pandemic.* Princeton, NJ: Princeton University Press.

Groisman, Pavel, Richard Knight, Thomas Karl, David Easterling, Bomin Sun, and Jay Lawrimore. 2004. Contemporary changes of the hydrological cycle over the contiguous United States: Trends derived from in situ observations. *Journal of Hydrometeorology* 5 (1): 64–85.

Groot, H. 1980. The reinvasion of Colombia by *Aedes aegypti:* Aspects to remember. *American Journal of Tropical Medicine and Hygiene* 29: 330–338.

Gross, J. E. 1866. Rough notes of the cholera epidemic at the government prison. *Medical Times and Gazette,* Gibraltar.

Gubler, D. J. 1987. Dengue and dengue hemorrhagic fever in the Americas. *Puerto Rico Health Sciences Journal* 6: 107–111.

———. 1989. *Aedes aegypti* and *Aedes aegypti*-borne disease control in the 1990s: Top down or bottom up. *American Journal of Tropical Medicine and Hygiene* 40: 571–578.

———. 1997. Dengue and dengue hemorrhagic fever: Its history and resurgence as a global public health problem. In *Dengue and dengue homorrhagic fever,* edited by D. J. Gubler and G. Kuno, 1–22. London: CAB International.

———. 1998. Dengue and dengue hemorrhagic fever. *Clinical Microbiology Reviews* 11: 480–496.

———. 2002. Epidemic dengue/dengue hemorrhagic fever as a public health, social and economic problem in the twenty-first century. *Trends in Microbiology* 10: 100–103.

———. 2004a. The changing epidemiology of yellow fever and dengue, 1900 to 2003: Full circle? *Comparative Immunology, Microbiology and Infectious Diseases* 27: 319–330.

———. 2004b. Cities spawn epidemic dengue viruses. *Nature Medicine* 10: 129–130.

———, and G. G. Clark. 1996. Community involvement in the control of *Aedes aegypti. Acta Tropica* 61: 169–179.

———, and D. W. Trent. 1993. Emergence of epidemic dengue/dengue hemorrhagic fever as a public health problem in the Americas. *Infectious Agents and Disease* 2: 383–393.

Guenter, C. D., K. Fonseca, D. M. Nielsen, V. J. Wheeler, and C. P. Pim. 2000. HIV prevalence remains low among Calgary's needle exchange program participants. *Canadian Journal of Public Health* 91 (2): 129–32.

Gusmão, H. H. 1982. Fighting disease-bearing mosquitoes through relentless field leadership. *American Journal of Tropical Medicine and Hygiene* 31: 705–710.

Guterman, Lila. 2005. Dead Iraqis: Why an estimate was ignored. *Columbia Journalism Review* 43 (6): 11.

Gutmann, Matthew C. 2003. *Changing men and masculinities in Latin America.* Durham, NC: Duke University Press.

Guzmán, M. G. 2001. Enfermedades virales emergentes. *Revista Cubana de Medicina Tropical* 53: 5–15.

————, V. Deubel, J. L. Pelegrino, D. Rosario, M. Marrero, C. Sariol, and G. Kourí. 1995. Partial nucleotide and amino acid sequences of the envelope and the envelope/nonstructural protein-1 gene junction of four dengue-2 virus strains isolated during the 1981 Cuban epidemic. *American Journal of Tropical Medicine and Hygiene* 52: 241–246.

————, and G. Kourí. 2002. Dengue: An update. *Lancet Infectious Diseases* 2: 33–42.

————, and G. Kourí. 2003. Dengue and dengue hemorrhagic fever in the Americas: Lessons and challenges. *Journal of Clinical Virology* 27 (1): 1–13.

————, G. Kourí, J. Bravo, M. Soler, S. Vázquez, and L. Morier. 1990. Dengue hemorrhagic fever in Cuba, 1981: A retrospective seroepidemiologic study. *American Journal of Tropical Medicine and Hygiene* 42: 179–184.

————, G. Kourí, J. Bravo, L. Valdés, S. Vázquez, and S. Halstead. 2002. Effect of age on outcome of secondary dengue 2 infection. *International Journal of Infectious Diseases* 6: 118–124.

————, G. Kourí, L. Valdés, J. Bravo, M. Álvarez, S. Vázques, I. Delgado, and S. B. Halstead. 2000. Epidemiologic studies on dengue in Santiago de Cuba, 1997. *American Journal of Epidemiology* 152: 793–799.

————, C. Triana, J. Bravo, and G. Kourí. 1992. Estimación de las afectaciones económicas causadas como consecuencia de la epidemia de dengue hemorrágico ocurrida en Cuba en 1981. *Revista Cubana de Medicina Tropical* 44: 13–17.

————, S. Vázquez, E. Martínez, M. Álvarez, R. Rodríguez, G. Kourí, J. de los Reyes, and F. Acevedo. 1996. [Dengue in Nicaragua, 1994: Reintroduction of serotype 3 in the Americas]. *Boletín de la Oficina Sanitaria Panamericana* 121: 102–110.

Hackett, Paul. 2005. From past to present: Understanding First Nations health patterns in a historical context. *Canadian Journal of Public Health* 96 (Supplement 1): S17–S21.

Haefner, James W. 2005. *Modeling biological systems: Principles and applications.* 2nd ed. New York: Springer.

Hage, G. 1998. *White nation: Fantasies of white supremacy in a multicultural society.* Annandale, Australia: Pluto Press.

Hahn, B. H., G. M. Shaw, K. M. Cock, and P. Sharp. 2000. AIDS as a zoonosis: Scientific and public health implications. *Science* 287 (5453): 607–614.

Haley, Nicole. 2008. When there's no accessing basic health care: Local politics and responses to HIV/AIDS at Lake Kopiago, Papua New Guinea. In *Making sense of AIDS: Culture, sexuality and power in*

Melanesia, edited by L. Butt and R. Eves, 24–40. Honolulu: University of Hawaii Press.

Hall, P., and U. Pfeiffer. 2000. *Background report on the World Report on the Urban Future.* Berlin: Federal Ministry of Transport, Building and Housing of the Federal Republic of Germany.

Hall, Roberta L., D. Wilder, P. Bodenroeder, and M. Hess. 1990. Assessment of AIDS knowledge, attitudes, behaviors, and risk level in northwestern American Indians. *American Journal of Public Health* 80: 875–877.

Hall, Stuart. 1985. Signification, representation, ideology: Althusser and the post-structuralist debates. *Critical Studies in Mass Communication* 2 (2): 91–114.

Halstead, S. B. 1988. Pathogenesis of dengue: Challenges to molecular biology. *Science* 239: 476–481.

———. 1997. Epidemiology of dengue and dengue hemorrhagic fever. In *Dengue and dengue hemorrhagic fever,* edited by D. J. Gubler and G. Kuno, 23–44. London: CAB International.

———, S. Nimmannitya, and S. N. Cohen. 1970. Observations related to pathogenesis of dengue hemorrhagic fever, 4: Relation of disease severity to antibody response and virus recovered. *Yale Journal of Biology and Medicine* 42: 311–328.

———, S. Nimmannitya, C. Yamarat, and P. K. Russell. 1967. Hemorrhagic fever in Thailand: Recent knowledge regarding etiology. *Japanese Journal of Medical Science and Biology* 20: 96–103.

———, T. G. Streit, J. G. Lafontant, R. Putvatana, K. Russell, W. Sun, N. Kanesa-Thasan, C. G. Hayes, and D. M. Watts. 2001. Haiti: Absence of dengue hemorrhagic fever despite hyperendemic dengue virus transmission. *American Journal of Tropical Medicine and Hygiene* 65: 180–183.

Hammar, Lawrence. 2007. Epilogue: Homegrown in PNG—Rural responses to HIV and AIDS. Special issue on HIV/AIDS in Rural Papua New Guinea, edited by A. Dundon and C. Wilde. *Oceania* 77 (1): 72–94.

Hammond, Evvelynn. 1997. Seeing AIDS: Race, gender and representation. In *The gender politics of HIV/AIDS in women: Perspectives on the pandemic in the United States,* edited by N. Goldstein and J. Manlowe, 113–126. New York: New York University Press.

Handcock, M. S., and J. H. Jones. 2004. Likelihood-based inference for stochastic models of sexual network formation. *Theoretical Population Biology* 65 (4): 413–422.

Harris, Cole. 2002. *Making Native space*. Vancouver: University of British Columbia Press.

Harrison, Λ. 2000. Tuberculosis in New Zealand: Why do we have twice as much as Australia? *New Zealand Medical Journal* 113: 68–69.

Hayner, Priscilla B. 2001. *Unspeakable truths: Confronting state terror and atrocity*. New York: Routledge.

Heath, K., Peter G. A. Cornelisse, Steffanie A. Strathdee, Anita Palepu, Mary-Lou Miller, Martin T. Schechter, Michael V. O'Shaughnessy, and Robert S. Hogg. 1999. HIV-associated risk factors among young Canadian Aboriginal and non-Aboriginal men who have sex with men. *International Journal of STD and AIDS* 10 (9): 582–587.

Herman, Edward S., and Noam Chomsky. 1988. *Manufacturing consent: The political economy of the mass media*. New York: Pantheon.

Hernández Llamas, Héctor, ed. 1984. *La atención médica rural en México, 1930–1980*. Mexico City: Instituto Mexicano del Seguro Social.

Heron, Melonie P., and Betty L. Smith. 2007. Deaths: Leading causes for 2003. *National Vital Statistics Reports* 55 (10). Hyattsville, MD: National Center for Health Statistics.

Herring, D. Ann. 2008. Viral panic, vulnerability and the next pandemic. In *Health, risk, and adversity: A contextual view from anthropology*, edited by C. Panter-Brick and A. Fuentes, 78–97. Oxford: Berghan.

———, and Lisa Sattenspiel. 2007. Social contexts, syndemics, and infectious disease in northern Aboriginal populations. *American Journal of Human Biology* 19 (2): 190–202.

Heymann, Jody. 2005. *Forgotten families: Ending the growing crisis confronting children and working parents in the global economy*. Oxford: Oxford University Press.

Hildreth, Martha L. 1991. The influenza epidemic of 1918–1919 in France: Contemporary concepts of etiology, therapy, and prevention. *Social History of Medicine* 4 (2): 277–294.

Hill, K., and L. R. Pebley. 1989. Child mortality in the developing world. *Population and Development Review* 15 (4): 657–687.

Hirano, A., L. T. Kurland, R. S. Krooth, and S. Lessell. 1961. PDC and endemic disease on the island of Guam, 2: Pathologic features. *Brain* 84: 622–679.

Hobfoll, Stevan E., Anita Bansal, Rebecca Schurg, Sarah Young, Charles A. Pierce, Ivonee Hobfoll, and Robert Johnson. 2002. The impact of perceived child physical and sexual abuse history on Native American women's psychological well-being and AIDS risk. *Journal of Consulting and Clinical Psychology* 70 (1): 252–257.

Hoffman, Frederick. 1930. Are the Indians dying out? *American Journal of Public Health* 20: 609–614.

Holbrooke, Richard C., and Laurie Garrett. 2008. When "sovereignty" risks global health. *Mmegi Online* 25 (139). Electronic document, www.mmegi.bw/index.php?sid=2&aid=19&dir=2008/September/Thursday18.

Hollenbeck, J. E. 2005. An avian connection as a catalyst to the 1918–1919 influenza pandemic. *International Journal of Medical Science* 2 (2): 97–90.

Holman, P. B., W. C. Jenkins, J. A. Gayle, C. Duncan, and B. K. Lindsey. 1991. Increasing the involvement of national and regional racial and ethnic minority organizations in HIV information and education. *Public Health Reports* 106 (6): 687–694.

Holman, Sheri. 2000. *The dress lodger.* New York: Ballantine Books.

Holmes, E. C., and S. S. Burch. 2000. The causes and consequences of genetic variation in dengue virus. *Trends in Microbiology* 8: 74–77.

———, and S. S. Twiddy. 2003. The origin, emergence and evolutionary genetics of dengue virus. *Infections, Genetics and Evolution* 3: 19–28.

Hota, Bala, Charlotte Ellenbogen, Mary Hayden, Alla Aroutcheva, Thomas Rice, and Robert Weinstein. 2007. Community-associated methicillin-resistant *Staphylococcus aureus:* Skin and soft tissue infections at a public hospital. *Archives of Internal Medicine* 167: 1026–1033.

Hotez, Peter J., Jeff Bethony, Maria Elena Botazzi, Simon Brooker, and Paolo Buss. 2005. Hookworm: The great infection of mankind. *PloS Medicine* 2 (3): 1–9.

Houghton, J., Y. Ding, and D. Griggs, eds. 2001. *Climate change 2001: The scientific basis. Contribution of Working Group I to the Third Assessment Report to the Intergovernmental Panel on Climate Change.* Cambridge: Cambridge University Press.

Houghton, P. 1980. *The first New Zealanders.* London: Hodder and Stoughton.

Houston, Stan. 2004. Sentinal surveillance of HIV and hepatitis C virus in two urban emergency departments. *Journal of Canadian Association of Emergency Physicians* 6 (2): 89–97.

Howard, H. H. 1919. *The control of hookworm disease by the intensive method.* New York: Rockefeller Foundation–International Health Board.

Howe, G. M. 1977. *A world geography of human diseases.* New York: Academic Press.

Hughes, Jenny. 1997. A history of sexually transmitted diseases in Papua New Guinea. In *Sex, disease, and society: A comparative history of sexually transmitted diseases and HIV/AIDS in Asia and the Pacific*, edited by M. Lewis, S.Bamber, and M. Waugh, 231–248. Westport, CT: Greenwood Press.

Humphreys, Margaret. 2002. No safe place: Disease and panic in American history. *American Literary History* 14 (4): 845–857.

Ingham, John M. 1984. Human sacrifices at Tenochitlan. *Comparative Studies in Society and History* 16: 379–400.

Inhorn, Marcia C., and Peter J. Brown. 1990. The anthropology of infectious disease. *Annual Review of Anthropology* 19: 89–117.

Institute of Medicine. 2000. *To err is human: Building a safer health system*. Washington, DC: National Academies Press.

Instituto Nacional Indigenista. 1955. *¿Que es el INI?* Mexico City: Instituto Nacional Indigenista.

———. 1994. *Diccionario enciclopédico de la medicina tradicional mexicana*. Mexico City: Instituto Nacional Indigenista.

International Cooperation Administration. 1956. *Technical cooperation in health*. Washington, DC: n.p.

Iraq Family Health Survey Study Group. 2008. Violence-related mortality in Iraq from 2002 to 2006. *New England Journal of Medicine* 358: 484–493.

Istúriz, R. E., D. J. Gubler, and J. Brea del Castillo. 2000. Dengue and dengue hemorrhagic fever in Latin America and the Caribbean. *Infectious Disease Clinics of North America* 14: 121–140, ix.

Ito, T., J. N. S. S. Couceiro, S. Kelm, L. G. Baum, S. Krauss, M. R. Castrucci, I. Donatelli, et al. 1998. Molecular basis for the generation in pigs of influenza A viruses with pandemic potential. *Journal of Virology* (September): 7367–7373.

Ito, Toshihiro, Hiroshi Kida, and Yoshihiro Kawaoka. 1996. Receptors of Influenza A viruses: Implications for the Role of pigs for the generation of pandemic human influenza strains. In *Options for the control of influenza*, edited by L. E. Brown, A. W. Hampson, and R. G. Webster, 516–519. Amsterdam: Elsevier.

Jacobs, Geert. 1999. *Preformulating the news: An analysis of the meta-pragmatics of press releases*. Amsterdam: John Benjamins.

Janabi, Ahmed. 2004. Iraqi group: Civilian toll over 37,000. Electronic document, http://english.aljazeera.net/archive/2004/07/200849155555897934.html.

Janes, Craig, Ron Stall, and Sandra M. Gifford, eds. 1986. *Anthropology and epidemiology: Interdisciplinary approaches to the study of disease*. Dordrecht, Netherlands: De. Reidel.

Johnson, Niall P. A. S. 2006. *Britain and the 1918–1919 influenza pandemic: A dark epilogue*. London: Routledge.

———, and Juergen Mueller. 2002. Updating the accounts: Global mortality of the 1918–1920 "Spanish" influenza pandemic. *Bulletin of the History of Medicine* 76 (1): 105–115.

Jones, David S. 2004. *Rationalizing epidemics: Meanings and uses of American Indian mortality since 1600*. Cambridge, MA: Harvard University Press.

Jones, Esyllt W. 2005. "Co-operation in all human endeavour": Quarantine and immigrant disease vectors in the 1918–1919 influenza pandemic in Winnipeg. *Canadian Bulletin of Medical History* 22 (1): 57–82.

Jones, J. H., and M. S. Handcock. 2003a. An assessment of preferential attachment as a mechanism for human sexual network formation. *Proceedings of the Royal Society of London, Series B, Biological Sciences* 270 (1520): 1123–1128.

———. 2003b. Sexual contacts and epidemic thresholds. *Nature* 423 (6940): 605–606.

Jordan, E. O. 1927. *Epidemic influenza: A survey*. Chicago: American Medical Association.

Joseph, Gilbert M., and Daniel Nugent, eds. 1994. *Everyday forms of state formation*. Durham, NC: Duke University Press.

Kabra, S. K., Y. Jain, R. M. Pandey, Madhulika, T. Singhal, P. Tripathi, S. Broor, P. Seth, and V. Seth. 1999. Dengue haemorrhagic fever in children in the 1996 Delhi epidemic. *Transactions of the Royal Society of Tropical Medicine and Hygiene* 93: 294–298.

Kalayanarooj, S., and S. Nimmannitya. 2005. Is dengue severity related to nutritional status? *Southeast Asian Journal of Tropical Medicine and Public Health* 36: 378–384.

Katz, Robert S. 1974. Influenza 1918–1919: A study in mortality. *Bulletin of the History of Medicine* 48 (3): 416–422.

———. 1977. Influenza 1918–1919: A further study in mortality. *Bulletin of the History of Medicine* 51 (4): 617–619.

Kaufman, Joan. 2008. China's health care system and avian influenza preparedness. *Journal of Infectious Disease* 197: S7–13.

Kawaoka, Yoshihiro. 2007. Aberrant innate immune response in lethal infection of macaques with the 1918 influenza virus. *Nature* 445 (18): 319–323.

Kelly, Isabel. 1955. El adiestramiento de parteras en México desde el punto de vista antropológico. *América Indígena* 15 (2): 109–117.

———. 1965. *Folk practices in North Mexico: Birth customs, folklore, medicine, and spiritualism in the Laguna zone*. Austin: University of Texas Press.

Kelm, Mary-Ellen. 1998. *Colonizing bodies: Aboriginal health and healing in British Columbia 1900–1950*. Vancouver: University of British Columbia Press.

———. 2004. Diagnosing the discursive Indian: Disease and sexuality in turn-of-the-century medical journals. *Ethnohistory* 52: 371–406.

Kermack, W. O., and A. G. McKendrick. 1927. A contribution to the mathematical theory of epidemics. *Proceedings of the Royal Society of London, Series A* 115: 700–721.

Kerr, A. 1972. TB and Polynesians (letter to the editor). *New Zealand Medical Journal* 76: 295.

Kilbourne, Edwin D. 1987. *Influenza*. New York: Plenum Medical Book Company.

———. 2006. Influenza pandemics of the 20th century. *Emerging Infectious Diseases* 12 (1): 9–14.

Killingray, David. 1994. The influenza pandemic of 1918–1919 in the British Caribbean. *Social History of Medicine* 7 (1): 59–87.

Kilpatrick, A. M., A. A. Chmura, D. Gibbons, R. Fleischer, P. Marra, and P. Daszak. 2006. Predicting the global spread of H5N1 avian influenza. *Proceedings of the National Academy of Sciences USA* 103 (51): 19368–19373.

Kinsella, Kevin, and Victoria A. Velkoff. 2001. *An aging world: 2001*. Washington, DC: US Census Bureau.

Kirchov, L. V. 1993. American trypasonomiasis (Chagas' disease). *New England Journal of Medicine* 329 (9): 639–644.

Kitagawa, Evelyn M., and Philip M. Hauser. 1973. *Differential mortality in the United States: A study in socioeconomic epidemiology*. Cambridge, MA: Harvard University Press.

Kliks, M. M. 1983. Parasitology: On the origins and impact of human-helminth relationships. In *Human ecology and infectious disease,* edited by N. A. Croll and J. H. Cross, 291–313. New York: Academic Press.

Klinenberg, Eric. 2002. *Heat wave: A social autopsy of disaster in Chicago*. Chicago: University of Chicago Press.

Knight, Alan. 1990. Racism, revolution and indigenismo: México, 1910–1940. In *The idea of race in Latin America*, edited by R. Graham, 71–113. Austin: University of Texas Press.

Knudsen, A., and R. Slooff. 1992. Vector-borne disease problems in rapid urbanization: New approaches to vector control. *Bulletin of the World Health Organization* 70: 1–6.

Kobasa, D., A. Takada, K. Shinya, M. Hatta, and P. Halfman. 2004. Enhanced virulence of influenza A viruses with the haemagglutinin of the 1918 pandemic virus. *Nature* 431 (7009): 703–707.

Kolata, Gina Bari. 1999. *Flu: The story of the great influenza pandemic of 1918 and the search for the virus that caused it.* New York: Farrar, Straus and Giroux.

Korns, John H. 1937. Comparative tuberculosis findings among Indians and white persons in Cattaraugus County, New York. *American Review of Tuberculosis* 34: 550–560.

Kourí, G., M. G. Guzmán, and J. R. Bravo. 1986. Hemorrhagic dengue in Cuba: History of an epidemic. *Bulletin of the Pan American Health Organization* 20: 24–30.

———, M. G. Guzmán, J. R. Bravo, and C. Triana. 1989. Dengue haemorrhagic fever/dengue shock syndrome: Lessons from the Cuban epidemic, 1981. *Bulletin of the World Health Organization* 67: 375–380.

Krause, Roland. 2006. The swine flu episode and the fog of epidemics. *Emerging Infectious Disease* 12: 40–43.

Kretzschmar, M., and M. Morris. 1996. Measures of concurrency in networks and the spread of infectious disease. *Mathematical Biosciences* 133 (2): 165–195.

Krieger, Nancy. 2000. Epidemiology and the social sciences: Toward a critical reengagement in the twenty-first century. *Epidemiological Reviews* 11: 155–163.

———. 2001. Theories for social epidemiology in the twenty-first century: An ecosocial perspective. *International Journal of Epidemiology* 30: 668–677.

———. 2007. Why epidemiologists cannot afford to ignore poverty. *Epidemiology* 18: 658–662.

———, and Stephen Sidney. 1996. Racial discrimination and blood pressure: The CARDIA study of young black and white adults. *American Journal of Public Health* 86: 1370–1378.

Kristensson, Krister. 2005. Avian influenza and the brain: Comments on the occasion of resurrection of the Spanish flu virus. *Brain Research Bulletin* 68 (6): 405–413.

Kroeger, A., U. Dehlinger, G. Burkhardt, W. Atehortua, H. Anaya, and N. Becker. 1995. Community based dengue control in Columbia: People's knowledge and practice and the potential contribution of the biological larvicide Bti (*Bacillus thuringiensis israelensis*). *Tropical Medicine and Parasitology* 46: 241–246.

———, M. Nathan, and J. Hombach. 2004. Focus: Dengue. *Nature Reviews Microbiology* 2 (5): 360–361.

Kuhn, K., D. Campbell-Lendrum, A. Haines, and J. Cox. 2005. *Using climate to predict infectious disease epidemics.* Geneva: World Health Organization.

Kuhn, Thomas S. 1962. *The structure of scientific revolutions*. Chicago: University of Chicago Press.

Kunitz, Stephen J. 1987. Explanations and ideologies of mortality patterns. *Population and Development Review* 13 (3): 379–408.

Kurland, Leonard T., and Donald W. Mulder. 1954. Epidemiological investigations of ALS, 1: Preliminary report on geographic distribution, with special reference to the Mariana Islands, including clinical and pathological observations. *Neurology* 4: 355–378, 438–448.

Lachmann, Mark. 2002. Human immunodeficiency virus: Emerging epidemic in Aboriginal people. *Canadian Family Physician* 48 (October): 1592–1593, 1600–1601.

Lange, R. 1999. *May the people live: A history of Maori health development, 1900–1920*. Auckland: University of Auckland Press.

Langford, Christopher. 2005. Did the 1918–1919 influenza pandemic originate in China? *Population and Development Review* 31 (3): 473–505.

Laranja, Francesco, Emannuel Dias, and G. Nobera. 1948. Clinica et terapeutica da doenca de Chaga. *Memorias do Instituto Oswaldo Cruz* 46 (2): 473–529.

Last, John, ed. 2001. *A dictionary of epidemiology*, 4th ed. Oxford: Oxford University Press.

Latour, Bruno. 1988. *The Pasteurization of France*. Translated by A. Sheridan and J. Law. Cambridge, MA: Harvard University Press.

———, and Stephen Woolgar. 1979. *Laboratory life: The social construction of scientific facts*. Beverly Hills, CA: Sage Publications.

Laumann, Edward O. 1994. *The social organization of sexuality: Sexual practices in the United States*. Chicago: University of Chicago Press.

Lawless, Jill. 2007. British backtrack on Iraq death toll. *The Independent*, 27 March, www.independent.co.uk/news/world/middle-east/british-backtrack-on-iraq-death-toll-442026.html.

Lawrence, J., R. Kearns, J. Park, L. Bryder, and H. Worth. 2008. Discourses of disease: Representations of tuberculosis within New Zealand newspapers. *Social Science & Medicine* 66: 727–739.

Layne, Scott P., Tony J. Beugelsdijk, C. Kumar, N. Patel, Jeffrey K. Taubenberger, Nancy J. Cox, Ian D. Gust, Alan J. Hay, Masato Tashiro, and Daniel Lavanchy. 2001. A global lab against influenza. *Science* 293 (5536): 1729.

Leatherman, Thomas, and Alan Goodman. 1998. Expanding the bio-cultural synthesis toward a biology of poverty. *American Journal of Physical Anthropology* 101 (1): 1–3.

Lebel, J. 2003. *Health: An ecosystem approach*. Ottawa, Canada: IDRC Books.

Lee, C. B., Robert C. Brunham, Elizabeth Sherman, and Godfrey K. M. Harding. 1987. Epidemiology of an outbreak of infectious syphilis in Manitoba. *American Journal of Epidemiology* 125 (2): 277–283.

León Portilla, Miguel. 1959. Panorama de la población indígena de México. *América Indígena* 19: 43–68.

———. 1962. México. *Indianist yearbook* (Mexico) 22: 65–82.

Lepani, Katherine. 2007. *Sovasova* and the problem of sameness: Converging interpretive frameworks for making sense of HIV and AIDS in the Trobriand Islands. Special issue on HIV/AIDS in rural Papua New Guinea, edited by A. Dundon and C. Wilde. *Oceania* 77 (1): 12–28.

———. 2008. Fitting condoms on culture: Rethinking approaches to HIV prevention in the Trobriand Islands of Papua New Guinea. In *Making sense of AIDS: Culture, power and sexuality in Melanesia,* edited by L. Butt and R. Eves, 246–266. Honolulu: University of Hawaii Press.

Leung, G. M., A. J. Hedley, L. M. H. P. Chau, I. Wong, T. Tach, A. Ghani, and C. A. Donnelly. 2004. The epidemiology of severe acute respiratory syndrome in the 2003 Hong Kong epidemic: An analysis of all 1755 patients. *Annals of Internal Medicine* 141 (9): 662.

Levinson, Jerome, and Juan de Onis. 1970. *The alliance that lost its way: A critical report on the Alliance for Progress.* Chicago: Quadrangle Books.

Levy, Barry S., and Victor W. Sidel, eds. 1997. *War and public health.* New York: Oxford University Press.

Lewinson, Rachel. 1979. Carlos Chagas (1879–1934), the discovery of *Trypanozoma cruzi* and of American trypanosomiasis. *Transactions of the Royal Society of Tropical Medicine and Hygiene* 73: 513–523.

Lewis, J. A., G. J. Chang, R. S. Lanciotti, R. M. Kinney, L. W. Mayer, and D. W. Trent. 1993. Phylogenetic relationships of dengue-2 viruses. *Virology* 197: 216–224.

Lieb, L. E. 1992. Racial miscalculation of American Indians with AIDS in Los Angeles County. *Journal of Acquired Immune Deficiency Syndromes* 5 (11): 1137–1141.

Liljeros, F., C. R. Edling, L. A. Amaral, H. E. Stanley, and Y. Aberg. 2001. The web of human sexual contacts. *Nature* 411 (6840): 907–908.

Lindenbaum, Shirley. 1971. Sorcery and structure in Fore society. *Oceania* 41: 277–288.

———. 1979. *Kuru sorcery: Disease and danger in the New Guinea highlands.* Palo Alto, CA: Mayfield.

———. 1982. Review of *Kuru: Early letters and fieldnotes from the collection of D. Carleton Gajdusek,* edited by J. D Farquar and D. C. Gajdusek. *Journal of Polynesian Society* 91 (1): 150–152.

———. 1991. Review of *A Continuing trial of treatment: Medical pluralism in Papua New Guinea,* edited by S. Frankel and G. Lewis. *Medical Anthropology Quarterly,* n.s., 5 (2): 175–177.

———. 2001. Kuru, prions, and human affairs: Thinking about epidemics. *Annual Review of Anthropology* 30: 363–385.

Linder, Forrest E., and Robert D. Grove. 1943. *Vital statistics rates in the United States, 1900–1940.* Washington, DC: Bureau of the Census, United States Department of Commerce.

Lindsay, James. 2001. Global warming heats up. *Brookings Review,* Fall, 26–29.

Littleton, J., and R. King. 2008. The political ecology of tuberculosis in Auckland: An interdisciplinary focus. In *Multiplying and dividing: Tuberculosis in Canada and Aotearoa New Zealand,* edited by J. Littleton, J. Park, A. Herring, and T. Farmer, 31–42. Research in Anthropology and Linguistics, e series. Auckland: Anthropology Department, University of Auckland.

Livingstone, David. 1999. Tropical climate and moral hygiene: The anatomy of a Victorian debate. *British Journal of the History of Science* 32: 93–110.

Lloberas, J., and A. Celada. 2002. Effect of aging on macrophage function. *Experimental Gerontology* 37 (12): 1325–1331.

Lloyd, L. 2003a. *Best practices for dengue control and prevention in the Americas.* Washington, DC: USAID Bureau for Latin Americas.

———. 2003b. *Strategic Report 7: Best practices for dengue control in the Americas.* Washington, DC: USAID/Environmental Health Project.

Lockerbie, Stacy. 2006. Diary of an ethnographer: Following fish from the local to the global. Master's thesis, Dalhousie University.

———, and D. Ann Herring. 2008. Global panic, local repercussions: Economic and nutritional effects of bird flu in Vietnam. In *Anthropology and public health: Bridging differences in culture and society,* 2nd ed., edited by R. A. Hahn and M. C. Inhorn, 566–587. Oxford: Oxford University Press.

Long, Esmond R. 1948. The decline of tuberculosis as the chief cause of death. *Proceedings of the American Philosophical Society* 92 (3): 139–143.

Longmate, N. 1966. *King cholera: The biography of a disease.* London: Hamish Hamilton.

Loss, Adolf. 1905. *The anatomy and the life history of* Ankylostoma duodenale: *A monograph.* London: Records of the School of Medicine.

Lowell, Anthony M., Lydia B. Edwards, and Carroll E. Palmer. 1969. *Tuberculosis.* Cambridge, MA: Harvard University Press.

Löwy, Ilana. 2003. Intervenir et representer: Campagnes sanitaires et élaboration des cartographies d'ankylostomiase. *History and Philosophy of Life Sciences* 25: 337–362.

Luk, J., P. Gross, and W. W. Thompson. 2001. Observations on mortality during the 1918 influenza pandemic. *Clinical Infectious Diseases* 33 (8): 1375–1378.

Lusso, P., R. Crowley, M. Malnati, C. Di Serio, M. Ponzoni, A. Biancotto, P. Markham, and R. Gallo. 2007. Human herpesvirus 6A accelerates AIDS progression in macaques. *Proceedings of the National Academy of Sciences USA* 104 (12): 5067–5072.

Lux, M. 1997. The Bitter Flats: The 1918 influenza epidemic in Saskatchewan. *Saskatchewan History* 49 (1): 3–13.

MacDougall, Heather. 2007. Toronto's health department in action: Influenza in 1918 and SARS in 2003. *Journal of the History of Medicine and Allied Sciences* 62 (1): 56–89.

Mackay, J. B. 1972. Tuberculosis in Polynesians (letter to the editor). *New Zealand Medical Journal* 76: 449.

———. 1991. Some aspects of tuberculosis in New Zealand and Western Samoa 1942–1985. In *History of tuberculosis in Australia, New Zealand and Papua New Guinea,* edited by A. J. Proust, 92–97. Canberra: Brolga Press.

Maclean, Neil. 1982. Is gambling "bisnis"? The economic and political functions of gambling in the Jimi Valley. *Social Analysis* 16: 44–59.

MacPherson, W. G. 1892. *Annual report on the health of Gibraltar 1891.* Gibraltar: Gibraltar Garrison Printing Press.

Madsen, Claudia. 1965. *A study in Mexican folk medicine.* New Orleans, LA: Middle American Research Institute, Tulane University.

Maher, Dermot, and Mario C. Raviglione. 2005. Global epidemiology of tuberculosis. *Clinics in Chest Medicine* 26 (2): 167–182.

Mair, Julie S., and Michael Mair. 2003. Violence prevention and control through environmental modifications. *Annual Review of Public Health* 24: 209–225.

Malamud, N., A. Hirano, and L. T. Kurland. 1961. Pathoanatomic changes in ALS of Guam. *Archives of Neurology* 5: 401–415.

Malinowski, Bronislaw. 1922. *Argonauts of the western Pacific.* London: Routledge.

———. 1929. *The sexual lives of savages in north-western Melanesia: An ethnographic account of courtship, marriage and family life among the natives of the Trobriand Islands, British New Guinea.* New York: Harcourt, Brace and World.

Mamelund, Svenn-Erik. 2003. Spanish influenza mortality of ethnic minorities in Norway, 1918–1919. *European Journal of Population* 19 (1): 83–102.

———. 2004. Can the Spanish influenza pandemic of 1918 explain the baby boom of 1920 in neutral Norway? *Population* 59 (2): 269–301.

———. 2006. A socially neutral disease? Individual social class, household wealth and mortality from Spanish influenza in two socially contrasting parishes in Kristiania, 1918–1919. *Social Science & Medicine* 62 (4): 923–940.

Mandavilla, A. 2005. Report on bird flu. 4 November. *Nature Medicine.* Electronic document, www.nature.com/news/2005/050912/full/050912-1.html.

Mandelbaum, David G. 1940. *The Plains Cree.* New York: American Museum of Natural History.

Mane, Purnima, and Peter Aggleton. 2001. Gender and HIV/AIDS: What do men have to do with it? *Current Sociology* 49 (6): 23–37.

Manuel, A. G., V. Goel, and I. Williams. 1998. The derivation of life tables for local areas. *Chronic Diseases in Canada* 19 (2) 1–8.

Marchoux, Emile, Albert Taurelli Salimbeni, and Paul Louis Simond. 1903. La fièvre jaune: Rapport de la mission française. *Annales de l'Institut Pasteur* 17: 665–731.

———, and Paul Louis Simond. 1906. Etudes sur la fièvre jaune: Troisième mémoire. *Annales de l'Institut Pasteur* 20: 104–148.

Maree, Cynthia, Robert Daum, Susan Boyle-Vavra, Kelli Matayoshi, and Loren Miller. 2007. Community-associated methicillin-resistant *Staphylococcus aureus* isolates causing healthcare-associated infections. *Emerging Infectious Diseases* 13 (2): 236–242.

Markel, H., H. B. Lipman, J. A. Navarro, A. Sloan, J. R. Michalsen, A. M. Stern, and M. S. Cetron. 2007. Nonpharmacological interventions implemented by cities during the 1918–1919 influenza pandemic. *Journal of the American Medical Association* 298 (6): 644–654.

Marshall, Mac. 2005. Carolina in the Carolines: A survey of patterns and meanings of smoking on a Micronesian island. *Medical Anthropology Quarterly* 19 (4): 354–382.

Martens, Willem, Louis Niessen, Jan Rotmans, Theo Jetten, and Anthony McMichael. 1995. Potential impact of global climate change on malaria risk. *Environmental Health Perspectives* 103: 458–464.

Martin, J. David, and Richard G. Matthias. 2002. HIV and hepatitis B surveillance in First Nations alcohol and drug treatment centers in British Columbia, Canada. *International Journal of Circumpolar Health* 61 (2): 104–109.

Martin, V., L. Sims, J. Lubroth, S. Kahn, J. Domenech, and C. Benino. 2006. History and evolution of HPAI viruses in Southeast Asia. *Annals of the New York Academy of Science* 1081: 153–162.

Martín Barbero, Jesús. 1987. *De los medios a las mediaciones: Comunicación, cultura y hegemonía*. Mexico City: Ediciones G. Gili.

Mas, P. 1979. Dengue fever in Cuba in 1977: Some laboratory aspects. In *Proceedings of Dengue in the Caribbean, 1977*, 40–42. Washington, DC: Pan American Health Organization.

Massachusetts Department of Health. 1918. *Third annual report of the State Department of Health of Massachusetts*. Boston: Wright and Potter.

———. 1919. *Fourth annual report of the State Department of Health of Massachusetts*. Boston: Wright and Potter.

———. 1920. *Fifth annual report of the State Department of Health of Massachusetts*. Boston: Wright and Potter.

Massachusetts Department of Public Health. 1921. *Sixth annual report of the Department of Public Health*. Boston: Wright and Potter.

Mathews, J. D. 1971. Kuru: A puzzle in culture and environmental medicine. PhD dissertation, University of Melbourne.

———. 2008. The changing face of kuru: A personal perspective. *Transactions of the Royal Philosophical Society, Series B* 363: 1510, 3679–3684.

———, R. M. Glasse, and S. Lindenbaum. 1968. Kuru and cannibalism. *Lancet* 2: 449–452.

Mattix, M. E., E. H. Zeman, R. Moeller, C. Jackson, and T. Larsen. 2006. Clinicopathologic aspects of animal and zoonotic diseases of bioterrorism. *Clinical Laboratory Medicine* 26 (2): 445–89.

Mawani, Renisa. 2001. The "savage Indian" and the "foreign plague": Mapping racial categories and legal geographies of race in British Columbia, 1871–1925. PhD dissertation, University of Toronto.

McCallum, Jane. 2005. This last frontier: Isolation and Aboriginal health. *Canadian Bulletin of Medical History* 22 (1): 103–120.

McClelland, R., L. Lavreys, C. Katingima, J. Overbaugh, V. Chohan, K. Mandaliya, J. Ndinya-Achola, and J. Baeten. 2005. Contribution of HIV-1 infection to acquisition of sexually transmitted disease: A 10-year prospective study. *Journal of Infectious Diseases* 191 (3): 333–338.

McCluskey, C. C., E. Roth, and P. Van Den Driessche. 2005. Implication of Ariaal sexual mixing on gonorrhea. *American Journal of Human Biology* 17 (3): 293–301.

McCullers, J., and J. Rehg. 2002. Lethal synergism between influenza virus and *Streptococcus pneumoniae*: Characterization of a mouse model and the role of platelet-activating factor receptor. *Journal of Infectious Diseases* 186: 341–350.

McGrew, R. E. 1965. *Russia and the cholera*. Madison: University of Wisconsin Press.

McKenna, Maryn. 2006a. Vietnam's success against avian flu may offer blueprint for others. Special report. University of Minnesota, Center for Infectious Disease Research and Policy. Electronic document, www.cidrap.umn.edu/cidrap/content/influenza/avianflu/news/oct2506vietsuccess.html.

———. 2006b. When avian flu control meets cultural resistance. Special report. University of Minnesota, Center for Infectious Disease Research and Policy. Electronic document, www.cidrap.umn.edu/cidrap/content/influenza/avianflu/news/oct2606vietculture.html.

McKenna, Neil. 1993. A disaster waiting to happen. *World AIDS* 27 (May): 5–9.

McKenney, David, Kathryn Brown, and David Allison. 1995. Influence of *Pseudomonas aeruginosa* exoproducts on virulence factor production in *Burkholderia cepacia:* Evidence of interspecies communication. *Journal of Bacteriology* 177 (23): 6989–6991.

McKeown, Iris, Sharon Reid, and Pamela Orr. 2004. Experiences of sexual violence and relocation in the lives of HIV infected Canadian women. *Circumpolar Health* 63 (2): 399–404.

McKeown, Thomas. 1976. *The modern rise of population*. London: Edward Arnold.

———. 1978. Determinants of health. *Human Nature* 1: 57–62.

McLaughlin, A. J. 1920. The Shattuck lecture: Epidemiology and etiology of influenza. *Boston Medical and Surgical Journal* 183: 1–23.

McLean, C. A., C. L. Masters, V. A. Vladimirtsev, et al. 1997. Viliuisk encephalomyelitis: Review of the spectrum of pathological changes. *Neuropathology and Applied Neurobiology* 23: 212–217.

McNaughton, A. D., Joyce Neal, Jianmin Li, and Patricia Fleming. 2005. Epidemiologic profile of HIV and AIDS among American Indians/Alaskan Natives in the USA through 2000. *Ethnicity and Health* 10 (1): 57–71.

McNeill, William H. 1976. *Plagues and peoples*. New York: Doubleday.

MediaLens 2006. *Lancet* report co-author responds to questions. October 31. Electronic document, http://medialens.org/alerts/06/061031_lancet_co_author.php.

Meindel, R. S., and A. C. Swedlund. 1977. Secular mortality trends in the Connecticut Valley, 1700–1850. *Human Biology* 49: 389–414.

Meltzer, M., J. Rigau-Pérez, G. Clark, P. Reiter, and D. Gubler. 1998. Using disability-adjusted life years to assess the economic impact of dengue in Puerto Rico: 1984–1994. *American Journal of Tropical Medicine and Hygiene* 59: 265–271.

Mendelsohn, J. Andrew. 1998. How epidemics became complex after World War I. In *Greater than the parts: Holism in biomedicine, 1920–1950*, edited by C. Lawrence and G. Weisz, 303–331. New York: Oxford University Press.

Miles, J. 1997. *Infectious diseases: Colonising the Pacific?* Dunedin, New Zealand: University of Otago Press.

Mill, Judy E. 1997. HIV risk behaviours become survival techniques for Aboriginal women. *Western Journal of Nursing Research* 19 (4): 466–489.

———. 2000. Describing an explanatory model of HIV illness among Aboriginal women. *Holistic Nurse Practitioner* 15 (1): 42–56.

Miller, Cari L. 2002. Females experiencing sexual and drug vulnerabilities are at elevated risk for HIV infection among youth who use injection drugs. *Journal of Acquired Immune Deficiency Syndromes* 30 (3): 335–341.

Miller, J. 2007. Interactions with TB by health providers. Research dissertation, School of Population Health, University of Auckland.

Miller, J. R. 1990. Owen Glendower, Hotspur and Canadian Indian policy. *Ethnohistory* 37 (4): 386–415.

Mills, Christina E., James M. Robins, and Marc Lipsitch. 2004. Transmissibility of the 1918 pandemic influenza. *Nature* 432: 904–906.

Mills, I. D. 1986. The 1918–19 influenza pandemic: The Indian experience. *Indian Economic and Social History Review* 23: 1–40.

Miniño, Arialdi M., Melonie P. Heron, Sherry L. Murphy, and Kenneth D. Kochanek. 2007. Deaths: Final data for 2004. *National Vital Statistics Reports* 55 (19). Hyattsville, MD: National Center for Health Statistics.

Ministry of Social Development. 2004. *The social report: Te purongo oranga tangata 2004*. Electronic document, www.socialreport.msd. govt.nz/2004/health/life-expectancy.html.

Mitchell, Christina M., Carol E. Kaufman, and the Pathways of Choice and Health Ways Project Team. 2002. Structure of HIV knowledge, attitudes, and behaviors among American Indian young adults. *AIDS Education and Prevention* 14 (5): 401–419.

———, Carol E. Kaufman, and Janette Beals. 2004. Identifying diverse HIV risk groups among American Indian young adults: The utility of cluster analysis. *AIDS and Behavior* 8 (3): 263–275.

Monath, T. P. 1994. Dengue: The risk to developed and developing countries. *Proceedings of the National Academy of Sciences USA* 91: 2395–2400.

Montet, Virginie. 2007. Smithsonian toned down global warming exhibit to please officials. *Seed Magazine*. Electronic document, www. seedmagazine.com/news/2007/05/smithsonian_toned_down_global. php.

Montgomery, L. G. 1933. Tuberculosis among Indian children. *Proceedings of the Staff Meetings of the Mayo Clinic* 7: 262–264.

———. 1934. Tuberculosis among pupils of a Canadian school for Indians. *American Review of Tuberculosis* 28 (4): 502–515.

Monto, A. S. 2005. The threat of an avian influenza pandemic. *New England Journal of Medicine* 352 (4): 323–325.

Moore, P. E. 1941. Tuberculosis control in the Indian population of Canada. *Canadian Journal of Public Health* 32: 13–17.

Moran, Emilio. 2006. *People and nature: An introduction to human ecological relations.* South Malden, MA: Blackwell.

Morbidity and Mortality Weekly Report. 1998. HIV/AIDS among American Indians and Alaskan Natives, United States, 1981–1997. *Morbidity and Mortality Weekly Report* 47 (8): 154–160.

Morgan, A. 2006. Avian influenza: An agricultural perspective. *Journal of Infectious Diseases* 194: S139–S146.

Morgan, Murray. 1958. *Doctors to the world.* New York: Viking Press.

Morier, L., G. Kourí, M. G. Guzmán, and M. Soler. 1987. Antibody-dependent enhancement of dengue 2 virus in people of white descent in Cuba. *Lancet* 1: 1028–1029.

Morris, M., and L. Dean. 1994. Effect of sexual behavior change on long-term human immunodeficiency virus prevalence among homosexual men. *American Journal of Epidemiology* 140 (3): 217–232.

———, and M. Kretzschmar. 1995. Concurrent partnerships and transmission dynamics in networks. *Social Networks* 17: 299–318.

———, and M. Kretzschmar. 1997. Concurrent partnerships and the spread of HIV. *AIDS* 11: 641–648.

Morse, Stephen S. 1993. Examining the origins of emerging viruses. In *Emerging Viruses,* edited by S. S. Morse, 10–28. Oxford: Oxford University Press.

Mounts, A. W., H. Wong, H. S. Izurieta, Y. Ho, T. Au, M. Lee, C. B. Bridges, et al. 1999. Case-control study of risk factors for avian influenza A (H5N1) disease, Hong Kong, 1997. *Journal of Infectious Diseases* 180 (2): 505–508.

MSAS (Ministerio de Sanidad y Asistencia Pública). 1991. Cólera. *Boletín Epidemiológico Semanal* 46: 66–75.

Mugusi, F., A. Swai, K. Alberti, and D. G. McLarty. 1990. Increased prevalence of diabetes-mellitus in patients with pulmonary tuberculosis in Tanzania. *Tubercle* 71 (4): 271–276.

Murray, C. J. L., A. D. Lopez, B. Chin, D. Feehan, and K. H. Hill. 2006. Estimation of potential global pandemic influenza mortality on the basis of vital registry data from the 1918–20 pandemic: A quantitative analysis. *Lancet* 368: 2211–2218.

Murray, Douglas L. 1994. *Cultivating crisis: The human cost of pesticides in Latin America.* Austin: University of Texas Press.

Murray, Stephen O., ed. 1995a. *Latin American male homosexualities.* Albuquerque: University of New Mexico Press.

———. 1995b. Modern male homosexuality in Mexico and Peru. In *Latin American male homosexualities,* edited by S. O. Murray, 145–149. Albuquerque: University of New Mexico Press.

Myers, T., S. L. Bullock, L. M. Calzavara, R. Cockerill, and V. W. Marshall. 1997. Differences in sexual risk-taking behavior with state of inebriation in an Aboriginal population in Ontario, Canada. *Journal of Studies in Alcohol* 58 (3): 312–322.

———, L. Calzavara, S. Bullock, R. Cockerill, and V. Marshall. 1994. Gender differences in the use and influence of alcohol and drugs upon sexual behaviour in an aboriginal population. Abstract. *International Conference on AIDS* 10: 59 (abstract no. 190D).

Myers, Ward P., Janice L. Westenhouse, Jennifer Flood, and Lee W. Riley. 2006. An ecological study of tuberculosis transmission in California. *American Journal of Public Health* 96 (4): 685–690.

Narro-Robles, J., and H. Gómez Dantes. 1995. El dengue en México: Un problema prioritario de salud pública [Dengue in Mexico: A priority problem of public health]. *Salud Pública de México,* Supplement 1995, S12–S20.

Nathan, M. B., and R. Dayal-Drager. 2007. Recent epidemiological trends, the global strategy and public health advances in dengue. In *Scientific working group report on dengue 2006,* 30–34. Geneva: Special Programme for Research and Training in Tropical Diseases.

National AIDS Council Secretariat (NACS). 2008. Papua New Guinea UNGASS 2008 Country Progress Report, 2006–2007. Waigani, PNG: NACS.

Nature. 2005. The 1918 flu virus is resurrected. *Nature* 437 (6): 794–795.

———. 2006. Web focus: Avian influenza. Electronic document, www.nature.com/nature/focus/avianflu/timeline.html.

———. 2007. Avian flu timelines. Electronic document, www.nature.com/avianflu/timeline.

———. 2009. Between a virus and a hard place. *Nature,* 7 May 2009.

Neel, J. V. 1982. The thrifty genotype revisited. In *Genetics of diabetes mellitus,* edited by J. Kobberling and R. Tattersall, 283–293. London: Academic Press.

Neustadt, Richard E., and Harvey Fineberg. 1983. *The epidemic that never was: Policy-making and the swine flu scare*. New York: Vintage Books.

Ng Shui, R. 2006. The place of tuberculosis: The lived experience of Pacific peoples in Auckland and Samoa. Master's thesis, University of Auckland.

Nguyen, T., T. Nguyen, H. Lei, Y. Lin, B. Le, K. Huang, C. Lin, et al. 2005. Association between sex, nutritional status, severity of dengue hemorrhagic fever, and immune status in infants with dengue hemorrhagic fever. *American Journal of Tropical Medicine and Hygiene* 72: 370–374.

Nichter, Mark. 2008. *Global health: Why cultural perceptions, social representations, and biopolitics matter*. Tucson: University of Arizona Press.

Nicolle, L. E., L. J. Strausbaugh, and R. A. Garibaldi. 1996. Infections and antibiotic resistance in nursing homes. *Clinical Microbiology Reviews* 9 (1): 1–17.

Nikiforuk, Andrew. 2005. *The fourth horseman: A short history of epidemics, plagues, famine and other scourges*. New York: M. Evans.

Noymer, Andrew. 2007. Contesting the cause and severity of the black death: A review essay. *Population and Development Review* 33 (3): 616–627.

———, and Michel Garenne. 2000. The 1918 influenza epidemic's effects on sex differentials in mortality in the United States. *Population and Development Review* 26 (3): 565–581.

———, and Michel Garenne. 2003. Long-term effects of the 1918 "Spanish" influenza epidemic on sex differentials of mortality in the USA. In *The Spanish Influenza Pandemic of 1918–19: New Perspectives*, edited by H. Phillips and D. Killingray, 202–221. London: Routledge.

Nunn, Paul, Brian Williams, Katherine Floyd, Christopher Dye, Gijs Elzinga, and Mario Raviglione. 2005. Tuberculosis control in the era of HIV. *Nature Reviews Immunology* 5 (10): 819–826.

Office of the Secretary of State of Massachusetts. 1915. *Seventy-fourth annual report on the vital statistics of Massachusetts: Births, marriages, divorces, and deaths*. Boston: Wright and Potter.

———. 1918. *Seventy-seventh annual report on the vital statistics of Massachusetts: Births, marriages, divorces and deaths*. Boston: Wright and Potter.

Oh, M. 2005. The Treaty of Waitangi principles in He korowai oranga–Maori health strategy: An effective partnership? A critique from the perspective of TB care. Master's thesis, University of Auckland.

Olsen, B., V. J. Munster, A. Wallenstein, J. Waldenstrom, A. Osterhaus, and R. Fouchier. 2006. Global patterns of influenza A virus in wild birds. *Science* 312 (5772): 384–388.

Olson, Donald R., Lone Simonsen, Paul J. Edelson, and Stephen S. Morse. 2005. Epidemiological evidence of an early wave of the 1918 influenza pandemic in New York City. *Proceedings of the National Academy of Sciences USA* 102 (31): 11059–11063.

Omran, A. R. 1971. The epidemiologic transition: A theory of the epidemiology of population change. *Millbank Memorial Fund Quarterly* 42 (4): 509–537.

O'Neil, John, and Javier Mignone. 2005. Social capital and youth suicide: Risk factors in First Nations communities. *Canadian Journal of Public Health* 96 (Supplement 1): S51–S54.

Organización Sanitaria Panamericana. 1955. *Actas de la decimocuarta Conferencia Sanitaria Panamericana, Sexta Reunión del Comité Regional de la Organización Mundial de la Salud para las Américas, Santiago, Chile, 7–22 octubre 1954.* Documentos Oficiales 14. Washington, DC: Oficina Sanitaria Panamericana.

Orr, P., E. Sherman, J. Blanchard, M. Fast, G. Hammond, and R. Brunham. 1994. Epidemiology of infection due to *Chlamydia trachomatis* in Manitoba, Canada. *Clinical Infectious Diseases* 19: 876–883.

Oshinsky, David M. 2005. *Polio: An American story.* Oxford: Oxford University Press.

Osterholm, Michael T. 2005. Preparing for the next pandemic. *New England Journal of Medicine* 352 (18): 1839–1842.

Otis, Laura. 1999. *Membranes: Metaphors of invasion in nineteenth-century literature, science, and politics.* Baltimore, MD: Johns Hopkins University Press.

Otte, Joachim, David Roland-Holst, and Dirk U. Pfeiffer. 2006. HPAI control measures and household incomes in Viet Nam. FAO, Pro-Poor Livestock Policy Initiative. Electronic document, www.fao.org/ag/pplpi.html.

Oxford, J. S., A. Sefton, R. Jackson, W. Innes, R. Daniels, and N. Johnson. 2002. World War I may have allowed the emergence of "Spanish" influenza. *Lancet Infectious Diseases* 2 (2): 111–114.

Packard, Randall M. 2007. *The making of a tropical disease: A short history of malaria.* Baltimore, MD: Johns Hopkins University Press.

Packenham, Robert A. 1992. *The dependency movement: Scholarship and politics in development studies.* Cambridge, MA: Harvard University Press.

Page Pliego, Jaime T. 2002. *Política sanitaria dirigida a los pueblos indígenas de México y Chiapas, 1857–1995.* Mexico City: Universidad Nacional Autónoma de México.

PAHO (Pan American Health Organization). 1985. Control and eradication of *Aedes aegypti:* Resolution XXVI of the XXXI meeting of the Directing Council of the Pan American Health Organization. Washington, DC: PAHO.

———. 2001. Blueprint for the next generation: Dengue prevention and control. Thirty-fifth session of the subcommittee of the Executive Committee on Planning and Programming. Washington, DC: PAHO.

———. 2007. Dengue outbreak continues to subside in Paraguay. *Emerging and Reemerging Infectious Diseases, Region of the Americas* 4 (8).

Palese, Peter. 1993. Evolution of influenza and RNA viruses. In *Emerging viruses*, edited by S. J. Morse, 226–233. Oxford: Oxford University Press.

———. 2004. Influenza: Old and new threats. *Nature Medicine Supplement* 10 (12): S82–S87.

———, Terrence M. Tumpey, and Adolfo Garcia-Sastre. 2006. What can we learn from reconstructing the extinct 1918 pandemic influenza virus? *Immunity* 24 (2): 121–124.

Palmer, Edwina, and Geoffrey W. Rice. 1992. A Japanese physician's response to pandemic influenza: Ijirō Gomibuchi and the "Spanish flu" in Yaita-Chō, 1918–1919. *Bulletin of the History of Medicine* 66 (4): 560–577.

Paluzzi, Joan E. 2004. A social disease/a social response: Lessons in tuberculosis from early 20th century Chile. *Social Science & Medicine* 59 (4): 763–773.

Pampana, Emilio J. 1963. *A textbook of malaria eradication*. Oxford: Oxford University Press.

Pandemics and Pandemic Threats since 1900. US Department of Health and Human Services. Electronic document, www.PandemicFlu.gov, accessed 23 May 2006.

Parker, Richard G. 1999. *Beneath the equator: Cultures of desire, male homosexuality, and emerging gay communities in Brazil*. New York: Routledge.

Parsons, Elsie C. 1931. Curanderos in Oaxaca, Mexico. *Scientific Monthly* 32 (1): 60–68.

Pastor, M. 1987. The effects of IMF programmes in the third world: Debate and evidence from Latin America. *World Development* 15 (2): 249–262.

Patterson, K. David. 1983. The influenza epidemic of 1918–1919 in the Gold Coast. *Journal of African History* 24 (4): 485–502.

———. 1985. Pandemic and epidemic influenza, 1830–1848. *Social Science & Medicine* 21 (5): 571–80.

———. 1986. *Pandemic influenza, 1700–1900: A study in historical epidemiology*. Totowa, NJ: Rowman and Littlefield.

———. 1994. Cholera diffusion in Russia, 1823–1923. *Social Science & Medicine* 38: 1171–1191.

———, and Gerald F. Pyle. 1983. The diffusion of influenza in sub-Saharan Africa during the 1918–1919 pandemic. *Social Science & Medicine* 17 (17): 1299–1307.

———, and Gerald F. Pyle. 1991. The geography and mortality of the 1918 influenza pandemic. *Bulletin of the History of Medicine* 65 (1): 4–21.

Patton, Cindy. 2002. *Globalizing AIDS*. Minneapolis: University of Minnesota Press.

Patz, Jonathan, Willem Martens, Dana Focks, and Theo Jetten. 1998. Dengue fever epidemic potential as projected by general circulation models of global climate change. *Environmental Health Perspectives* 106: 147–153.

Peard, Julyan. 1999. *Race, place and medicine: The idea of tropics in nineteenth-century Brazilian medicine*. Durham, NC: Duke University Press.

Pearl, Raymond. 1919. Influenza studies, 1: On certain general statistical aspects of the 1918 epidemic in American cities. *Public Health Reports* 34 (32): 1743–1783.

Peinado, J., S. M. Goodreau, P. Goicochea, J. Vergara, N. Ojeda, M. Casapia, A. Ortiz, V. Zatnalloa, R. Galvan, and J. R. Sanchez. 2007. Role versatility among men who have sex with men in urban Peru. *Journal of Sex Research* 44 (3): 233–239.

Pelling, M. 1978. *Cholera, fever and English medicine, 1825–1865*. Oxford: Oxford University Press.

Pennington, S. 1995. Global warming and disease. *Geographic Magazine* 67: 7.

People's Daily Online. 2007. Bird flu returns in Vietnam. Electronic document, http://English.people.com.cn.

Pereira, Marguerite S. 1980. The effects of shifts and drifts on the epidemiology of influenza in man. *Proceedings of the Royal Society of London, Series B: Biological Sciences* 288 (1029): 423–432.

Perrin, Edward, and Michele Ver Ploeg, eds. 2004. *Eliminating health disparities: Measurement and data needs*. Washington, DC: National Research Council.

Petraglia Kropf, Simone. 2005. Science health and development: Chagas' disease in Brazil, 1943–1962. *Parassitologia* 47: 379–386.

———, Nara Azavedo, and Luis Octavio Ferreira. 2003. Biomedical research and public health in Brazil: The case of Chagas' disease, 1909–1950. *Social History of Medicine* 16 (1): 111–129.

Pettipas, Katherine. 1994. *Severing the ties that bind: Government repression of indigenous religious ceremonies on the prairies.* Winnipeg, Canada: University of Manitoba.

Pfeiffer, Dirk U. 2006. Avian influenza in Viet Nam. In *Socio-economic impact assessment of selected control strategies for avian influenza in Viet Nam and Thailand,* 15–18. Meeting report, FAO, Pro-Poor Livestock Policy Initiative, Bangkok, 29 June 2005.

Phillips, Howard. 2004. The re-appearing shadow of 1918: Trends in the historiography of the 1918–19 influenza pandemic. *Canadian Bulletin of Medical History* 21 (1): 121–134.

Pichainarong, N., N. Mongkalangoon, A. S. Kalayanarooj, and W. Chaveepojnkamjorn. 2006. Relationship between body size and severity of dengue hemorrhagic fever among children aged 0–14 years. *Southeast Asian Journal of Tropical Medicine and Public Health* 37: 283–288.

Pinheiro, F. P. 1989. Dengue in the Americas, 1980–1987. *Epidemiological Bulletin* 10: 1–8.

———, and S. Corber. 1997. Global situation of dengue and dengue haemorrhagic fever, and its emergence in the Americas. *World Health Statistics Quarterly* 50: 161–169.

Plato, C. C., and D. C. Gajdusek. 1972. Genetic studies in relation to kuru, 4: Dermatoglyphics of the Fore and Anga populations of the eastern highlands of Papua New Guinea. *American Journal of Human Genetics* 24 (Supplement): S86–S94.

Platt, A. 1995. Global warming and disease. *World Watch* 8: 26–32.

Pollitzer, R. 1959. *Cholera.* Geneva: World Health Organization.

Ponce-De-Leon, A., M. Garcia, M. Garcia-Sancho, F. Gomez-Perez, J. Gomez, G. Fernandez, R. Rojas, et al. 2004. Tuberculosis and diabetes in southern Mexico. *Diabetes Care* 27 (7): 1584–1590.

Pool, I. 1991. *Te Iwi Maori: A New Zealand population, past, present and projected.* Auckland: Auckland University Press.

Poovey, Mary. 1998. *A History of the modern fact: Problems of knowledge in the sciences of wealth and society.* Chicago: University of Chicago Press.

Porter, Dorothy. 1992. Changing disciplines: John Ryle and the making of social medicine in twentieth-century Britain. *History of Science* 30: 119–147.

Preston, Samuel H. 1975. The changing relation between mortality and level of economic development. *Population Studies* 29 (2): 231–248.

———. 1990. Sources of variation in vital rates: An overview. In *Convergent issues in genetics and demography,* edited by J. Adams, D. A. Lam, A. I. Hermalin, and P. E. Smouse, 335–350. New York: Oxford University Press.

———, and Etienne van de Walle. 1978. Urban French mortality in the nineteenth century. *Population Studies* 32 (2): 275–297.

Prison Report. 1861. Bermuda and Gibraltar for the year 1860. Manuscript, National Archives of London.

Pyle, Gerald F. 1986. *The diffusion of influenza: Patterns and paradigms.* Totowa, NJ: Rowman and Littlefield.

Rabbani, G. H., and W. B. Greenough. 1992. Pathophysiology and clinical aspects of cholera. In *Cholera*, edited by D. Barua and W. B. Greenough, 209–228. New York: Plenum Medical Book Company.

Rabe, Stephen G. 1988. *Eisenhower and Latin America: The foreign policy of anticommunism.* Chapel Hill: University of North Carolina Press.

Rajan, Kaushik Sunder. 2006. *Biocapital: The constitution of postgenomic life.* Durham, NC: Duke University Press.

Ramirez, J. R, W. D. Crano, R. Quist, M. Burgoon, E. M. Alvaro, and J. Grandpre. 2002. Effects of fatalism and family communication on HIV/AIDS awareness variations in Native American and Anglo parents and children. *AIDS Education and Prevention* 14 (1): 29–40.

Ranger, Terence, and Paul Slack. 1992. *Epidemics and ideas: Essays on the historical perception of pestilence.* Cambridge: Cambridge University Press.

Raufman, J. P. 1998. Cholera. *American Journal of Medicine* 104: 386–394.

Rawlings, J. A., K. A. Hendricks, C. R. Burgess, R. M. Campman, G. G. Clark, L. J. Tabony, and M. A. Patterson. 1998. Dengue surveillance in Texas, 1995. *American Journal of Tropical Medicine and Hygiene* 59: 95–99.

Ray, Arthur. 2002. *I have lived here since the world began.* Toronto: University of Toronto Press.

Reed, Adam. 1997. Contested images and common strategies: Early colonial sexual politics in the Massim. In *Sites of desire, economies of pleasure: Sexualities in Asia and the Pacific,* edited by L. Manderson and M. Jolly, 48–71. Chicago: University of Chicago Press.

Reed, D. M., and J. A. Brody. 1975. ALS and PDC of Guam, 1945–1972, 1: Descriptive epidemiology. *American Journal of Epidemiology* 101: 287–301.

Reed, Walter, and James Carroll. 1901. The etiology of yellow fever: A supplemental note. Communication during a conference of the American Association of Bacteriologists, Chicago, 31 December 1901–1 Januuary 1902. Reprinted in *Yellow fever: Compilation of various publications,* edited by M. Owen, 149–160. Washington, DC: Government Printing Office, 1911.

———, James Carrol, and Aristides Agramonte. 1901. The etiology of yellow fever: An additional note. *Journal of the American Medical*

Association 36: 431–440. Reprinted in *Yellow fever: Compilation of various publications,* edited by M. Owen, 79–89. Washington, DC: Government Printing Office.

————, James Carroll, and Jesse W. Lazear. 1900. The etiology of yellow fever: A preliminary note. Communication at the 28th Congress of the American Public Health Association, Indianapolis, 22–26 October. Reprinted in *Yellow fever: Compilation of various publications,* edited by M. Owen, 57–69. Washington, DC: Government Printing Office, 1911.

Reeder, L. G. 1972. Social epidemiology: An appraisal. In *Patients, physicians and illness,* 2nd ed., edited by E. G. Jaco, 97–101. New York: Free Press.

Reid, A. H., T. G. Fanning, J. V. Hultin, and J. K. Taubenberger. 1999. Origin and evolution of the 1918 "Spanish" influenza virus hemagglutinin gene. *Proceedings of the National Academy of Sciences USA* 96 (4): 1651–1656.

Reid, Alice. 2005. The effects of the 1918–1919 influenza pandemic on infant and child health in Derbyshire. *Medical History* 49 (1): 29–54.

Reid, Elizabeth. 1994. *Approaching the epidemic.* Issues paper 14, HIV and Development Programme. New York: United Nations Development Programme.

Reid, Lucy Hamilton, and D. Carleton Gajdusek. 1969. Nutrition in the kuru region 11: A nutritional evaluation of traditional Fore diet in Moke Village in 1957. *Acta Tropica* 26 (4): 331–345.

Reid, Roddy. 2005. *Globalizing tobacco control: Anti-smoking campaigns in California, France, and Japan.* Bloomington: Indiana University Press.

Reinberg, Steven. 2007. Global warming poses health threats. *Washington Post,* 2 February, 1.

Reisen, William, Hugh Lothrop, Robert Chiles, Minoo Madon, Cynthia Cossen, Leslie Woods, Stan Husted, Vicki Kramer, and John Edman. 2004. West Nile virus in California. *Emerging Infectious Diseases* 10 (8).

Reiter, P., and D. J. Gubler. 1997. Surveillance and control of urban dengue vectors. In *Dengue and dengue hemorrhagic fever,* edited by D. J. Gubler and G. Kuno, 425–462. London: CAB International.

Rhodes, Richard. 1997. *Deadly feasts: Tracking the secrets of a terrifying new plague.* New York: Simon and Schuster.

Rice, L. 1923. Dengue fever: Clinical report of the Galveston epidemic of 1922. *American Journal of Tropical Medicine and Hygiene* 3 (2): 73–89.

Richards, W. G. 1932. Tuberculosis among the Indians of Montana. *American Review of Tuberculosis* 26: 492–497.

Richardson, S. H. 1994. Host susceptibility. In *Vibrio cholerae and cholera: Molecular to global perspectives*, edited by I. K. Wachsmuth, P. A. Blake, and O. Olsvik, 273–289. Washington, DC: ASM Press.

Richerson, Peter J., and Robert Boyd. 1987. Simple models of complex phenomena: The case of cultural evolution. In *The latest on the best: Essays on evolution and optimality*, edited by J. Dupré, 27–52. Cambridge, MA: MIT Press.

Rickard, E. R. 1937a. The organization of the visceroctomy service. *Annual Report of the Rockefeller Foundation, 1937*. New York: Rockefeller Foundation.

———. 1937b. The organization of the visceroctome service of the Brazilian cooperative Yellow Fever Service. *American Journal of Tropical Medicine* 17: 163–190.

Rickerts, Volker, Hans Reinhard Brodt, Bernd Schneider, Eckhart Weidmann, and Kai Uwe Chow. 2006. Host factors and disease severity in two patients with SARS. *LaboratoriumMedizin* 30 (1): 18–22.

Rico-Hesse, R. 1990. Molecular evolution and distribution of dengue viruses type 1 and 2 in nature. *Virology* 174: 479–493.

———, L. M. Harrison, R. A. Salas, D. Tovar, A. Nisalak, C. Ramos, J. Boshell, M. T. de Mesa, R. M. Nogueira, and A. T. da Rosa. 1997. Origins of dengue type 2 viruses associated with increased pathogenicity in the Americas. *Virology* 230: 244–251.

Rigau-Pérez, J., A. Ayala-López, E. García-Rivera, S. Hudson, et al. 2002. The reappearance of dengue-3 and a subsequent dengue-4 and dengue-1 epidemic in Puerto Rico in 1998. *American Journal of Tropical Medicine and Hygiene* 67: 355–362.

———, D. J. Gubler, A. V. Vorndam, and G. G. Clark. 1994. Dengue surveillance: United States, 1986–1992. *Morbidity and Mortality Weekly Reports, Surveillance Summaries* (Centers for Disease Control) 43: 7–19.

———, A. Vorndam, and G. Clark. 2001. The dengue and dengue hemorrhagic fever epidemic in Puerto Rico, 1994–1995. *American Journal of Tropical Medicine and Hygiene* 64: 67–74.

Riley, James C. 2001. *Rising life expectancy: A global history*. Cambridge: Cambridge University Press.

———. 2005. The timing and pace of health transitions around the world. *Population and Development Review* 31 (4): 741–764.

Rivière-Cinnamond, A., N. T. K. Cuc, and C. Wollny. 2005. Support policy strategy for avian influenza emergency recovery and rehabilitation of the poultry sector in Vietnam. *Conference on International Agricultural Research for Development*, Stuttgart-Hohenheim, October 11–13. Electronic document, www.tropentag.de/2005/abstracts/full/311.

pRizk, Marlene. 1991. Sin cólera tenemos mil muertes por diarrhea. *El Nacional,* 3 December 1991, C-3.

Robbins, Joel. 2004. *Becoming sinners: Christianity and moral torment in a Papua New Guinea society.* Berkeley: University of California Press.

Roberts, B. 1995. *The making of citizens: Cities of peasants revisited.* New York: Arnold Publishers.

Roberts, E. 1866. Report on the Sanitary Commissioners of Gibraltar for the year 1866. Gibraltar: Gibraltar Garrison Printing Press.

Roberts, Les, Riyadh Lafta, Richard Garfield, Jamal Khudhairi, and Gilbert Burnham. 2004. Mortality before and after the 2003 invasion of Iraq: Cluster sample survey. *Lancet* 364: 1857–1864.

Romanowski, B., R. Sutherland, E. J. Love, and D. Mooney. 1991. Epidemiology of an outbreak of infections of syphilis in Alberta. *International Journal of STD and AIDS* 2: 424–427.

Romero Sa, Magali. 2005. The discovery of *Trypanosoma cruzi* by Carlos Chagas and the German school of protozoology. *Parassitologia* 47: 309–317.

Romo, V. C. 2003. *Decomposition methods in demography.* Amsterdam: Rozenberg.

Root, H. F. 1934. The association of diabetes and tuberculosis. *New England Journal of Medicine* 210: 1–13.

Rosenberg, Charles E. 1962. *The cholera years: The United States in 1832, 1849, and 1866.* Chicago: University of Chicago Press.

———. 1966. Cholera in nineteenth-century Europe: A tool for social and economic analysis. *Comparative Studies in Society and History* 8: 452–463.

———. 1989. Disease in history: Frames and framers. *Milbank Memorial Fund Quarterly* 67 (Supplement 1): 1–15.

———. 1992a. *Explaining epidemics and other studies in the history of medicine.* Cambridge: Cambridge University Press.

———. 1992b. What is an epidemic? AIDS in historical perspective. In *Explaining epidemics and other studies in the history of medicine,* by C. E. Rosenberg, 278–292. Cambridge: Cambridge University Press.

———. 1992c. Explaining epidemics. In *Explaining epidemics and other studies in the history of medicine,* by C. E. Rosenberg, 293–304. Cambridge: Cambridge University Press.

———. 1992d. Framing disease: Illness, society and history. In *Framing disease: Studies in cultural history,* edited by C. E. Rosenberg and J. Golden, xiii–xxvi. New Brunswick, NJ: Rutgers University Press.

———. 2008. Siting epidemic disease: Three centuries of American history. *Journal of Infectious Disease* 197 (Supplement 1): S4–6.

Ros Romero, María del Consuelo. 1992. *La imagen del Indio en el discurso del Instituto Nacional Indigenista*. Mexico City: Centro de Investigaciones y Estudios Superiores en Antropología Social, Secretaría de Educación Pública.

Rothman, A. L. 2004. Dengue: Defining protective versus pathologic immunity. *Journal of Clinical Investigation* 113: 946–951.

————, and F. A. Ennis. 1999. Immunopathogenesis of dengue hemorrhagic fever. *Virology* 257: 1–6.

Rothman, David. 2003. *Strangers at the bedside: A history of how law and bioethics transformed medical decision making*. New York: Aldine de Gruyter.

Rothman, Sheila M. 1994. *Living in the shadow of death: Tuberculosis and the social experience of illness in America*. New York: Basic Books.

Rubottom, Roy, Jr. 1958. Communism in the Americas. *Department of State Bulletin* 38: 180–185.

Russell, Edmund. 2001. *War and nature: Fighting humans and insects with chemicals from World War I to* Silent Spring. Cambridge: Cambridge University Press.

Russell, Paul F. 1977. Obituary: Fred Lowe Soper. *Transactions of the Royal Society of Tropical Medicine and Hygiene* 71 (3): 272–273.

Rutherford, Major W. 1866. General report upon the cholera epidemic in Gibraltar during the summer and autumn of 1865. *House of Commons Parliamentary Papers* 28: 378–468.

Ruzicka, L., and P. Kane. 1990. Health transition: The course of morbidity and mortality. In *What we know about health transition: The cultural, social, and behavioral determinants of health,* edited by J. Caldwell, S. Findley, P. Caldwell, G. Santow, W. Cosford, J. Braid, and D. Broers Freeman, 1–24. Canberra: Health Transition Centre.

Santos, Ricardo Augusto dos, Wanda Latmann Weltman, Eduardo Vilela Thielen, Fernando Antonio Pires Alves, Jaime Larry Benchimol, and Marli Brito de Albuquerque. 1991. *Science heading for the backwoods: Images of the expeditions conducted by the Oswaldo Cruz Institute scientists to the Brazilian hinterland, 1911–1913*. Rio de Janeiro: Casa Oswaldo Cruz.

Sariol, C. A., J. L. Pelegrino, A. Martínez, E. Arteaga, G. Kourí, and M. G. Guzmán. 1999. Detection and genetic relationship of dengue virus sequences in seventeen-year-old paraffin-embedded samples from Cuba. *American Journal of Tropical Medicine and Hygiene* 61: 994–1000.

Sattenspiel, Lisa. 1987a. Epidemics in nonrandomly mixing populations: A simulation. *American Journal of Physical Anthropology* 73 (2): 251–265.

———. 1987b. Population structure and the spread of disease. *Human Biology* 59 (3): 411–438.

———. 1990. Modeling the spread of infectious disease in human populations. *Yearbook of Physical Anthropology* 33: 245–276.

———, and C. Castillo-Chavez. 1990. Environmental context, social interactions, and the spread of HIV. *American Journal of Human Biology* 2 (4): 397–417.

———, and K. Dietz. 1995. A structured epidemic model incorporating geographic mobility among regions. *Mathematical Biosciences* 128 (1–2): 71–91.

———, and D. Ann Herring. 1998. Structured epidemic models and the spread of influenza in the central Canadian subarctic. *Human Biology* 70 (1): 91–115.

———, and D. Ann Herring. 2003. Simulating the effect of quarantine on the spread of the 1918–1919 flu in central Canada. *Bulletin of Mathematical Biology* 65 (1): 1–26.

———, J. Koopman, C. Simon, and J. A. Jacquez. 1990. The effects of population structure on the spread of the HIV infection. *American Journal of Physical Anthropology* 82 (4): 421–429.

———, A. Mobarry, and D. A. Herring. 2000. Modeling the influence of settlement structure on the spread of influenza among communities. *American Journal of Human Biology* 12 (6): 736–748.

Sawchuk, Lawrence A. 2001. *Deadly visitations in dark times: A social history of Gibraltar in the time of cholera.* Monograph 2. Gibraltar: Gibraltar Government Heritage Publications.

———, and S. D. A. Burke. 2003. The ecology of a health crisis: Gibraltar and the 1865 cholera epidemic. In *Human biologists in the archives,* edited by D. A. Herring and A. C. Swedlund, 178–215. Cambridge: Cambridge University Press.

Sawyer, Wilbur. 1951. Medicine as a social instrument: Tropical medicine. *New England Journal of Medicine* 244 (6): 221–224.

———, and Wray Lloyd. 1931. The use of mice in test of immunity against yellow fever. *Journal of the American Medical Association* 54 (2): 533–555.

Scheiblauer, H., M. Reinacher, M. Tashiro, and R. Rott. 1992. Interactions between bacteria and influenza A virus in the development of influenza pneumonia. *Journal of Infectious Diseases* 166: 783–791.

Scheper-Hughes, Nancy. 1992. *Death without weeping: The violence of everyday life in Brazil.* Berkeley: University of California Press.

———, and Margaret Lock. 1987. The mindful body: A prolegomenon to future work in medical anthropology. *Medical Anthropology Quarterly,* n.s., 1 (1): 6–41.

Schieffelin, Bambi B., Kathryn Woolard, and Paul V. Kroskrity, eds. 1998. *Language ideologies: Practice and theory*. Oxford: Oxford University Press.

Scholtissek, C. 1992. Cultivating a killer virus. *Natural History* 101 (1): 3–6.

———. 1994. Source for influenza pandemics. *European Journal of Epidemiology* 4: 455–458.

Scott, James C. 1998. *Seeing like a state: How certain schemes to improve the human condition have failed*. New Haven, CT: Yale University Press.

Scrimshaw, Nevin S. 2003. Historical concepts of interactions, synergism, and antagonism between nutrition and infection. *Journal of Nutrition* 133 (Supplement): 316S–321S.

Searle, A. 2004. Having TB: The experience of Pakeha in Auckland. Master's thesis, University of Auckland.

———. 2008. Pakeha and tuberculosis in New Zealand: Not the other. In *Multiplying and dividing: Tuberculosis in Canada and Aotearoa New Zealand*, edited by J. Littleton, J. Park, A. Herring, and T. Farmer, 187–195. Research in Anthropology and Linguistics, e series. Auckland: Anthropology Department, University of Auckland.

Seidel, Gill, and Laurent Vidal. 1997. The implications of "medical," "gender and development" and "culturist" discourses for HIV/AIDS policy in Africa. In *Anthropology of policy: Critical perspectives on governance and power*, edited by S. Cris and S. Wright, 59–87. London: Routledge.

Senft, Gunter. 1998. "Noble savages" and the "Islands of Love": Trobriand Islanders in "popular publications." In *Pacific answers to Western hegemony: Cultural practices of identity construction*, edited by J. Wassmann, 119–140. Oxford: Berg.

Setel, Philip W. 1999. *A plague of paradoxes: AIDS, culture and demography in northern Tanzania*. Chicago: University of Chicago Press.

Sethi, S. 2002. Bacterial pneumonia: Managing a deadly complication of influenza in older adults with comorbid disease. *Geriatrics* 57 (3): 56–61.

Sherertz, R. J., D. R. Reagan, K. D. Hampton, K. L. Robertson, S. A. Streed, H. Hoen, R. Thomas, and G. Jack. 1996. A cloud adult: The *Staphylococcus aureus*–virus interaction revisited. *Annals of Internal Medicine* 124 (6): 539–547.

Shilts, Randy. 1987. *And the band played on: Politics, people, and the AIDS epidemic*. New York: St. Martin's.

Shinya, K., M. Ebina, S. Yamada, M. Ono, et al. 2006. Avian flu: Influenza virus receptors in the human airway. *Nature* 440: 435–436.

Shope, R. E. 1936. The incidence of neutralizing antibodies for swine influenza virus in the sera of human beings of different ages. *Journal of Experimental Medicine* 63 (5): 669–684.

Shortridge, K. F., J. K. Peiris, and Y. Guan. 2003. The next influenza pandemic: Lessons from Hong Kong. *Journal of Applied Microbiology* 94 (Supplement): 70S–79S.

Silverstein, Michael. 2004. Cultural concepts and the language-culture nexus. *Current Anthropology* 45 (5): 621–652.

Simoni, J. M., S. Sehgal, and K. L. Walters. 2004. Triangle of risk: Urban American Indian women's sexual trauma, injection drug use, and HIV sexual risk behaviors. *AIDS and Behavior* 8 (1): 33–46.

Simonsen, L., M. J. Clarke, L. B. Schonberger, N. H. Arden, N. Cox, and K. Fukuda. 1998. Pandemic versus epidemic influenza mortality: A pattern of changing age distribution. *Journal of Infectious Diseases* 178 (1): 53–60.

Singer, Merrill. 2009. *Introduction to syndemics: A systems approach to public and community health.* San Francisco: Jossey-Bass.

———, and Scott Clair. 2003. Syndemics and public health: Reconceptualizing disease in bio-social context. *Medical Anthropology Quarterly* 17 (4): 423–441.

———, D. Ann Herring, Judith Littleton, and Melanie Rock. n.d. Syndemics in public health. In *Medical anthropology companion,* edited by M. Singer and P. Erickson. San Francisco: Wiley. In press.

Slack, Paul. 1992. Introduction. In *Epidemics and ideas: Essays on the historical perception of pestilence,* edited by T. Ranger and P. Slack, 1–20. Cambridge: Cambridge University Press.

Slosek, J. 1986. *Aedes aegypti* mosquitoes in the Americas: A review of their interactions with the human population. *Social Science and Medicine* 23: 249–257.

Slots, J. 2007. Herpesviral-bacterial synergy in the pathogenesis of human periodontitis. *Current Opinion in Infectious Disease* 20 (3): 278–283.

Smallman-Raynor, Matthew, and Andrew D. Cliff. 1998. The Philippines insurrection and the 1902–4 cholera epidemic, part 2: Diffusion patterns in war and peace. *Journal of Historical Geography* 24: 188–210.

———, Niall Johnson, and Andrew D. Cliff. 2002. The spatial anatomy of an epidemic: Influenza in London and the county boroughs of England and Wales, 1918–1919. *Transactions of the Institute of British Geographers* 27 (4): 452–470.

Smith, D. P. 2004. *Survival 9.2: A program for life tables and related measures.* Austin: University of Texas, School of Public Health.

Smith, Peter H. 2000. *Talons of the eagle: Dynamic of US–Latin American relations.* New York: Oxford University Press.

Smith, P. W. 2000. Microbiologic survey of long-term care facilities. *American Journal of Infection Control* 28 (1): 8–13.

Smith, R. L. 2003. Invited commentary: Timescale-dependent mortality effects of air pollution. *American Journal of Epidemiology* 157: 1066–1070.

Smith, Theobald. 1917. Certain aspects of natural and acquired resistance to tuberculosis, and their bearing on preventive measures. *Journal of the American Medical Association* 68: 669–674, 764–769.

———. 1934. *Parasitism and disease.* Princeton, NJ: Princeton University Press.

Smoyer-Tomic, Karen, Justine Klaver, Colin Soskolne, and Donald Spady. 2004. Health consequences of drought on the Canadian prairies. *EcoHealth* 1 (Supplement 2): 144–154.

Snowden, F. M. 1995. *Naples in the time of cholera, 1884–1911.* Cambridge: Cambridge University Press.

Sontag, Susan. 2001. *Illness as metaphor* and *AIDS and its metaphors.* New York: Picador.

Soper, Fred L. 1957. El concepto de la erradicación de las enfermedades transmisibles. *Boletín de la Oficina Sanitaria Panamericana* 42 (1): 1–5.

———. 1960. The epidemiology of a disappearing disease: Malaria. *American Journal of Tropical Medicine and Hygiene* 8: 357–366.

———. 1965a. The 1964 status of *Aedes aegypti* eradication and yellow fever in the Americas. *American Journal of Tropical Medicine and Hygiene* 14: 887–891.

———. 1965b. Rehabilitation of the eradication concept in prevention of communicable diseases. *Public Health Reports* 80: 855–869.

———, E. R. Rickard, and P. J. Crawford. 1934. The routine post mortem removal of liver tissue from rapidly fatal fever cases for the discovery of isolated yellow fever foci. *American Journal of Hygiene* 19 (3): 549–556.

Sorenson, E. Richard. 1976. *The edge of the forest: Land, childhood, and change in a New Guinea protoagricultural society.* Washington, DC: Smithsonian Institution Press.

———, and D. Carleton Gajdusek. 1969. Nutrition in the kuru region 1: Gardening, food handling and diet of the Fore people. *Acta Tropica* 26 (4): 281–330.

Spencer, Peter S., Peter B. Nunn, Jacques Hugon, et al. 1987. Guam amyotrophic lateral sclerosis–Parkinsonism–dementia linked to a plant excitant neurotoxin. *Science* 237: 517–522.

Spittal, Patricia, Kevin J. P. Craib, Evan Wood, Nancy Laliberte, Kathy Li, Mark W. Tyndall, Michael V. O'Shaughnessy, and Martin T. Schechter. 2002. Risk factors for elevated HIV incidence rates among female injection drug users in Vancouver. *Journal of the Canadian Medical Association* 166 (7): 894–899.

Stall, Ron, M. Friedman, and J. Catania. 2007. Interacting epidemics and gay men's health: A theory of syndemic production among urban gay men. In *Unequal opportunity: Health disparities affecting gay and bisexual men in the United States*, edited by R. J. Wolitski, R. Stall, and R. O. Valdiserri, 251–274. Oxford: Oxford University Press.

Steain, Megan, Bin Wang, Dominic Dwyer, and Nitin Saksena. 2004. HIV-1 co-infection, superinfection and recombination. *Sexual Health* 1 (4): 239–250.

Steinhauer, David A., and John J. Skehel. 2002. Genetics of influenza viruses. *Annual Review of Genetics* 36: 305–332.

Stepan, Nancy. 1978. The interplay between socio-economic factors and medical science: Yellow fever research, Cuba, and the United States. *Social Studies of Science* 8: 397–423.

———. 1998. Tropical medicine and public health in Latin America. *Medical History* 42 (1): 104–112.

———. 2001. Apparences and disapparances. In *Picturing tropical medicine*, 180–207. London: Reaktion Books.

Sternberg, George. 1889. Resultado de los experimentos hechos sobre el micrococcus *Tetragenus versatilis* para los doctores Finlay y Delgado. *Annales de la Academia de Ciencias Médicas, Físicas y Naturales de la Habana* 29: 134–147.

Stiles, C. W. 1902. A new species of hookworm (*Urcinaria maericanis*) parasitic in man. *American Medicine* 3: 777–778.

Stillwaggon, Eileen. 2003. Racial metaphors: Interpreting sex and AIDS in Africa. *Development and Change* 34 (5): 809–832.

Stöhr, K. 2005. Avian influenza and pandemics: Research needs and opportunities. *New England Journal of Medicine* 352 (4): 405–407.

Stokes, Adrien, Johannes Bauer, and Paul Hudson. 1928. The transmission of yellow fever to *Macacus rhesus*. *Journal of the American Medical Association* 90 (4): 243–254.

Stokes, H. 1867. *Report of the officer of health of the sanitary commissioners of Gibraltar for the year 1866*. Gibraltar: Gibraltar Garrison Printing Press.

Stone, Richard. 2002. Siberia's deadly stalker emerges from the shadows. *Science* 296: 642–645.

Straw, Jack. 2004. Written ministerial statement responding to a *Lancet* study on Iraqi casualty figures, Rt. Hon. Jack Straw MP, November 17, Hansard. Electronic document, www.fco.gov.uk/servlet/Front?pagename=OpenMarket/Xcelerate/ShowPage percent20&c=Page&cid=1007029391629&a=KArticle&aid=1100183680513.

Struck, Doug. 2006. Climate change drives disease to new territory. *Washington Post*, 5 May, A16.

Sullivan, Carol. 1991. Pathways to infection: AIDS vulnerability among the Navajo. *AIDS Education and Prevention* 3 (3): 241–257.

Sutherland, J. 1867. *Report on the sanitary condition of Gibraltar with reference to the epidemic cholera in the year 1865.* London: George Edward Eyre and William Spottiswode.

Swedlund, Alan C. 1978. Historical demography as population ecology. *Annual Review of Anthropology* 7: 137–173.

———. 1997. Diabetes as a disease of civilization: The impact of culture change on peoples. *Medical Anthropology Quarterly* 11 (1): 118–120.

———. 2010. *Shadows in the Valley: A cultural history of illness, death, and loss in New England, 1840–1916.* Amherst: University of Massachusetts Press.

———, and Helen L. Ball. 1998. Nature, nurture, and the determinants of infant mortality: A case study from Massachusetts, 1830–1920. In *Building a new biocultural synthesis: Political-economic perspectives on human biology,* edited by A. H. Goodman and T. L. Leatherman, 191–228. Ann Arbor: University of Michigan Press.

———, and Alison Donta. 2003. Scarlet fever epidemics of the nineteenth century: A case of evolved pathogenic virulence? In *Human biologists in the archives: Demography, health, nutrition, and genetics in historical populations,* edited by D. A. Herring and A. C. Swedlund, 159–177. Cambridge: Cambridge University Press.

Sweeney, A. W. 1999. Prospects for control of mosquito-borne diseases. *Journal of Medical Microbiology* 48: 879–881.

Sydenstricker, Edgar. 1931. The incidence of influenza among persons of different economic status during the epidemic of 1918. *Public Health Reports* 46 (4): 154–70.

Taubenberger, J. K. 2005. The virulence of the 1918 pandemic influenza virus: Unraveling the enigma. *Archives of Virology Supplementa* 19: 101–115.

———, A. H. Reid, R. M. Lourens, R. Wang, G. Jin, and T. G. Fanning. 2005. Characterization of the 1918 influenza virus polymerase genes. *Nature* 437 (6): 889–893.

Taylor, C. 1943. Notifications of tuberculosis in New Zealand. *New Zealand Medical Journal* 42: 151–154.

Teixeira, M., M. Barreto, M. Costa, L. Ferreira, P. Vasconcelos, and S. Cairncross. 2002. Dynamics of dengue virus circulation: A silent epidemic in a complex urban area. *Tropical Medicine and International Health* 7: 757–762.

Tellier, Raymond. 2006. Review of aerosol transmission of influenza A virus. *Emerging Infectious Diseases* 12 (11): 1657–1662.

Theiler, Max. 1930. Suceptibility of white mice to the yellow fever virus. *Science* 71: 367–369.

Theilmann, John, and Frances Cate. 2007. A plague of plagues: The problem of plague diagnosis in medieval England. *Journal of Interdisciplinary History* 37 (3): 371–393.

Thieren, Michel. 2005. Health information systems in humanitarian emergencies. *Bulletin of the World Health Organization* 83: 584–589.

———. 2007. Health and foreign policy in question: The case of humanitarian action. *Bulletin of the World Health Organization* 85: 218–224.

Thisyakorn, U., and S. Nimmannitya. 1993. Nutritional status of children with dengue hemorrhagic fever. *Clinical Infectious Diseases* 16: 295–297.Thomas, M., and R. Ellis-Pegler. 2006. Tuberculosis in New Zealand: Poverty casts a long shadow. *New Zealand Medical Journal* 119: 1–3.

Thompson, W. W., L. Comanor, and D. K. Shay. 2006. Epidemiology of seasonal influenza: Use of surveillance data and statistical models to estimate the burden of disease. *Journal of Infectious Diseases* 194: S82–S91.

———, D. K. Shay, E. Weintraub, L. Brammer, N. Cox, L. Anderson, and K. Fukuda. 2003. Mortality associated with influenza and respiratory syncytial virus in the United States. *Journal of the American Medical Association* 289 (2): 179–186.

Thornley, C., and K. Pikholz. 2008. Patterns of tuberculosis epidemiology in Auckland, 1995–2006. In *Multiplying and dividing: Tuberculosis in Canada and Aotearoa New Zealand*, edited by J. Littleton, J. Park, A. Herring, and T. Farmer, 10–21. Research in Anthropology and Linguistics, e series. Auckland: Anthropology Department, University of Auckland.

Tipps, Dean C. 1973. Modernization theory and the comparative study of societies: A critical perspective. *Comparative Studies in Society and History* 15 (2): 199–226.

Tiruviluamala, Parvathi, and Lee B. Reichman. 2002. Tuberculosis. *Annual Review of Public Health* 23: 403–426.

Tognotti, E. 2003. Scientific triumphalism and learning from facts: Bacteriology and the "Spanish flu" challenge of 1918. *Social History of Medicine* 16 (1): 97–110.

Tomes, Nancy. 1998. *The gospel of germs: Men, women, and the microbe in American life*. Cambridge, MA: Harvard University Press.

———. 2000. The making of a germ panic, then and now. *American Journal of Public Health* 90 (2): 191–198.

———. 2002. Epidemic entertainments: Disease and popular culture in early-twentieth-century America. *American Literary History* 14 (4): 625–652.

Tomkins, Sandra M. 1992a. The failure of expertise: Public health policy in Britain during the 1918–1919 influenza epidemic. *Social History of Medicine* 5 (3): 435–454.

———. 1992b. The influenza epidemic of 1918–1919 in Western Samoa. *Journal of Pacific History* 27 (2): 181–197.

Torres Escobar, E. 1994. Will Central America's farmers survive the export boom? *NACLA Report on the Americas* 28: 28–33.

Toulemon, L., and M. Barbieri. 2008. The mortality impact of the August 2003 heat wave in France: Investigating the "harvesting" effect and other long-term consequences. *Population Studies* 62: 39–53.

Treas, J., and B. Logue. 1986. Economic development and the older population. *Population and Development Review* 12 (4): 645–673.

Treichler, Paula A. 1999. *How to have theory in an epidemic: Cultural chronicles of AIDS*. Durham, NC: Duke University Press.

Trennert, Robert. 1998. *White man's medicine: Government doctors and the Navajo*. Albuquerque: University of New Mexico Press.

Trombly, Maria. 2003. *Geneva Conventions: A reference guide*. Indianapolis, Ind.: Society of Professional Journalists.

Trostle, James A. 1986. Anthropology and epidemiology in the twentieth century: A selective history of collaborative projects and theoretical affinities, 1920 to 1970. In *Anthropology and epidemiology: Interdisciplinary approaches to the study of health and diseases*, edited by C. R. Janes, R. Stall, and S. M. Gifford, 59–94. Dordrecht, Netherlands: Reidel.

———. 2005. *Epidemiology and culture*. Cambridge: Cambridge University Press.

Trust for Health. 2006. Covering the pandemic flu threat: Tracking articles and some key events, 1997 to 2005. Electronic document, http://healthyamericans.org/reports/flumedia/CoveringReport.pdf.

Tseng, Alice Lin-In. 1996. Anonymous HIV testing in the Canadian Aboriginal population. *Canadian Family Physician* 42: 1734–1740.

Tsing, Anna Lowenhaupt. 2005. *Friction: An ethnography of global connection*. Princeton, NJ: Princeton University Press.

Tuckel, Peter, Sharon Sassler, Richard Maisel, and Andrew Leykam. 2006. The diffusion of the influenza pandemic of 1918 in Hartford, Connecticut. *Social Science History* 30 (2): 167–196.

Turbott, H. 1935. *Tuberculosis in the Maori, East Coast, New Zealand*. Wellington, New Zealand: Department of Health.

UNAIDS. 2008. *Report on the global AIDS epidemic 2008*. Geneva: UNAIDS.

UNDP (United Nations Development Programme). 1995. *Human development report*. New York: UNDP.

UNFPA (United Nations Population Fund). 2007. *State of world population 2007*. New York: United Nations Population Fund.

Ungar, S. 1998. Hot crises and media reassurance: A comparison of emerging diseases and Ebola Zaire. *British Journal of Sociology* 49 (1): 36–56.

United Nations Human Settlements Programme. 2003. *The challenge of slums: Global report on human settlements*. London: Earthscan.

US Bureau of the Census. 1920. Mortality statistics 1918: Nineteenth annual report. Vital statistics report. Washington, DC: Government Printing Office.

US Department of Health, Education, and Welfare. 1956. Death rates by age, race, and sex, United States, 1900–1953: Selected causes. Vital Statistics, Special Reports 1–31. Washington DC: National Office of Vital Statistics.

US Environmental Protection Agency. 2007. Sea level changes. Electronic document: www.epa.gov/climatechange/science/recentslc.html#ref.

Valdés, L., M. G. Guzmán, G. Kourí, J. Delgado, I. Carbonell, M. V. Cabrera, D. Rosario, and S. Vázquez. 1999. [Epidemiology of dengue and hemorrhagic dengue in Santiago, Cuba 1997]. *Revista Panamericana de Salud Pública* 6: 16–25.

Valverde, C., and C. Smeja. 1993. Reflections on an Aboriginal AIDS awareness programme in the UN Year of the Indigenous Person. Abstract. *International Conference on AIDS* 9: 811 (abstract no. PO-D05-3558).

van der Oest, A. C., R. Kelly, and D. Hood. 2004. The changing face of tuberculosis control in a rural district of New Zealand. *International Journal of Tuberculosis and Lung Disease* 8: 969–975.

Van Gerven, D. 1990. Nutrition, disease, and the human life cycle: A bioethnography of a medieval Nubian community. In *Primate life history and evolution*, edited by C. J. deRousseau, 297–324. New York: Wiley-Liss.

van Hartesveldt, Fred R., ed. 1992. *The 1918–1919 pandemic of influenza: The urban impact in the western world.* Lewiston, NY: Edwin Mellen Press.

Vargas, Luís. 1958. Consideraciones generales sobre la epidemiología de la malaria evanescente en México. *Gaceta Médica de México* 88: 613–633.

———. 1963. La interpretación epidemiológica del paludismo, con énfasis en campañas de erradicación. *Revista Venezolana de Sanidad y Asistencia Social* 28 (4): 339–509.

———. 1965. Realizaciones del programa de erradicación. *Salud Pública de México* 7: 737–740.

———, and A. Almaraz Ugalde. 1963. Evaluación epidemiológica de la erradicación del paludismo en 1959, tercer año de cobertura integral. *Salud Pública de México* 5: 257–269.

Varia, Monali, Samantha Wilson, Shelly Sarwal, Allison McGeer, Effie Gournis, Eleni Galanis, and Bonnie Henry. 2003. Investigation of a nosocomial outbreak of severe acute respiratory syndrome (SARS) in Toronto, Canada. *Canadian Medical Association Journal* 169 (4): 285–292.

Vaughan, Kay. 1997. *Cultural politics in revolution: Teachers, peasants, and schools in Mexico, 1930–1940.* Tucson: University of Arizona Press.

Vaughn, D. W. 2000. Invited commentary: Dengue lessons from Cuba. *American Journal of Epidemiology* 152: 800–803.

Vernon, Irene. 2001. *Killing us quietly: Native Americans and HIV/AIDS.* Lincoln: University of Nebraska Press.

Vladimirtsev, V. A., R. S. Nikitina, Neil Renwick, et al. 2007. Family clustering of Viliuisk encephalomyelitis in traditional and new geographic regions. *Emerging Infectious Diseases* 13: 1321–1326.

Wald, Priscilla. 2008. *Contagious: Cultures, carriers, and the outbreak narrative.* Durham, NC: Duke University Press.

Waldram, James. 2004. *Revenge of the Windigo.* Toronto: University of Toronto Press.

———, D. Ann Herring, and T. Kue Young. 2006. *Aboriginal health in Canada.* Toronto: University of Toronto Press.

Wall, J. J. 1934. Trachoma among the Indians of western Canada. *Canadian Public Health Journal* 25 (6): 524–532.

Walters, K. L., J. M. Simoni, and C. Harris. 2000. Patterns and predictors of HIV risk among urban American Indians. *American Indian and Alaskan Native Mental Health Research* 9 (2): 1–21.

Waltner-Toews, David. 1995. Changing patterns of communicable disease: Who's turning the kaleidoscope? *Perspectives in Biology and Medicine* 39: 43–55.

————. 2007. *The chickens fight back: Pandemic panics and deadly diseases that jump from animals to humans*. Vancouver: Greystone Books.

Waltz, E. 2006. Pandemic prevention schemes threaten diversity, experts warn. *Nature Medicine* 12: 598.

Wang, Fu-Lin. 2005. Potential factors that may affect acceptance of routine prenatal HIV testing. *Canadian Journal of Public Health* 96 (1): 60–65.

Wardlow, Holly. 2002. Giving birth to *Gonolia*: "Culture" and sexually transmitted disease among the Huli of Papua New Guinea. *Medical Anthropology Quarterly* 16 (2): 151–175.

————. 2006. *Wayward women: Sexuality and agency in a New Guinea society*. Berkeley: University of California Press.

Warner, Michael. 2002. *Publics and counterpublics*. New York: Zone Books.

Waters, W. 2001. Globalization, socioeconomic restructuring, and community health. *Journal of Community Health* 26 (2): 79–92.

Watkins, K. 1995. *The Oxfam poverty report*. Oxford: Oxfam.

Watkins, R. E., and A. J. Plant. 2006. Does smoking explain sex differences in the global tuberculosis epidemic? *Epidemiology and Infection* 134 (2): 333–339.

Watts, Charlotte H., and Robert M. May. 1992. The influence of concurrent partnerships on the dynamics of HIV/AIDS. *Mathematical Biosciences* 108: 89–104.

Watts, S. J. 1997. *Epidemics and history: Disease, power and imperialism*. New Haven, CT: Yale University Press.

Webby, R. J., and R. G. Webster. 2001. Emergence of influenza A viruses. *Philosophical Transactions of the Royal Society of London, Series B, Biological Sciences* 356 (1416): 1817–1828.

Webster, R., S. Plotkin, and B. Dodet. 2005. Emergence and control of viral respiratory diseases (conference summary). Electronic document, www.cdc.gov/ncidod/EID/vol11no04/05-0076.htm.

Weiner, Annette B. 1976. *Women of value, men of renown*. Austin: University of Texas Press.

————. 1988. *The Trobrianders of Papua New Guinea*. New York: Holt, Rinehart and Winston.

Weiner, Jonathan. 2005. The tangle: Searching for the cause of a brain disease. *New Yorker*, April 11, 42–51.

Weir, Erica. 2005. The ecology of avian influenza. *Canadian Medical Association Journal* 173 (8): 869–870.

Weiss, R. A. 2001. The Leeuwenhoek Lecture 2001: Animal origins of human infectious disease. *Philosophical Transactions of the Royal Society of London, Series B, Biological Sciences* 356 (1410): 957–977.

Wells, A. 1991. Tuberculosis in New Zealand Maoris. In *History of tuberculosis in Australia, New Zealand and Papua New Guinea*, edited by A. J. Proust, 97–102. Canberra: Brolga Press.

White, P. J., H. Ward, J. A. Cassell, C. H. Mercer, and G. P. Garnett. 2005. Vicious and virtuous circles in the dynamics of infectious disease and the provision of health care: Gonorrhea in Britain as an example. *Journal of Infectious Diseases* 192 (5): 824–836.

Whiteford, Michael B. 1999. Homeopathic medicine in the city of Oaxaca, Mexico: Patients' perspectives and observations. *Medical Anthropology Quarterly* 13 (1): 69–78.

White House. 2006. Press conference by the President, 11 October 2006, www.pierretristam.com/Bobst/library/wf-397.htm.

Whiting, M. G. 1963. Toxicity of cycads. *Economic Botany* 17: 271–302.

Whitman, S., G. Good, E. Donoghue, N. Benbow, W. Shou, and S. Mou. 1997. Mortality in Chicago attributed to the July 1995 heatwave. *American Journal of Public Health* 87: 1515–1551.

WHO (World Health Organization). 1969. *Twenty-second World Health Assembly, Boston, Massachusetts, 8–25 July 1969, Part 2: Plenary meetings, committees, summary records and reports.* Geneva: WHO.

———. 1999. *Influenza pandemic plan: The role of WHO and guidelines for national and regional planning.* Geneva: WHO.

———. 2002. *Reducing risks and promoting health life.* Vienna: WHO.

———. 2004. *Dengue: Burdens and trends.* Geneva: WHO.

———. 2006. Epidemiology of WHO-confirmed human cases of avian influenza A (H5N1) infection. *Weekly Epidemiological Record* 26 (81): 249–260.

———. 2007. H5N1 avian influenza: Timeline. Electronic document, www.who.int/csr/disease/avian_influenza/timeline.pdf.

———. 2008. World malaria report 2008. Electronic document, www.who.int/malaria/wmr2008/.

———. 2009. Cumulative number of confirmed human cases of avian influenza A/(H5N1) reported to WHO. Electronic document, www.who.int/csr/disease/avian_influenza/country/cases_table_2009_05_06/en/index.html.

———. n.d. Areas of confirmed cases of H5N1 avian influenza since 2003. Electronic document, http://gamapserver.who.int/mapLibrary/Files/Maps/Global_H5N1inHumanCUMULATIVE_FIMS_20090506.png, accessed 14 May 2009.

Wilcox, Francis O. 1957. International organizations: Aid to world trade and prosperity. *Department of State Bulletin* 37: 749–754.

Wolf, Eric. 1974. *Anthropology.* New York: W. W. Norton.

Wolfe, N. D., P. Daszak, A. M. Kilpatrick, and D. S. Burke. 2005. Bushmeat hunting deforestation and prediction of zoonoses emergence. *Emerging Infectious Diseases* 11 (12): 1822–1827.

———, W. Switzer, J. Carr, V. Bhullar, V. Shanmugam, U. Tamoufe, A. Prosser, J. Torimiro, A. Wright, and E. Mpoudi-Ngole. 2004. Naturally acquired simian retrovirus infections in central African hunters. *Lancet* 363 (9413): 932–937.

Wong, Brandon. 2007. Iraqi doctor who disputes official death tolls is denied visa to visit UW. *Seattle Post-Intelligencer,* 20 April, B3.

Wong, Samson S. Y., and Kwok-yung Yuen. 2006. Avian influenza virus infections in humans. *Chest* 129 (1): 156–168.

Wong, T. W., C. Lee, T. Lau, T. Yu, S. Lui, P. Chan, Y. Li, J. Bresee, J. Sung, and U. Parashar. 2004. Cluster of SARS among medical students exposed to single patient, Hong Kong. *Emerging Infectious Diseases* 10 (2): 269–276.

Worboys, Michael. 1976. The emergence of tropical medicine: A study in the establishment of a scientific specialty. In *Perspectives on the emergence of scientific disciplines,* edited by G. Lemaine, R. MacLeod, M. Mulkay, and P. Weingart, 75–98. The Hague: Mouton.

World Bank. 1994. *Averting the old age crisis: Policies to protect the old and promote growth.* Oxford: Oxford University Press.

Wright, Peter F., and Robert G. Webster. 2001. Orthomyxoviruses. In *Fields' virology,* edited by D. M. Knipe and P. M. Howley, 1533–1579. Philadelphia: Lippincott Williams and Wilkins.

Yang, J., Y. Feng, M. Yuan, S. Yuan, H. Fu, B. Wu, G. Sun, et al. 2006. Plasma glucose levels and diabetes are independent predictors for mortality and morbidity in patients with SARS. *Diabetic Medicine* 23 (6): 623–628.

Yost, D. 1998. HIV/AIDS and STD prevention in a rural Arizona Indian tribe. Abstract. *International Conference on AIDS* 12: 879 (abstract no. 43162).

Zanotto, P. M., E. A. Gould, G. F. Gao, P. H. Harvey, and E. C. Holmes. 1996. Population dynamics of flaviviruses revealed by molecular phylogenies. *Proceedings of the National Academy of Sciences USA* 93: 545–546.

Zigas, V., and D. C. Gajdusek. 1959. Kuru: Clinical, pathological and epidemiological study of a recently discovered acute progressive degenerative disease of the central nervous system among natives of the eastern highlands of New Guinea. *Papua New Guinea Medical Journal* 3: 1–24.

Index